UPDATE:
DERMATOLOGY IN
GENERAL MEDICINE

UPDATE: DERMATOLOGY IN GENERAL MEDICINE

Thomas B. Fitzpatrick, M.D., Ph.D.

Edward Wigglesworth Professor of Dermatology
Chairman, Department of Dermatology
Harvard Medical School
Chief, Dermatology Service
Massachusetts General Hospital, Boston

Arthur Z. Eisen, M.D.

Professor of Medicine
Head, Division of Dermatology
Washington University School of Medicine
Dermatologist-in-Chief
Barnes Hospital, St. Louis

Klaus Wolff, M.D.

Professor and Chairman, Department of Dermatology I
University of Vienna Medical School, Vienna

Irwin M. Freedberg, M.D.

George Miller MacKee Professor of Dermatology
Chairman, Department of Dermatology
New York University School of Medicine, New York

K. Frank Austen, M.D.

Theodore Bevier Bayles Professor of Medicine
Harvard Medical School
Chairman, Department of Rheumatology and Immunology
Brigham and Women's Hospital, Boston

McGraw-Hill Book Company

New York   St. Louis   San Francisco   Auckland   Bogotá   Guatemala   Hamburg   Johannesburg
Lisbon   London   Madrid   Mexico   Montreal   New Delhi   Panama   Paris
San Juan   São Paulo   Singapore   Sydney   Tokyo   Toronto

UPDATE: DERMATOLOGY IN GENERAL MEDICINE

1 2 3 4 5 6 7 8 9 0   HDHD   8 9 8 7 6 5 4 3 2

ISBN 0-07-021198-1

This book was set in Times Roman by Monotype Composition Company, Inc.; the editors were Richard S. Laufer and Donna McIvor; the production supervisor was Jeanne Skahan; the designer was Murray Fleminger.
Halliday Lithograph Corporation was printer and binder.

Library of Congress Cataloging in Publication Data
Main entry under title:

Update—dermatology in general medicine.

  1. Dermatology.   2. Cutaneous manifestations of general diseases.   I. Fitzpatrick, Thomas B.
[DNLM: 1. Skin diseases.   2. Skin manifestations.
WR 100 U66]
RL71.U63 1983   616.5   82-9995
ISBN 0-07-021198-1

CONTENTS

LIST OF
CONTRIBUTORS

John P. Atkinson, M.D.

Investigator, Howard Hughes Medical Institute; Associate Professor, Division of Rheumatology, Department of Medicine, Washington University School of Medicine, St. Louis.

K. Frank Austen, M.D.

Theodore Bevier Bayles Professor of Medicine, Harvard Medical School; Chairman, Department of Rheumatology and Immunology, Brigham and Women's Hospital, Boston.

Calvin L. Day, Jr., M.D.

Research Fellow in Dermatology, Department of Dermatology, Harvard Medical School, Massachusetts General Hospital, Boston.

Richard L. Edelson, M.D.

Assistant Director, Columbia-Presbyterian General Clinical Research Center; Associate Professor, Columbia University, College of Physicians & Surgeons, New York.

Evan R. Farmer, M.D.

Assistant Professor of Dermatology, Johns Hopkins University School of Medicine; Director, Division of Dermatopathology, Johns Hopkins Medical Institutions, Baltimore.

Thomas B. Fitzpatrick, M.D., Ph.D.

Edward Wigglesworth Professor of Dermatology and Chairman, Department of Dermatology, Harvard Medical School; Chief, Dermatology Service, Massachusetts General Hospital, Boston.

Irwin M. Freedberg, M.D.

George Miller MacKee Professor and Chairman, Department of Dermatology, New York University School of Medicine, New York.

Franz Greiter, Ph.D.

Professor, Technical University, Vienna.

Harley A. Haynes, A.B., M.D.

Associate Professor of Dermatology, Harvard Medical School; Director, Dermatology Division, Brigham and Women's Hospital; Chief, Dermatology, West Roxbury Veterans Administration Hospital, Boston.

Herbert Hönigsmann, M.D.

Associate Professor of Dermatology, Department of Dermatology I, University of Vienna Medical School, Vienna.

Antoinette F. Hood, M.D.

Assistant Professor, Department of Dermatology, Johns Hopkins Medical Institutions, Baltimore.

Stephen I. Katz, M.D., Ph.D.

Chief, Dermatology Branch, National Cancer Institute, National Institutes of Health, Bethesda.

Kenneth H. Kraemer, M.D.

Research Scientist, Laboratory of Molecular Carcinogenesis, National Cancer Institute, National Institutes of Health, Bethesda.

Robert A. Lewis, M.D.

Assistant Professor of Medicine, Harvard Medical School; Assistant Physician, Robert B. Brigham Division and Junior Associate in Medicine, Peter B. Brigham Division, Brigham and Women's Hospital, Boston.

Martin C. Mihm, Jr., B.A., M.D.

Professor of Pathology, Chief, Dermatopathology Unit, Harvard Medical School; Pathologist, Assistant Dermatologist, Massachusetts General Hospital, Boston.

David B. Mosher, M.D.

Instructor in Dermatology, Harvard Medical School; Clinical Fellow, Massachusetts General Hospital, Boston.

Jan E. Muhlbauer, M.D.

Chief Resident in Dermatopathology, Harvard Medical School, Massachusetts General Hospital, Boston.

John A. Parrish, B.S., M.D.

Associate Professor of Dermatology, Harvard Medical School; Assistant Dermatologist, Massachusetts General Hospital, Boston.

Madhu A. Pathak, B.Sc. (Hon.), M.S. (Tech.), M.B., M.S., Ph.D.

Senior Associate in Dermatology, Harvard Medical School, Massachusetts General Hospital, Boston.

Gary L. Peck, M.D.

Senior Investigator, Dermatology Branch, National Cancer Institute, National Institutes of Health, U.S. Public Health Service, Bethesda.

Stephanie H. Pincus, M.D.

Assistant Professor of Dermatology, Departments of Medicine and Dermatology, Tufts University School of Medicine, Boston.

Arthur R. Rhodes, M.D., M.P.H.

Chief, Division of Dermatology, Department of Medicine, Children's Hospital Medical Center; Assistant Professor, Department of Dermatology, Harvard Medical School, Boston.

Susan Bromberg Schneider, M.D.

Clinical Fellow, Division of Allergy and Immunology, and Instructor in Medicine, Department of Internal Medicine, Washington University School of Medicine, St. Louis.

Arthur J. Sober, M.D.

Associate Professor of Dermatology, Harvard Medical School, Massachusetts General Hospital, Boston.

Georg Stingl, M.D.

Associate Professor of Dermatology, Department of Dermatology I, University of Vienna Medical School, Vienna.

Dorothy B. Windhorst, M.D.

Director, Biomedical Data Systems, Hoffmann–La Roche Inc., Nutley, New Jersey; Clinical Professor of Dermatology, College of Physicians & Surgeons, Columbia University, New York.

Klaus Wolff, M.D.

Professor and Chairman, Department of Dermatology I, University of Vienna Medical School, Vienna.

Sheldon M. Wolff, M.D.

Physician-in-Chief, New England Medical Center Hospital; Endicott Professor and Chairman, Department of Medicine, Tufts University School of Medicine, Boston.

PREFACE

"The art of being wise is the art of knowing what to overlook," said William James. In the Second Edition of *Dermatology in General Medicine* (*DIGM*) there were some omissions and too-brief discussions of important topics. A one-volume text necessarily restricts space and prohibits complete coverage of all subjects. We tried to include the important topics of general interest, yet there is a real need for more extended discussions; this can only be accomplished by an appendix to the main volume.

DIGM Update is therefore not only an update but a "tidying up" of *DIGM*: (1) more detailed presentations of diseases incompletely covered (e.g., pyoderma gangrenosum, graft-versus-host disease, erythema elevatum diutinum, variegate porphyria); (2) presentations of subjects in which recent knowledge has considerably altered our understanding (e.g., cutaneous T-cell lymphoma, the prognosis of Stage I primary melanoma of the skin, the pivotal role of the Langerhans cell in immunologic reactions of the skin); and (3) considerations of new therapies such as the retinoids, a series of pharmacologic agents that have proved to be effective in cystic acne and disorders of keratinization and which offer some promise in the chemoprevention of cutaneous and other organ cancers.

There can be no doubt that in 1982 most patients with skin disease receive far better care than they did three decades ago. This change is directly related to medical research; there have emerged new diagnostic techniques and approaches to therapy. A critical mass of dermatologist-scientists has now been established in the medical schools and hospitals of Europe, Japan, and the United States. This flowering of academic dermatology is important for the practicing physician because teachers and researchers provide for the future.

The principal aim of *DIGM* and the *DIGM Update* is to help the busy physician keep abreast of this progress.

We wish to acknowledge the cooperation of the McGraw-Hill Book Company staff, most especially Donna McIvor, Steven Tenney, and Richard Laufer. The editors are again grateful to Patricia Novak, who prepared the book for publication.

Thomas B. Fitzpatrick
Arthur Z. Eisen
Klaus Wolff
Irwin M. Freedberg
K. Frank Austen

UPDATE: DERMATOLOGY IN GENERAL MEDICINE

THE LANGERHANS CELL

Georg Stingl

Klaus Wolff

Definition

Langerhans cells (LCs) are immunocompetent, dendritic cells of bone marrow derivation that reside within the epidermis, where they represent roughly 4 percent of the total cell population; they also occur in certain mucosal epithelia, the dermis, lymph nodes, and thymus and, thus, have a wide tissue distribution. Langerhans cells carry receptors for complement components and for the Fc portion of IgG and synthesize Ia antigens, which are encoded for by the I region of the major histocompatibility complex. Langerhans cells are the only epidermal cells capable of presenting antigens to immune T cells and of serving as stimulator cells in the syngeneic and the allogeneic mixed leukocyte reaction. They represent the most peripheral outpost of the afferent limb of the immune system, being responsible for antigen recognition, processing, and presentation, but probably also fulfill other functional capacities which yet have to be clarified.

Historical Aspects

In 1868, the medical student Paul Langerhans [1] discovered a population of dendritic cells in the suprabasal regions of the epidermis which he and others considered to be a part of the nervous system. During the 1950s and 1960s another hypothetical concept postulated a relationship between LCs and melanocytes, but both the neural and melanocyte theory have been disproved [2,3]. The finding by Birbeck et al. [4] that LCs display a unique ultrastructural morphology led to the discovery that these cells are not confined to the skin but also reside in various mesodermal tissues and make up a sizable portion of the cellular infiltrate in histiocytosis X [3,5]. These findings provided suggestive evidence for a mesenchymal origin of LC, renewed the interest in these cells, and stimulated experimental studies which in the past few years have resulted in the elucidation of their origin and several of their functional capacities.

Identification of Langerhans Cells

Light Microscopy

Langerhans cells are not apparent in routinely fixed and stained paraffin-embedded sections of mammalian skin. Although a series of special staining methods exists which allows their visualization, the LC specificity of these procedures holds true only for the epidermis as they also stain a variety of mesodermal cells in the dermis or other tissues. Among the many staining procedures available [3,6] histochemical and immunologic methods have proved to be particularly reliable.

Histochemical Techniques. Langerhans cells contain various hydrolytic enzymes which can be demonstrated by histochemical techniques. Since these procedures reveal only weak or no reactions with other epidermal cells, they permit a selective visualization of LCs not only in frozen skin sections, but also on epidermal sheet preparations, thus providing a useful tool to assess quantitatively the epidermal LC population. Depending on the species to be investigated, staining for either nucleosidephosphatase, alkaline phosphatase, aminopeptidase, or nonspecific esterase activities results in LC labeling [3,7]. In humans, guinea pigs, rhesus monkeys, and mice the demonstration of a membrane-bound, formalin-resistant, and sulfhydryl-dependent adenosinetriphosphatase (ATPase) is a highly reliable and widely used procedure for the identification of epidermal LCs [3] (Figs. 1 and 2).

Immunologic Techniques. IMMUNOGLOBULIN AND COMPLEMENT RECEPTORS. In the process of investigating whether or not human epidermal cells possess surface marker characteristics of immunocompetent cells, Stingl et al. [8] made the observation that LCs—but no other epidermal cells—express receptor sites for the Fc portion of the IgG molecule (Fc-IgG receptors) and the third component of complement but lack classical T- and B-cell markers. These studies were later extended to other species and the presence of Fc-IgG and complement receptors on mouse and guinea pig Langerhans cells has now been unequivocally demonstrated [9–11]. Rosette assays are most commonly employed to detect the respective receptor sites on epidermal LCs (Fig. 3). IgG antibody–coated bovine red blood cells (EA-

Fig. 1. Suprabasal dendritic Langerhans cells in human epidermis as revealed by the ATPase technique. Arrows denote the dermal-epidermal junction. × 800. [*From Wolff K: Arch Klin Exp Dermatol 229:54–101, 1976, with permission.*]

Fig. 2. Histochemical (ATPase technique) demonstration of the Langerhans cell population in sheet preparation of guinea-pig epidermis. × 100. [*From Wolff K et al: Proceedings of the 13th International Congress on Dermatology, Munich, 1967, vol. 2. Springer, Berlin/Heidelberg/New York, 1968, pp 1502–1504.*]

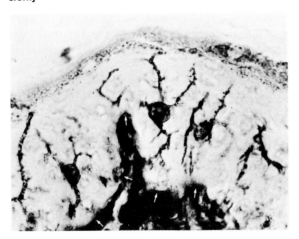

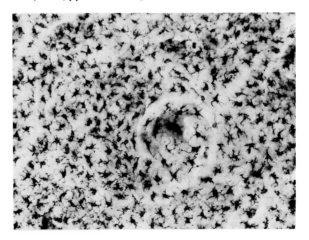

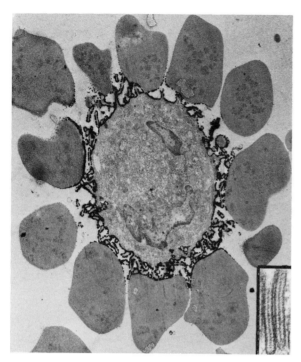

Fig. 3. Low-power electron micrograph of a rosetted human epidermal Langerhans cell. A suspension of single epidermal cells was incubated with IgG antibody–coated bovine red cells and then processed for the ultrastructural demonstration of ATPase activity. The rosetted Fc-IgG receptor–bearing cell exhibits a folded nucleus, dendritic and villous surface projections, ATPase reaction product on its membrane, and typical Langerhans cell granules in its cytoplasm (inset). *[From Stingl et al [8], with permission.]*

IgG) serve as indicator reagent for Fc-IgG receptors whereas IgM antibody– and complement–coated bovine red cells (EAC) allow the detection of complement receptor sites. These rosette assays are reliable tools for LC identification and enumeration in single epidermal cell suspensions but cannot be used for LC labeling on tissue sections.

IMMUNE RESPONSE–ASSOCIATED (Ia) ANTIGENS. In most species so far investigated the major histocompatibility complex (MHC) consists of several gene regions which encode for the production of membrane-bound alloantigens which serve as crucial recognition structures in both the afferent and the efferent limb of the immune response [12].

One set of MHC-encoded alloantigens are termed H-2K and H-2D antigens in mice, GPLA-B antigens in guinea pigs, and HLA-A, -B, and -C antigens in humans. These classical serologically detectable antigens are membrane-bound glycoproteins composed of two subunits, the smaller one being β_2 microglobulin, and are present on virtually all nucleated cells. For many years, their only recognizable role was to provide strong trans-

plantation antigens, but, clearly, their evolutionary development was not designed for this purpose. In the last few years, it has become evident that they are important recognition structures in cytotoxic T-cell reactions toward hapten-modified, virus-modified, and tumor antigen-bearing target cells.

Another region within the MHC, the I region, contains immune response (Ir) genes which control the capacity to respond to certain defined synthetic antigens, proteins, and alloantigens. In addition, I-region genes exist which code for the predominant determinants stimulating proliferation in the mixed leukocyte reaction (MLR) whereas another I subregion controls suppressor T-cell function. Ia antigens are the serologically detectable I-region products. Ia antigens are glycoproteins and consist of two components with molecular weights of 33,000 and 25,000, respectively. In contrast to the H-2K and H-2D antigens, Ia antigens have a restricted tissue distribution in that they are expressed only on immunocompetent cells.

Using alloantisera or, more recently, monoclonal antibodies directed against the various MHC-subregion products it has been convincingly shown that in all species so far investigated (humans, guinea pigs, mice) essentially all epidermal cells bear HLA-A, -B, and -C or GPLA-B and H-2K/H-2D antigens, respectively, whereas only LCs bear and synthesize Ia antigens [9,10,13–16].

The immunofluorescent detection of Ia antigens can be used as a marker for epidermal LCs both in tissue sections, where they appear as highly dendritic cells at a suprabasal level, and in epidermal sheet preparations, which permit studies of the distribution of the entire LC population [17]. Also, the incubation of isolated epidermal cells with a specific anti-Ia serum in an indirect immunofluorescence (IF) procedure produces a rimlike membrane fluorescence of 3 to 4 percent of the cells, which, by double-labeling procedures, have been shown to represent the LC population (Fig. 4). The latter procedure permits quantitative assessments and is used as a control in functional studies.

ANTIGENS DEFINED BY HYBRIDOMA-DERIVED MONOCLONAL ANTIBODIES. In the past few years, hybridoma technology has been successfully used by several investigators to produce monoclonal antibodies against a variety of antigenic specificities expressed on immunocompetent cells. So far, two laboratories have succeeded in producing monoclonal antibodies recognizing antigenic determinants on LCs. Fithian et al. [18] provided evidence that OKT 6, a monoclonal antibody

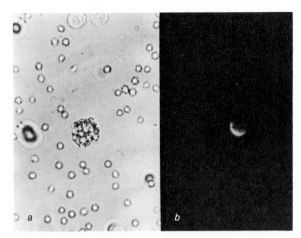

Fig. 4. Strain 2 guinea-pig epidermal cells were initially rosetted with IgG antibody–coated bovine red cells and then reacted with an anti-Ia.2,4 serum (detecting Ia specificities on strain 2 cells) in an indirect immunofluorescence procedure. (a) Low-power view of four epidermal cells. The cell in the center exhibits Fc-IgG rosette formation. (Phase contrast microscopy) ×54. (b) The same area viewed by fluorescence microscopy. Membrane fluorescence is visible only on the single Fc-IgG rosette-forming epidermal cell in the center of the field. *[From Stingl et al [10], with permission.]*

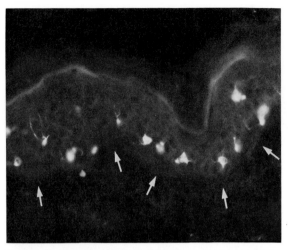

Fig. 5. Immunofluorescent detection of epidermal Langerhans cells on cryostat section of normal human skin using a monoclonal antibody (VI-CY1) [19]. Arrows denote the dermal-epidermal junction. ×40.

reactive with 70 percent of thymocytes but unreactive with peripheral blood B cells, T cells, and monocytes, strongly binds to human epidermal LC cytoplasmic membranes. Majdic et al. [19] characterized a monoclonal antibody reactive with a cytoplasmic antigenic specificity present in human B cells, a subpopulation of monocytes, Kupffer cells, and epidermal LCs. These two reagents represent valuable tools for immunohistologic identification of LCs (Fig. 5) and can be expected to facilitate their characterization in disease states.

Electron Microscopy

The major disadvantage of light microscopic techniques is that they allow LC identification only within the epidermis. It was electron microscopy that gave the LC its morphologic identity and led to the discovery that LCs are not restricted to the epidermis but also occur in other tissues. In 1961, Birbeck et al. [4] established the criteria which now allow the recognition and identification of LCs at *any* location (Fig. 6): (1) a clear cytoplasm devoid of tonofilaments and a membrane devoid of desmosomes; (2) a lobulated, frequently convoluted nucleus; (3) the presence of a distinctive cytoplasmic organelle—termed *Langerhans cell granule* or *Birbeck granule* (Fig. 7). It usually appears as a rod-shaped organelle of variable

length with a central periodically striated density and an occasional bleb at one end which gives this structure a tennis-racket appearance. Three-dimensional reconstructions of the Langerhans cell granule suggest that it is a flat, platelike, occasionally twisted or cup-shaped structure with a vesicular protrusion [3,20]. The function of this granule is unknown. In addition, LCs are fully equipped to act as metabolically active cells in that they exhibit a considerable number of mitochondria, centrioles, lysosomes, endoplasmic reticulum, and a well-developed Golgi apparatus [3].

Distribution of Langerhans Cells

Using either light microscopic or electron microscopic criteria, LCs have so far been identified only in mammals, including humans, guinea pigs, rhesus monkeys, various Lorisidae, sheep, mice, rats, hamsters, rabbits, and bats. The distribution of LCs within epithelial tissues is essentially confined to stratified squamous epithelia, including the epidermis, skin appendages, the oral mucosa, esophagus, and the stratified epithelium of the uterine cervix (for review, see [3]). However, LCs also occur in mesodermal tissues, such as dermis, thymus, and lymph nodes (for review, see [3]).

The application of LC-specific histochemical and IF staining techniques to epidermal sheets has provided a reliable technique for quantitative assessments of the epidermal LC population. Whereas in the guinea pig the density of the LC population is almost identical in different regions of the body

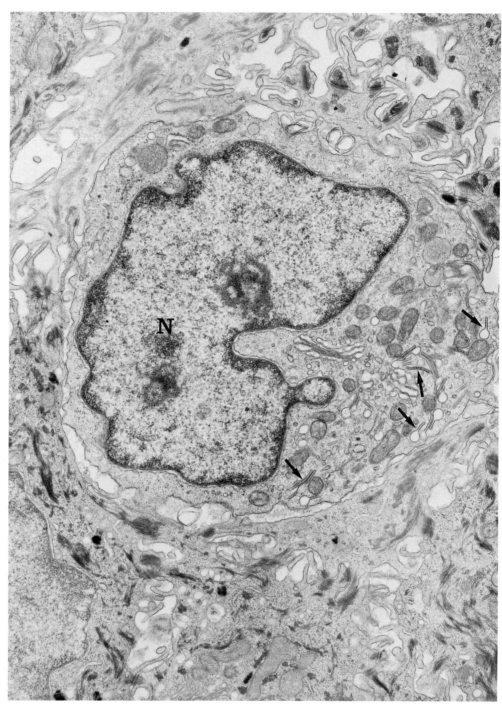

Fig. 6.   Electron micrograph of a Langerhans cell in human epidermis. Arrows denote Birbeck granules. N = nucleus. ×15,000. *[From Stingl G: Int J Dermatol 19:189–213, 1980, with permission.]*

[21], there exist regional differences in other species [21,22]. In humans, LC counts range from 460 to 1000 cells per square millimeter, and in the mouse, there is a considerable difference in LC densities between tail skin and the rest of the body [22]. LC paucity in the mouse tail is due to the structural patterning of this particular region in that LCs are virtually absent from scale regions but are present in interscale areas. In addition, there exist strain-specific variations in murine epidermal LC numbers in that C57Bl/6 mice have a considerably smaller LC population than other mouse strains [22]. Certain epithelia either contain only few LCs (e.g., hamster cheek pouch) or are

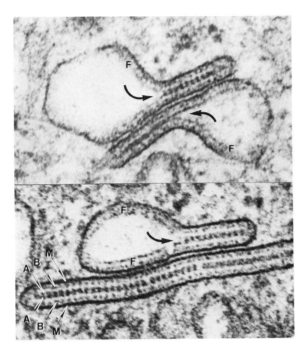

Fig. 7. High-power electron micrograph of Birbeck granules. The curved arrows indicate the zipperlike fusion of the fuzzy coats (F) of the vesicular portion of the granule. The delimiting membrane (M) envelopes two sheets of particles (B) attached to it and a central lamella composed of two linear arrays of particles (A). *[From Wolff K: J Cell Biol 35:466–473, 1967, with permission.]*

completely devoid of LCs (e.g., the central portion of the cornea) [22]. As will be discussed later in this chapter, LC paucity, or even absence, may contribute to the "immunologic privilege" that has been observed for mouse tail skin, hamster cheek pouch, and cornea.

Derivation of Langerhans Cells

In the past few years, the concept of a mesenchymal origin of LCs as originally put forward by Wolff [3] has gained strong support by the observation that surface marker characteristics (Fc-IgG receptors, complement receptors, Ia antigens) of LCs resemble those of monocytes and macrophages. Very recently, Katz et al. [23] directly addressed the question of LC origin. They transplanted sex-matched skin of mouse A (donor) onto an A × B hybrid mouse (recipient) and then determined after variable time periods whether the H-2 and Ia antigens of LCs and of other epidermal cells were those of the donor or the recipient. As early as 3 weeks after transplantation, most LCs isolated from the transplanted skin of mouse A were of recipient (A × B) origin, whereas the

residual epidermal cells still had donor characteristics, which suggested that the LCs of transplanted skin were derived from a mobile pool of recipient cells. In a second set of experiments, mice A were made chimeric by irradiation with 750 to 800 R and subsequent reconstitution with semiallogeneic (A × B) or allogeneic (B) bone marrow cells. After variable time periods, the H-2 and Ia specificities of keratinocytes and LCs, respectively, were determined and it was found that 7 days after chimerization both keratinocytes and LCs were still of recipient origin; after about 3 months, however, most LCs proved to be of donor origin whereas keratinocytes still bore H-2 specificities of the recipient. In accordance with these results, Frelinger et al. [24], using immunoprecipitation techniques, demonstrated that in x-irradiated bone marrow–reconstituted chimeric mice the epidermal Ia molecules are synthesized by bone marrow–derived cells. These findings clearly show that epidermal LCs originate from and are continuously repopulated by a mobile pool of bone marrow–derived precursor cells. The differentiation pathway, however, i.e., the exact nature of the precursor cell, is still unknown. It must be remembered at this point that the homeostasis of the epidermal LC is not only maintained by this reservoir of bone marrow–derived precursors, but also by a small population of resident epidermal LCs capable of mitotic activity [25].

Functional Properties of Langerhans Cells

Although it is conceivable that LCs play a vital role in a variety of physiologic and pathologic processes of the skin, the only functional capacity of LCs for which experimental proof is currently available is the immunologic function of this cell type. The idea that LCs might perform immunologic functions is not new and had been already speculatively proposed in the 1960s. It was with the work of Silberberg et al. [26] that this purely speculative concept gained experimental support. These authors investigated the cellular events occurring in cutaneous delayed-type hypersensitivity reactions at the level of the electron microscope. In both humans and guinea pigs actively or passively sensitized to a variety of substances (dinitrochlorobenzene, mercuric chloride), they observed a close apposition of LCs to lymphocytes only a few hours after antigenic challenge, whereas, at the peak of the response, LCs were reduced in number and exhibited signs of damage. These phenomena were not observed in primary irritant dermatitis. On the basis of these findings, Silberberg et al. [26] proposed that LCs serve as important induction and target structures in cutaneous delayed-type hypersensitivity reactions.

Experimental evidence for an immunologic role of LCs was obtained when it was found that these cells are the only epidermal cells that possess surface characteristics of immunocompetent cells [8–10,13–16]. The presence of Fc-IgG receptors, complement receptors, and Ia antigens as opposed to the absence of E receptors and membrane-incorporated intrinsic immunoglobulins suggested an ontogenic and, more importantly, a functional relationship between LCs and cells from the monocyte-macrophage-histiocyte series. Considering the fact that LCs are located in the most peripheral tissue of the organism, i.e., the epidermis, it seemed conceivable that they play a functional role in the afferent limb of the immune response in a manner similar to that of Ia-bearing macrophages.

Antigen Presentation Function of Epidermal Langerhans Cells

It is established that recognition of soluble protein and haptenized antigens by the T lymphocyte requires an initial uptake and "processing" of these antigens by a macrophage-like cell [27,28] and that the subsequent functional interaction between antigen-exposed macrophage and T lymphocyte—which finally results in marked T-cell proliferation—is regulated by gene products encoded for by the I region of the MHC [28,29]. Evidence available to date indicates that the serologically detectable Ia antigens represent the relevant I-region products responsible for immunocompetent cell interaction [30].

Stingl and coworkers, using both the guinea pig [31] and the mouse system [32], investigated the antigen-presenting capacity of LCs by using an in vitro system that previously had been used successfully for the elucidation of macrophage antigen-presenting function [28,29]. They incubated purified T cells sensitized to either soluble protein antigens or simple chemical haptens with a variety of antigen-exposed stimulator cells and after a 3-day culture period determined the extent of T-cell proliferation. LCs, but not other epidermal cells, proved to be as potent stimulators of antigen-specific T-cell proliferation as were macrophages and, in furthering the analogy, LC-lymphocyte interactions exhibited all signs of I region–mediated genetic restriction. Similar results recently have been obtained in the human system [33].

Langerhans Cells Stimulate Allogeneic and Syngeneic T-Cell Activation

Histocompatibility has been found a fundamental in vitro tool in the study of the interactions that take place in cultures of allogeneic lymphocytes, collectively called the *mixed leukocyte reaction* (MLR). Increased macromolecule synthesis and vigorous cell proliferation represent the major events occurring in such cultures. The phenomenon of the MLR depends on two major properties of the mixed lymphocyte populations, i.e., the expression of cell surface-incorporated stimulatory determinants and the presence of recognition structures for these determinants; the responder cells belong to specific T-cell subpopulations [34,35]. It is now generally agreed that certain mononuclear phagocytes or cells somehow related to them are the principal stimulator cells of allogeneic T-cell activation [36,37]. The finding that monoclonal antibodies directed against Ia specificities expressed on the stimulator cell prevent allosensitization [30] strongly implies that Ia antigens themselves are the critical stimulatory determinants.

Furthering the analogy between certain Ia-positive macrophages and epidermal LCs, conclusive evidence has been provided in both guinea pigs and humans [31,33] that LCs are the only epidermal cells capable of substantially stimulating allogeneic T-cell activation. Most recently, these studies were extended to the mouse system and it was observed that LCs not only stimulate allogeneic T-cell activation but also initiate considerable activation of syngeneic T cells [38]. The phenomenon of T-cell activation by syngeneic non-T cells is termed *syngeneic mixed leukocyte reaction* and appears to be a good in vitro correlate for the "self recognition" capacity of T cells and, thus, for the capacity of the immune system to mount T cell–dependent immune responses.

These in vitro data strongly suggest that LCs are the most peripheral outpost of the immune apparatus and play a decisive role in the afferent limb of the immune response. It appears likely that cutaneously applied antigen is taken up by a variety of cells, including keratinocytes, but that only LCs have the capacity of processing the antigen and, more importantly, of presenting immunologically relevant determinants to the T lymphocyte, an event that triggers a strong sensitizing signal to the immune apparatus. The fact that LCs have the capacity to initiate antigen-specific and allogeneic T-cell activation does by no means exclude the possibility that they also have other immunologic functions. Most recent data from Pehamberger et al. [38a] indicate that LCs fulfill a critical accessory cell function in the generation of cytotoxic T cells and, although experimental evidence is lacking, it is even conceivable that antigen-modified LCs represent preferential target structures in hapten- and virus-specific cytotoxic T-cell reactions affecting the skin. However, a cytotoxic potential of LCs per se has so far not been demonstrated and most recent investigations addressing this question indicate that LCs are neither cytotoxic in an antibody-dependent cellular cytotoxicity assay nor do they mediate mitogen-induced cellular cytotoxicity [39].

A potentially important aspect of LC function has so far not been systematically investigated, i.e., possible secretory capacities of these cells. A critical prerequisite for these investigations is to obtain LC suspensions virtually devoid of contaminating epidermal symbionts. Although the ideal tool for the investigation of LC functions, a Langerhans cell line, has not yet been successfully established, techniques are now available that allow the preparation of epidermal cell suspensions either highly enriched for or essentially depleted of LCs, respectively [40]. It is hoped that these techniques will enable us to determine whether or not LCs synthesize and secrete similar products as do mononuclear phagocytes, i.e., complement components [41], prostaglandins [42,43], interferon [44,45], and a variety of enzymes [46–49]. Mononuclear phagocytes, when activated by certain agents, produce soluble factors—termed *monokines* [50]—that modulate a number of lymphocyte activities. One particular monokine— termed *lymphocyte activating factor* (LAF) or *interleukin I*— is directly mitogenic for thymocytes, augments lymphoproliferative responses to lectins, and also promotes T cell–dependent in vitro antibody responses of murine B lymphocytes. Recently performed studies [51,52] indicate that epidermal cells have the capacity to secrete a thymocyte activating factor which displays physicochemical and functional properties similar to interleukin I. Surprisingly enough, the cellular source of this factor appears to be the keratinocyte rather than the LC, which may suggest that immune reactions initiating in the epidermis depend upon a close functional interaction between LCs and keratinocytes. This brings back the old concept of the "epidermal Langerhans cell unit" [3] which postulated that each LC and those keratinocytes that surround it and are in physical contact with its dendrites function in symbiotic union.

Another important issue that needs to be clarified is the question concerning the endocytotic capacities of LCs, i.e., whether or not these cells fulfill the requirements of mononuclear phagocytes. Although their capacity to phagocytose large molecules appears to be rather poor as compared to conventional macrophages or, even, surrounding keratinocytes [3], it may well be that LCs are capable of receptor-mediated phagocytosis, i.e., either the internalization of opsonized particles via their Fc-IgG and C3b receptor sites [53] or the binding of selected extracellular proteins or peptides to specific cell surface receptors and their subsequent uptake [54]. One may express the hope that in the course of such investigations one of the enigmas in LC research, i.e., derivation, fate, and function of the unique trilaminar LC granules, will be unraveled and finally resolved.

Effects of Physical and Chemical Agents on Langerhans Cells and Langerhans Cell Function

Ultraviolet (UV) Light

The effect of UV irradiation on the epidermal LC population was investigated many years ago, but the results obtained were conflicting, and, because of considerable differences in experimental design, methods of LC identification, light sources, and energy doses applied, these older data do not allow valid conclusions as to the fate of epidermal LCs following UV irradiation. The increasing understanding of the preeminent significance of LCs in epidermal cell biology and the fact that these cells reside in the only tissue that is naturally exposed to UV light prompted several investigators to reinvestigate this issue using well-defined parameters. Unfortunately, the data obtained by different groups are again somewhat divergent. Whereas Bergstresser et al. [55] and Aberer et al. [56] found that small doses of short-wave UVB sufficed to decrease dramatically the number of ATPase- and/or Ia-positive cells in murine or human epidermis, respectively, Nordlund and Ackles [57] reported an increase of Ia-positive epidermal cells after single or multiple applications of short-wave UV. The situation is further complicated by studies from our laboratory [56] which have shown that UVB irradiation depletes LCs of their surface markers but does not induce a significant destruction of the LC population itself. Most recently, in vitro studies investigating the effect of UVB on I region–mediated LC functions have been undertaken. Results obtained demonstrated that exposure of murine epidermal cells to 10 to 20 mJ/cm² UVB leads to an abrogation of the LC-induced antigen-specific and allogeneic T-cell activation without producing lethal cell damage to the majority of the residual cells [32,38]. This particular UV susceptibility of LC I-region functions may have important biologic and pathophysiologic implications which will be discussed further below. In the case of long-wave UVA, 100 to 200 J/cm² are needed to deplete the epidermis from ATPase- or Ia-positive cells. These extremely high doses are far beyond what one may encounter under conditions of solar irradiation and are, therefore, of only negligible biologic significance [56].

Psoralen and UVA (PUVA)

Nordlund and Ackles [57] exposed C3H/He mice to topical 8-methoxypsoralen (100 μL of a 0.5% solution) and UVA (3.6 J/cm²) 3 times per week for a total of 3 weeks. After 1 week of PUVA, the number of Ia-positive epidermal cells had decreased by approximately 50 percent, after 3 weeks by 64 percent, and after 6 weeks, i.e., 3 weeks after stopping PUVA, Ia-positive cells were reduced to 12 percent of the original density. Two weeks later, their number had returned to normal.

Contact Allergens

When murine skin is exposed to a sensitizing regimen of either dinitrofluorobenzene (DNFB) or oxazolone [55,58], the numbers of ATPase- or Ia-positive cells transiently decrease but return to normal after 24 hr. After application of the challenging dose [58], however, a transient increase of ATPase- and Ia-positive epidermal cells has been observed followed by a sharp decrease 48 to 120 hr postchallenge; 7 days after challenge, the cell numbers have been reported to rebound to normal.

Corticosteroids

After either topical or systemic application of triamcinolone acetonide for 10 or 5 consecutive days, respectively, the number of Ia-positive murine epidermal cells has been reported to decrease sharply to approximately 5 percent of the original value. This effect seems to be long lasting as normal densities of Ia-positive cells were only encountered after 5 weeks [57]. Similar observations were made in the guinea-pig system where it was demonstrated that a variety of corticosteroid preparations not only produce a decrease in number of ATPase- and Ia-positive cells, but also induce structural alterations in LCs [59].

Melanocytotoxins

Agents like pyrocatechol and p-tert-butylphenol reportedly cause a substantial increase in the density and size of Ia-positive epidermal cells. These phenomena are reversed by 2 weeks after discontinuation of the treatment [58]. These observations are in partial disagreement with reports from the older literature [3].

Implications in Immune Reactions

The data presented above may be relevant for a new understanding of immune reactions involving the skin.

Contact Hypersensitivity

The finding that hapten-modified LCs but not hapten-modified keratinocytes stimulate activation of hapten-sensitized T lymphocytes strongly suggests that LCs play an important role in the inductive phase of contact hypersensitivity. It seems likely that a variety of contactants, particularly chemical haptens, bind to the majority of epidermal cells but that only Ia-bearing LCs are capable of modifying or processing the allergen in such a way that immunologically relevant determinants are presented to the T lymphocyte and, thus, cause sensitization. Once the sensitizing signal has occurred, interleukin I-like keratinocyte factors may provide important ancillary signals for augmenting the ongoing T-cell response. The mechanism of in vivo interaction between antigen-bearing LCs and T cells is still a matter of speculation but it has been proposed that antigen-laden LCs migrate across the dermal-epidermal junction and initiate T-cell sensitization either in the dermis or the regional lymph node [60].

Another body of evidence pointing to an important role for LCs in contact hypersensitivity stems from the observation that skin relatively deficient in LCs (such as mouse tail epidermis) is resistant to sensitization to DNFB. More importantly, mice whose first exposure to DNFB occurred through the tail skin were unable subsequently to become specifically sensitized when immunization was attempted through the conventional route using normal body-wall skin [61]. Similar phenomena were observed when sensitization was attempted on normal body-wall skin treated with UV irradiation.

Elicitation reactions could be easily provoked in normal control mice sensitized with DNFB on abdominal-wall skin, but not in UV-irradiated mice. Again, these irradiated mice were unresponsive to attempts to immunize them with DNFB through normal skin in the conventional fashion. However, they responded to sensitization with other antigens [61]. It is likely that this UV-induced antigen-specific unresponsiveness is due to a UV-induced loss or modulation of LC membrane markers such as membrane-bound nucleosidetriphosphatases and, more importantly, Ia antigens [56]. It is conceivable that it is this loss or modulation of LC-Ia antigens that is responsible for an alteration in immune responsiveness as related to contact hypersensitivity. Recent studies indicate that the response of the immune system to highly reactive molecules, such as DNFB, is delicately balanced and that given different experimental circumstances, either sensitization or tolerance occurs [62]. One might postulate that the association of hapten with LC membrane–Ia moieties provides the "altered self" signal which induces specific sensitization. When Ia molecules are lacking or modified (e.g., by UV), the message delivered to the immune apparatus may no longer be that of sensitization but rather that of specific unresponsiveness. This hypothesis gains support from the observation that UV irradiation of epidermal cells in vitro renders LCs incapable of acting as antigen-presenting cells [32]. Activation of precursors and, finally, effector cells of delayed-type hypersensitivity may no longer occur and stimulation of T suppressor cells may, thus, be the predominating event.

While the above data attribute to LCs an important role in the inductive phase of contact hypersensitivity, much less information is available on the possible participation of these cells in the effector phase of this reaction. It is interesting to note that the earliest histologic epidermal changes in contact allergic reactions occur in the suprabasal layers of the epidermis where LCs are known to reside. The early findings of Silberberg et al. [26], who observed in allergic contact dermatitis (i.e., in the sensitized host), but not in primary irritant dermatitis, a close apposition of LCs to lymphocytes and, finally, LC damage, indicated that LCs represent important target structures in contact hypersensitivity reactions. The injured LCs themselves, in turn, may release the substances they contain (perhaps prostaglandins and lysosomal enzymes) and thus initiate further inflammatory changes in the surrounding epidermis and dermis.

Viral Diseases, Photocarcinogenesis

The antigen-presenting capacity of LCs is by no means restricted to simple chemical haptens. It is also conceivable that LCs account for the effective immunogenic presentation of viral and tumor-associated antigens and thus play a crucial role in the prevention of the devastating spread of viruses infecting the skin and also in the elimination of neoplastic epidermal cell clones. Though speculative, this concept is in keeping with the clinical experience that UV irradiation results in activation of herpes virus infection and that chronically UV-exposed epidermis is more prone to undergo malignant transformation than light-protected skin.

Graft Rejection

In the induction of skin graft rejection, the role of the "passenger leukocyte" has been a widely debated issue [63] and it is generally accepted that transient cellular constituents, namely leukocytes trapped in allografts when the grafts were taken from donors, are substantial contributors to allograft immunogenicity. This, of course, may also hold true for skin allografts. The allosensitizing capacities of leukocytes reside mainly in their expression of H-2 encoded alloantigens. According to the model proposed by Sollinger and Bach [64] two populations of T lymphocytes are generated in response to an alloantigenic stimulus in vitro. One population composed of proliferating T helper cells responds primarily to I-region differences (probably Ia antigens) whereas cytotoxic T cells are more strongly activated by K/D-region products. There is some evidence that, in the absence of I-region differences, the generation of cytotoxic T cells is less efficient. In the case of epidermal allografts, it seems conceivable that the Ia-positive LCs represent "resident leukocytes" and provide the necessary stimulus required for allosensitization. Streilein et al. [65] probed this assumption by investigating the fate of mouse corneal grafts on body-wall skin. The reason for using cornea was that this tissue is obviously completely devoid of Ia-positive LCs. Using different inbred mouse strains they found that corneal grafts from animals which were only I-region different from the recipient enjoyed as good a survival as did syngeneic grafts. By contrast, skin grafts containing normal LC numbers were readily rejected even if there was only an I-region difference between donor and recipient. These findings imply that LCs are critical factors in epidermal allosensitization provided that only I-region differences exist between donor and recipient. In keeping with these data is the recent observation that murine skin grafts that had been depleted of LCs by vigorous tape stripping [66] enjoy a prolonged survival on I region–disparate recipients [67].

Miscellaneous

Apart from the fact that certain histiocytic cells in histiocytosis X contain LC granules (for review, see [3]), there exists a plethora of data on quantitative and qualitative changes of epidermal LCs in several disease states, e.g., mycosis fungoides [68,69], atopic dermatitis [70], cutaneous lupus erythematosus [71], vitiligo [4,72–74] and many others. Although each of these observations may be relevant for our understanding of the respective disease process, they allow, at the moment, only the construction of highly speculative concepts of pathogenesis and are therefore not included.

Conclusion

We have reviewed the more recent developments in LC research relevant for our understanding of the role of these cells in skin biology. Because of the major progress made in the past few years, this long-neglected cell type has become one center of research interest not only for dermatologists, but also for biochemists, immunologists, and microbiologists, who will certainly focus their large repertoire of in vitro techniques on the further exploration of LC functions.

References

1. Langerhans P: Über die Nerven der menschlichen Haut. *Virchows Arch [Pathol Anat]* **44**:325–337, 1868
2. Breathnach AS et al: Langerhans cells in mouse skin experimentally deprived of its neural crest component. *J Invest Dermatol* **50**:147–160, 1968
3. Wolff K: The Langerhans cell. *Curr Probl Dermatol* **4**:79–145, 1972
4. Birbeck MS et al: An electron microscope study of basal melanocytes and high-level clear cell (Langerhans cell) in vitiligo. *J Invest Dermatol* **37**:51–64, 1961
5. Basset F, Turiaf J: Identification par la microscopie électronique de particules de nature probablement virale dans les lésions granulomateuses d'une histiocytose ''X'' pulmonaire. *C R Acad Sci (Paris)* **261**:3701–3703, 1965
6. Symposium: The Langerhans cell and contact dermatitis. *Acta DermVenereol (Stockh)* **79s**:1–76, 1977
7. Berman B, Francis DS: Histochemical analysis of Langerhans cells. *Am J Dermatopathol* **1**:215–221, 1979
8. Stingl G et al: Epidermal Langerhans cells bear Fc and C3 receptors. *Nature* **258**:245–246, 1977
9. Tamaki K et al: Ia antigens in mouse skin are predominantly expressed on Langerhans cells. *J Immunol* **123**:784–787, 1979
10. Stingl G et al: Detection of Ia antigens on Langerhans cells in guinea pig skin. *J Immunol* **120**:570–578, 1978
11. Burke KE, Gigli I: Receptors for complement on Langerhans cells. *J Invest Dermatol* **75**:46–51, 1980
12. Dorf ME (ed): *The Role of the Major Histocompatibility Complex.* Garland STPM, New York, 1980
13. Rowden G et al: Ia antigen expression on human epidermal Langerhans cells. *Nature* **268**:247–248, 1977
14. Klareskog L et al: Epidermal Langerhans cells express Ia antigens. *Nature* **268**:248–250, 1977
15. Stingl G et al: Immunofluorescent detection of human B cell alloantigens on S-Ig-positive lymphocytes and epidermal Langerhans cells. *J Immunol* **120**:661–664, 1978
16. Rowden G et al: Visualization of Ia antigen localization in murine keratinizing epithelia. *Immunogenetics* **7**:465–478, 1978
17. Nordlund JJ, Ackles AE: A specific method for quantifying cells bearing Ia antigens in murine epidermis. *J Invest Dermatol* **74**:248A, 1980
18. Fithian E et al: Reactivity of Langerhans cells with hybridoma antibody. *Proc Natl Acad Sci USA* **78**:2541–2544, 1981
19. Majdic O et al: Monoclonal antibody reactive with a cytoplasmic determinant present in B-cells and certain mononuclear phagocytes, in *Leukemia Markers.* Edited by W Knapp. Academic, London, 1981, pp 125–127
20. Caputo R et al: Freeze-fracture of Langerhans granules. A comparative study. *J Invest Dermatol* **66**:297–301, 1976
21. Wolff K, Winkelmann RK: Quantitative studies on the Langerhans cell population of guinea pig epidermis. *J Invest Dermatol* **48**:504–513, 1967
22. Bergstresser P et al: Surface densities of Langerhans cells in relation to rodent epidermal sites with special immunologic properties. *J Invest Dermatol* **74**:77–80, 1980
23. Katz SI et al: Epidermal Langerhans cells are derived from cells originating in the bone marrow. *Nature* **282**:324–326, 1979
24. Frelinger JG et al: Mouse epidermal Ia molecules have a bone marrow origin. *Nature* **282**:321–323, 1979
25. Schellander F, Wolff K: Zur autoradiographischen Markierung von Langerhans-Zellen mit ³H-Thymidin. *Arch Klin Exp Dermatol* **230**:140–145, 1967
26. Silberberg I et al: The role of Langerhans cells in allergic contact hypersensitivity. A review of findings in man and guinea pigs. *J Invest Dermatol* **66**:210–217, 1976
27. Rosenthal AS et al: Macrophage-lymphocyte interaction and antigen recognition. *Fed Proc* **34**:1743–1748, 1975
28. Thomas DW et al: T lymphocyte stimulation by hapten-conjugated macrophages: a model system for the study of immunocompetent cell interactions. *Immunol Rev* **40**:181–204, 1978
29. Schwartz RH et al: Interaction between antigen-presenting cells and primed T lymphocytes: an assessment of Ir gene expression in the antigen-presenting cell. *Immunol Rev* **40**:153–180, 1978
30. Burger R, Shevach EM: Monoclonal antibodies to guinea pig Ia antigens. II. Effect on alloantigen-, antigen-, and mitogen-induced T lymphocyte proliferation in vitro. *J Exp Med* **152**:1011–1023, 1980
31. Stingl G et al: Immunologic functions of Ia-bearing epidermal Langerhans cells. *J Immunol* **121**:2005–2013, 1978

32. Stingl G et al: Antigen presentation by murine epidermal Langerhans cells and its alteration by ultraviolet B light. *J Immunol* **127:**1707–1713, 1981

33. Braathen LR, Thorsby E: Studies on human epidermal Langerhans cells. I. Allo-activating and antigen-presenting capacity. *Scand J Immunol* **11:**401–408, 1980

34. Cantor H, Boyse EA: Functional subclasses of T lymphocytes bearing different Ly antigens. I. The generation of functionally distinct T cell subclasses is a differentiative process independent of antigen. *J Exp Med* **141:**1376–1389, 1975

35. Cantor H, Boyse EA: Functional subclasses of T lymphocytes bearing different Ly antigens. II. Cooperation between subclasses of Ly⁺ cells in the generation of killer activity. *J Exp Med* **141:**1390–1399, 1975

36. Greineder DK, Rosenthal AS: Macrophage activation of allogeneic lymphocyte proliferation in the guinea pig mixed leukocyte culture. *J Immunol* **114:**1541–1547, 1975

37. Steinman RM, Nussenzweig MC: Dendritic cells: features and functions. *Immunol Rev* **53:**127–148, 1980

38. Aberer W et al: UV-induced abrogation of the murine Langerhans cell—lymphocyte reaction (Abstr). *J Invest Dermatol* **76:**414, 1981

38a. Pehamberger H et al: Generation of alloreactive cytotoxic T lymphocytes by epidermal cells: requirement for Langerhans cells. *Clin Res*, in press

39. Pehamberger H et al: Epidermal Langerhans cells are not cytotoxic in antibody dependent cellular cytotoxicity. *J Invest Dermatol* **76:**325A, 1981

40. Belter S et al: A new method for Langerhans cell enrichment (Abstr). *J Invest Dermatol* **76:**427, 1981

41. Brade V, Bentley C: Synthesis and release of complement components by macrophages, in *Mononuclear Phagocytes.* Edited by R van Furth. Martinus Nijhoff, The Hague, 1980

42. Wahl LM et al: Prostaglandin regulation of macrophage collagenase production. *Proc Natl Acad Sci USA* **74:**4955–4958, 1977

43. Davies P et al: Secretion of arachidonic acid oxygenation products by mononuclear phagocytes: their possible significance as modulators of lymphocyte function, in *Macrophage Regulation of Immunity.* Edited by ER Unanue, AS Rosenthal. Academic, New York/London, 1980, pp 347–360

44. Neumann Ch, Sorg C: Immune interferon. I. Production by lymphokine-activated murine macrophages. *Eur J Immunol* **7:**719–725, 1977

45. Neumann Ch et al: Interferon production by *Corynebacterium parvum* and BCG-activated murine spleen macrophages. *Immunobiology* **157:**12–23, 1980

46. Gordon S et al: In vitro synthesis and secretion of lysozyme by mononuclear phagocytes. *J Exp Med* **139:**1228–1248, 1974

47. Werb Z, Gordon S: Elastase secretion by stimulated macrophages. Characterization and regulation. *J Exp Med* **142:**361–377, 1975

48. Wahl LM et al: Collagenase production by lymphokine activated macrophages. *Science* **187:**261–263, 1975

49. Unkeless JC et al: Secretion of plasminogen activator by stimulated macrophages. *J Exp Med* **139:**834–850, 1974

50. Oppenheim JJ et al: Role of cytokine- and endotoxin-induced monokines in lymphocyte proliferation, differentiation, and immunoglobulin production, in *Macrophage Regulation of Immunity.* Edited by ER Unanue, AS Rosenthal. Academic, New York/London, 1980, pp 379–398

51. Luger TA et al: Epidermal cell (keratinocyte)-derived thymocyte-activating factor (ETAF). *J Immunol* **127:**1493–1498, 1981

52. Sauder DN et al: Epidermal cell production of thymocyte activating factor. *Clin Res* **29:**285A, 1981

53. Griffin FM Jr: Effects of soluble immune complexes on Fc-receptor and C3b-receptor-mediated phagocytosis by macrophages. *J Exp Med* **152:**905–919, 1980

54. Goldstein JL et al: Coated pits, coated vesicles, and receptor-mediated endocytosis. *Nature* **279:**679–685, 1979

55. Bergstresser PR et al: Natural and perturbed distributions of Langerhans cells: responses to ultraviolet light, heterotopic skin grafting, and dinitrofluorobenzene sensitization. *J Invest Dermatol* **75:**73–77, 1980

56. Aberer W et al: Ultraviolet light depletes surface markers of Langerhans cells. *J Invest Dermatol* **76:**202–210, 1981

57. Nordlund JJ, Ackles AE: The effects of ultraviolet light and certain drugs on murine epidermal Langerhans cells (LC). *J Invest Dermatol* **76:**325A, 1981

58. Nordlund JJ, Ackles AE: Response of Ia bearing cells in murine skin to contact allergens and melanocytotoxins. *J Invest Dermatol* **76:**308A, 1981

59. Belsito DV et al: Effects of topical steroids on epidermal Langerhans cells. *J Invest Dermatol* **76:**325A, 1981

60. Silberberg-Sinakin I et al: Antigen-bearing Langerhans cells in skin, dermal lymphatics and in lymph nodes. *Cell Immunol* **25:**137–151, 1976

61. Toews GB et al: Epidermal Langerhans cell density determines whether contact sensitivity of unresponsiveness follows skin painting with DNFB. *J Immunol* **124:**445–453, 1980

62. Claman HN et al: Suppressive mechanisms involving sensitization and tolerance in contact allergy. *Immunol Rev* **50:**105–132, 1980

63. Steinmuller D: Passenger leukocytes and the immunogenicity of skin allografts. *J Invest Dermatol* **75:**107–115, 1980

64. Sollinger HW, Bach FH: Collaboration between in vivo responses to LD and SD antigens of major histocompatibility complex. *Nature* **259:**487–488, 1976

65. Streilein JW et al: Corneal allografts fail to express Ia antigens. *Nature* **282:**326–327, 1979

66. Lessard R et al: Induced shedding of the epidermal Langerhans cells. *Nature* **212:**628, 1966

67. Bergstresser PR, Streilein JW: Tape stripping of murine skin removes epidermal Langerhans cells and permits prolonged allograft survival. *J Invest Dermatol* **76:**334A, 1981

68. Rowden G et al: Target role of Langerhans cells in mycosis fungoides. Transmission and immuno-electron microscopy. *J Cutan Pathol* **6:**364–382, 1979

69. Chu A et al: Dermal Langerhans cells in cutaneous lymphoma: an in situ study using monoclonal antibodies. *J Invest Dermatol* **76:**324A, 1981

70. Uno H, Hanifin JM: Langerhans cells in acute and chronic epidermal lesions of atopic dermatitis, observed by L-dopa histofluorescence, glycol methacrylate thin section, and electron microscopy. *J Invest Dermatol* **75:**52–60, 1980

71. Sontheimer RD et al: Langerhans cell involvement in the epidermal pathology of cutaneous lupus erythematosus. *J Invest Dermatol* **76:**309A, 1981

72. Niebauer G: Über die Dendritenzellen bei Vitiligo. *Dermatologica* **130:**317–324, 1965

73. Brown J et al: Langerhans cells in vitiligo: a quantitative study. *J Invest Dermatol* **49:**386–390, 1967

74. Zelickson AS, Mottaz JH: Epidermal dendritic cells. *Arch Dermatol* **98:**652–659, 1968

DERMATOLOGIC DISEASES ASSOCIATED WITH EOSINOPHILIA

Stephanie H. Pincus

Sheldon M. Wolff

It has been just over 100 years since the eosinophil was described by Paul Ehrlich. Since that time, peripheral blood eosinophilia has been associated with a wide variety of diseases but is most frequently associated with allergic and parasitic diseases [1]. Despite considerable speculation, the biologic role of the eosinophil remains uncertain. Some recent experiments have concentrated on the eosinophil as an effector cell causing actual destruction of the organisms in parasitic diseases [2,3]. It has been shown that eosinophils can kill larval forms of *Schistosoma mansoni* and *Trichinella spiralis* in vitro [3–5]. A distinctive feature of the eosinophil is the presence of a strongly basic protein (major basic protein) with a molecular weight of approximately 9000 in the unique eosinophil granule [6]. This protein is released when the eosinophil comes in contact with a parasite and may contribute to killing of the organism [7]. Additionally, this protein may be a cause of tissue damage during allergic reactions [8]. Serum levels of major basic protein may be elevated in patients with hypereosinophilia of diverse causes and may also be elevated in some patients with skin disease and normal peripheral blood eosinophil counts [9].

Recently, it has been recognized that certain diseases are associated with peripheral blood or tissue eosinophilia without evidence of parasitic disease or hypersensitivity reactions. These conditions suggest a unique role for the eosinophil in the pathophysiology of these diseases. Some conditions, such as the hypereosinophilic syndrome

1 Hypeeosinophilic syn.

2 Eosin. fasciitis

3 Wells

4 Angiolym. hyperplasia c̄ eosin.

5. Eosinophilia pustrulr folliculitis
   Eos. Leuk

13

and eosinophilic fasciitis, are systemic diseases with cutaneous manifestations and others appear to be predominantly cutaneous such as Well's syndrome or angiolymphoid hyperplasia with eosinophilia (Kimura's disease). This review will concern new findings related to diseases characterized by peripheral and tissue eosinophilia.

Hypereosinophilic Syndrome

For many years, a debate existed as to the existence of a unique disease associated with eosinophilia in the absence of other systemic illness. It is now accepted that there is a unique condition which is called the *hypereosinophilic syndrome* [10]. There is another distinct group of hypereosinophilic patients who have a true eosinophilic leukemia associated with an increase in blast cells in the peripheral blood and/or bone marrow, and these patients should not be included in hypereosinophilic syndrome. These leukemic patients can be distinguished from those with marked persistent eosinophilia, diffuse organ infiltration, and *normal bone marrow morphology*. Unfortunately, the distinctness of the syndrome becomes difficult since patients with other causes of hypereosinophilia (such as eosinophilic leukemia) may develop complications such as Loeffler's fibroplastic endocarditis, a common occurrence in the hypereosinophilic syndrome.

A recent review by Chusid et al. [10] provides convincing evidence of a distinct hypereosinophilic syndrome not related to collagen vascular disease, bone marrow abnormalities, or known allergic or parasitic disease. Fourteen patients seen at the National Institutes of Health (NIH) were compared with patients described in the literature. Criteria for the diagnosis of hypereosinophilic syndrome included (1) a persistent eosinophilia of greater than 1500 eosinophils per cubic millimeter for greater than 6 months, (2) a lack of evidence for parasitic, allergic, or other disease associated with eosinophilia, and (3) signs and symptoms consistent with organ infiltration. Criteria for evidence of organ infiltration included hepatosplenomegaly, heart murmurs, congestive heart failure, neurologic dysfunction, and/or pulmonary disease. There is a marked male predominance; 91 percent of those patients reported in the literature and all of patients described by Chusid et al. were males. Most commonly the patients are middle-aged and the presenting complaints include fever, weight loss, fatigue, malaise, and skin rash. In the group of patients under review, weight loss was the most

common sign (71 percent) and rash and neurologic abnormalities were noted in 57 percent of the patients. Common findings included splenomegaly, hepatomegaly, cardiac murmurs, fever, diarrhea, edema, cough, arthralgia, and abdominal pain. Though all patients had peripheral blood eosinophilia, there was marked variation in the percentage of eosinophils, ranging from 17 to 90 percent. In addition, many patients had eosinophils with a decreased number of granules, hypersegmentation of the nucleus, or cytoplasmic vacuolization.

There was evidence of multiple-organ involvement in all the patients studied. The cardiovascular system was involved in 93 percent of the patients studied at the NIH. A subsequent study by Parillo et al. in 1979 [11] described the cardiovascular manifestations in 26 patients (including the previously described NIH patients) with hypereosinophilic syndrome. Cardiovascular symptoms such as cough, chest pain, or dyspnea were present in 58 percent of the patients, and signs of cardiovascular disease including mitral regurgitation, and congestive failure, were found in 65 percent of the patients. In addition, approximately half the patients had cardiomegaly or congestive failure on chest x-ray and approximately two-thirds of the patients had abnormal EKG findings including T-wave inversion (35 percent) and left atrial enlargement (28 percent). The most sensitive test demonstrating cardiovascular involvement was the echocardiogram, which was abnormal in 82 percent of the patients studied. The most common echocardiographic abnormalities were thickening of the left ventricular free wall (68 percent), septal thickening (59 percent), or an increase in left ventricular mass (73 percent). Prospective echocardiographic examination revealed that some untreated patients or patients with progressive disease had increases in left ventricular wall thickness throughout the course of study. In patients with long-standing hypereosinophilic syndrome, cardiac disease is a major cause of morbidity and mortality. Congestive heart failure due to a restrictive cardiomyopathy is characterized histopathologically by endocardial fibrosis, myocardial inflammation, and mural thrombus formation.

Dermatologic manifestations are frequently seen in the hypereosinophilic syndrome. Fifty-seven percent of the NIH patients had cutaneous disease, as described in a report by Kazmierowski et al. [12]. The lesions seen in the hypereosinophilic syndrome are not specific and can have differing morphologic appearances. The majority of patients had either a pruritic erythematous papular eruption or an urticarial eruption with angioedema. Dermographia was present in greater than 75 percent of the patients [13]. However, in each biopsy of the eight patients studied, perivascular infiltration with eosinophils was a common finding. In addition, some patients had mild-to-moderate mononuclear and neutrophilic infiltrates in a perivascular distribution. In general, the course of the skin eruption paralleled the course of the systemic disease. Thus, the skin biopsy may provide an easily accessible confirmation of organ involvement.

Multiple-organ involvement may include neurologic, pulmonary, or gastrointestinal disease. Patients with hypereosinophilic syndrome frequently have neurologic abnormalities; both central defects and peripheral neuropathies have been described. It was initially suspected that the neuropathy might be on the basis of embolic vascular occlusion or eosinophilic infiltration of peripheral nerves. However, recent investigations suggest that the eosinophils contain a potentially neurotoxic substance [14,15]. Although it is relatively uncommon to find serologic evidence of hepatic involvement, in six hypereosinophilic patients who had liver biopsies all specimens demonstrated organ damage defined as periportal eosinophilic infiltrate or eosinophilic triaditis [10]. Transient pulmonary infiltrates and episodic diarrhea were found in many patients, and presumably reflect tissue infiltration with eosinophils.

Laboratory diagnosis of the hypereosinophilic syndrome requires a persistently elevated total eosinophil count, greater than 1500 mm³. Although many patients have an elevated sedimentation rate, it is not a consistent finding. The majority of laboratory tests including serum electrolytes, blood sugar, calcium, alkaline phosphatase, iron, total protein, and protein electrophoresis are usually within normal limits. A more thorough study of immunologic parameters in patients with the hypereosinophilic syndrome was performed in 21 patients [13]. Elevated IgE levels were present in 38 percent of the patients, but IgG, IgA, and IgM levels were normal or only slightly elevated in a small proportion of the patients. Patients with increased serum IgE are more likely to have angioedema [16]. Some patients had elevated C4 or C1q measurements. Though there was a statistically significant decrease in T cells as measured by rosetting techniques, T-cell function as measured by lymphocyte response to mitogens or cutaneous delayed-hypersensitivity testing was normal. An elevated histamine level was found in only two patients who also had pressure urticaria.

The diagnosis of hypereosinophilic syndrome requires a high clinical suspicion because of the variety of signs and symptoms. An absolute requirement is persistent eosinophilia, and it is essential that there be no evidence of allergic, or parasitic, disease or of the other conditions sometimes associated with eosinophilia. Diagnosis depends on the exclusion of other diseases, rather than on any positive findings. Histopathologic evidence of tissue infiltration of eosinophils may be useful.

The cause of death in hypereosinophilic syndrome is frequently difficult to identify. However, in a survey of the literature [10] where a cause of death could be identified, it was most commonly related to cardiovascular disease. In approximately 65 percent of the cases reported in the literature death was ascribed to congestive heart failure. Infections, bleeding, renal disease, and liver failure have also been identified as causes of death. Despite the fact that it is difficult to identify clearly the cause of death, there is significant morbidity associated with hypereosinophilic syndrome. In one study a 77 percent mortality in 3 years was observed [16].

Autopsy studies confirm that all patients had some type of cardiac abnormality such as an increase in heart size. Other findings included endocardial thrombi and fibrosis, valvular damage, myocardial necrosis, myocardial fibrosis, and, rarely (13 percent), eosinophilic infiltration of the myocardium. In general, left ventricular involvement was more prominent, and thrombus formation and endocardial fibrosis were more commonly seen at the cardiac apex. Pulmonary involvement, typically interstitial eosinophilic infiltrates, were seen in approximately 40 percent of autopsied cases. Though hepatic and splenic infiltration by eosinophils was frequently seen on autopsy, there was little to suggest that this was related to the cause of death. Vasculitis was rarely seen despite careful search.

Because cardiovascular disease, if present, progresses in the absence of treatment, it is important to treat certain patients with hypereosinophilic syndrome. Factors correlated with a poor prognosis include a high peripheral leukocyte count greater than 90 to 100,000 leukocytes per cubic millimeter, the appearance of myeloblasts in the peripheral blood, and the development of congestive heart failure. Indications for treatment include documentation of organ involvement and progression of the disease [16]. A group of patients appear to be responsive to prednisone. Usually, the patients are given daily prednisone (up to 60 mg/day) and then switched to every-other-day therapy.

These patients are characterized by an elevated serum IgE, frequent angioedema, and a prolonged decrease in circulating eosinophils following a single dose challenge with prednisone. Prednisone should be mantained as long as necessary to control the hypereosinophilia. Patients who respond to prednisone have not become refractory to treatment. Those patients not responsive to prednisone are often responsive to hydroxyurea. The usual dose is 1 to 2 g daily. In the most recent study six of eight patients who were unresponsive to corticosteroids had an excellent response to hydroxyurea [16]. The decline in peripheral eosinophilia was correlated with an improvement in the cardiac status. Indeed, in their prospective study [10], treated patients had a decrease in left ventricular wall thickness as measured by echocardiography and a decrease in left ventricular mass. This suggests that aggressive early treatment of hypereosinophilic syndrome may minimize the cardiovascular complications. It is of note that patients with congestive heart failure due to eosinophilic cardiomyopathy may be refractory to treatment with digitalis and/or diuretics in the absence of antihypereosinophilic treatment. Though the pathophysiology of this disease remains unclear, the presence of myocardial damage and other conditions associated with hypereosinophilia raises the question of possible direct cardiac toxicity [17]. It is also noteworthy that certain patients with hypereosinophilia with little or no evidence of organ involvement, save for a pruritic dermatitis, may require no therapy at all.

Eosinophilic Fasciitis

In 1974, two patients with a syndrome resembling acute-onset scleroderma associated with peripheral blood eosinophilia were described by Shulman [18]. Since that time, this condition has been called *Shulman's syndrome* or eosinophilic fasciitis. There has been considerable debate as to whether or not it is a variant of scleroderma or deserves its own category. However, because of its unique clinical presentation, this syndrome will be described separately.

Four patients, described in detail by Shulman in 1975 [19], presented with acute onset of firm, tight bound-down skin involving the legs and arms. There was no history of Raynaud's phenomenon. Several of the patients gave a history of having substantially increased their level of activity immediately prior to development of the syndrome. Peripheral blood eosinophilia and hypergamma-globulinemia were noted in the patients. Because of the deep indurated nature of the lesions, initial biopsies included muscle and fat. There was marked thickening of the fascia with edema, an infiltrate of plasma cells, lymphocytes, and the development of lymphoid follicles. Despite the findings of peripheral blood eosinophilia, there was little evidence of infiltration by eosinophils. A most striking and clinically unique feature of these cases was clear-cut improvement following prednisone treatment with a demonstrable reduction in the muscular and subcutaneous induration.

Since these original descriptions, over 50 patients have been reported in the literature. As is the case with most diseases characterized by eosinophilia, the majority of the patients are male. Again, similar to hypereosinophilic syndrome, the mean age at diagnosis was 44 years and 42 years, respectively, in two recent series [20,21]. In recent reviews approximately 50 percent of the patients with eosinophilic fasciitis noted the onset of symptoms following excessive physical exertion [20,22]. Typically, the acute onset of swelling, stiffness, and tenderness occurred in the forearms and/or hands. Frequently, the process involved the legs and appeared simultaneously in all affected areas. Face and trunk involvement were much less frequent. In a small proportion of patients synovitis or arthralgias were noted, and low-grade fever was reported. The involved extremities were edematous, with marked induration and (frequently) "orange peel" wrinkling and puckering of the skin.

Laboratory studies confirmed that approximately 90 percent of the patients had eosinophilia which ranged from 4 to 49 percent, though sometimes the eosinophilia spontaneously resolved. Though total eosinophil counts were frequently elevated, they were not ascertained in all cases. Hypergammaglobulinemia was present in 60 to 74 percent of the patients and an elevated sedimentation rate was present in 40 to 68 percent of the patients [20–22]. There was little evidence of immunologic disease; only 12 to 15 percent of the patients had anti-DNA or antinuclear antibodies [20]. No evidence was found for a decrease in circulating complement, and cryoglobulins were not detected.

Deep incisional biopsies extending to muscle consistently were abnormal. In a series of 20 cases in which careful histologic examination was performed using both standard hematoxylin and eosin as well as special stains, the pathologic picture was more clearly delineated [19]. On gross examination the fascia was 2 to 15 times thicker than normal. It was sclerotic and firmly adherent to the overlying subcutaneous tissue. On microscopic examination the epidermis was normal in most cases (80 percent); when abnormal, the epidermis demonstrated slight atrophy thought to be due to dermal sclerosis. In about 65 percent of the biopsy specimens there was mild to moderate fibrosis of the reticular dermis and a patchy infiltrate of lymphocytes, plasma cells, histiocytes, and occasional eosinophils. In cases with more severe fibrosis, the reticular dermis was thick and hyalinized. The subcutaneous tissue was involved in all cases, with changes varying from edema and inflammation of the fibrous septa to marked fibrosis. As the disease progressed, there was increasing fibrosis with eventual fusion of the septum to the fascia and entrapment of the fat cells. As a net effect, the thickness of the subcutaneous tissue was decreased. The changes in the fascia varied from marked thickening and fibrosis to inflammation and edema. The cellular composition of inflammatory infiltrates was similar to the dermal infiltrates. Though about 20 percent of the patients may have histologically normal muscle tissue, the remainder demonstrate mild-to-moderate perivascular infiltration of lymphocytes, plasma cells, histiocytes, and eosinophils. Mild focal interstitial fibrosis was frequently noted. There was no actual vasculitis, although occasionally endothelial cell proliferation was noted. In only 13 of the 20 cases studied was the number of tissue eosinophils increased, and in about half of these cases the eosinophils were distributed in focal aggregates. Immunofluorescent studies were done in eight patients. Of the five patients with IgG, IgM, and/or C3 in the skin, there was no consistent pattern which could be correlated with disease activity. Other associated findings include synovitis and muscle involvement as evidenced by an elevated CPK (creatine phosphokinase) or an abnormal EMG.

Thus, the diagnosis of eosinophilic fasciitis is made on the basis of the clinical history and histologic examination of the skin, subcutaneous tissue, and muscle fascia. Though an increase in circulating eosinophils or hypergammaglobulinemia is confirmatory, their presence is not required for diagnosis. Because of the responsiveness of this condition to therapy, it is important to be alert for the possibility of making this diagnosis.

A striking feature of this syndrome is the rapid objective response to adrenal corticosteroid treatment. Prednisone in doses ranging from 40 to 100 mg per day resulted in moderate-to-substantial improvement in the majority of patients. Therapeutic responses include objective improvement in cutaneous edema and induration as well as a decrease in circulating eosinophils, a decrease in the sedimentation rate, and a reduction in hypergammaglobulinemia. Within weeks of beginning therapy most patients note decreased induration, tightness, and improvement of clinical symptoms.

The clinical features and response to steroid therapy might suggest that this disease may be clearly distinguished from scleroderma. However, caution is required since some authors report cases that are histologically and clinically indistinguishable from scleroderma but appear to have passed through a stage consistent with eosinophilic fasciitis. Though further experience may lead to categorization as a variant of scleroderma, the unique clinical features and responsiveness to treatment should be emphasized. The fact that over 50 cases have appeared in the literature since the initial description in 1974 suggests that eosinophilic fasciitis may be more common than initially supposed and may not have been previously recognized.

Well's Syndrome

By way of contrast, Well's syndrome, acute nonbacterial cellulitis with eosinophilia, has been infrequently reported since the initial description in 1971 [23]. About one dozen patients have been described as of 1980 [23–25]. Each of the original four patients gave a history of recurrent localized swelling of the extremities over a period of years. The initial lesions began with a burning sensation or itching associated with redness and local induration. The most common cutaneous signs were persistent urticarial eruptions or infiltrated erythemas with an annular or circinate pattern. Over the course of several days, the eruption spread outward rapidly to involve an extremity, and central clearing developed. The area had the clinical appearance of cellulitis. Typically there was a sharp rosy or violaceous border. Some cases developed a central bulla. The eruption gradually subsided without treatment of the lesion. A brawny bluish (slate) discoloration and edema persisted for several weeks and faded slowly from the center outward. A third clinical phase of local atrophy similar to morphea follows but gradually resolves without treatment. During the phase of initial onset and local persistence, eosinophilia is present. Eosinophilia of 13 to 44 percent was noted in half the recent cases [24,25].

Histopathologic examination of the acute stage reveals marked infiltration of the dermis with eosinophils and dermal edema. Eosinophils accumulate in a perivascular distribution. In those cases where bullae developed, eosinophils were present in a subepidermal distribution. During the more chronic. subacute stage biopsies show infiltration of the connective tissue bundles with eosinophils and histiocytes. The granulomatous infiltrate develops focal "flame figures" which have a unique histologic appearance. The distinctive flame figures are aggregates within the dermis which consist of a central collagen bundle and eosinophilic debris [24,25]. Over the next few weeks, correlating with gradual clinical improvement, the biopsy shows fewer eosinophils but histiocytes persist. Despite the perivascular distribution of eosinophils, there is no histologic evidence that Well's syndrome represents a vasculitis or is in any way related to the granulomatous vasculitis described by Churg and Strauss [26]. The possible etiology of Well's syndrome, which also goes by the name of *recurrent granulomatous dermatitis with eosinophilia*, is completely unknown. Fortunately, prednisone may be effective in some patients.

Angiolymphoid Hyperplasia with Eosinophilia (Kimura's Disease)

In the late 1940s, several case reports from Japan and other Asian countries described patients with acute onset of flesh-colored nodules of the head and neck [27]. The patients were predominantly male, and histologic examination showed lymphoid hyperplasia eosinophilic infiltration and a variable degree of endothelial hyperplasia. The disease is called *Kimura's disease*. By 1966, it was noteworthy that approximately 150 cases had been described in the Orient [28]. Similar cases in the English literature were first described by Wells and Whimster in 1969 [29]. They reported a group of nine young adults equally distributed between male and female who had slowly growing nodular lesions, multiple or singular, of the head and neck. Blood eosinophilia was present in seven patients. Though the clinical appearance of the lesions was not distinctive, histologic examination led to grouping the cases together. In all cases, the main histologic abnormality lay in the subcutaneous fat, where there was a poorly demarcated area of vascular proliferation with masses of endothelial cells and an angiomatous appearance. In addition, there was a heavy infiltrate of eosinophils and focal lymphocytic infiltration with lymphoid folli-

cle and germinal center development. There was some variability in histology, with some patients having greater predominance of lymphocytic changes and lymphoid follicle development. Because several patients had serial biopsies, it was possible to outline the sequence of development. Earliest lesions showed exuberant angioid proliferation with massive eosinophilia in the tissues. Aggregates of lymphocytes were present in earlier lesions, and these seemed to develop into lymphoid follicles with germinal centers in more advanced lesions. There appeared to be an increase in mast cells throughout the process. Histologically, these lesions must be distinguished from eosinophilic granuloma, benign lymphocytic infiltrates of the skin, atypical pyogenic granuloma, angioid lymphoid hematomas, and persistent insect-bite reactions. The marked angioid hyperplasia would be unusual in a prolonged bite reaction, which may otherwise have a similar histologic appearance [30]. A group of patients described as having pseudopyogenic granuloma [30] have clinically and histologically very similar lesions; however, the infiltrate is distributed more in the dermis than the subcutaneous tissue. The course is slowly progressive and treatments have included topical steroids and low-dose x-ray with variable results.

Eosinophilic Pustular Folliculitis

This syndrome, originally recognized in Japan in 1970 [31], is characterized by mildly pruritic follicular or perifollicular 1- to 3-mm papules and pustules in annular or polycyclic array on an erythematous base. Typically, the patient is a young adult (there is a marked male predominance) and the eruption begins on the face or upper arms [31,32]. The condition waxes and wanes. The mucosa is not involved and there are no systemic signs. Biopsy shows eosinophilic exocytosis of the epidermis with small eosinophilic intraepidermal abscesses. The eosinophilic abscesses involve the hair follicles and the sebaceous glands. There may be a perivascular or perifollicular dermal mononuclear infiltrate with a variable number of eosinophils. Immunofluorescent studies were unrevealing [32,33]. Peripheral blood eosinophils ranging from 5 to 40 percent were present in 15 of 18 cases [32]. Treatment has included sulfones, antibiotics, and griseofulvin without significant improvement; however, most patients respond well to systemic steroid treatment.

References

1. Beeson PB, Bass DA: *The Eosinophil in Major Problems in Internal Medicine*. Edited by LH Smith. Saunders, Philadelphia, 1977
2. Kazura JW: Protective role of eosinophils, 1977, in *The Eosinophil in Health and Disease*. Edited by AAF Mahmoud, KF Austen. Grune & Stratton, New York, 1980, pp 231–252
3. Butterworth AD et al: Mechanisms of eosinophil-mediated helminthotoxicity, in *The Eosinophil in Health and Disease*. Edited by AAF Mahmoud, KF Austen. Grune & Stratton, New York, 1980, pp 253–271
4. Bass DA, Szejda P: Mechanisms of killing of newborn larvae of *Trichinella spiralis* by neutrophils and eosinophils: killing by generators of hydrogen peroxide *in vitro*. *J Clin Invest* **64:**558–564, 1979
5. Bass DA, Szejda PA: Eosinophils versus neutrophil in host defense: killing of newborn larvae of *Trichinella spiralis* by human granulocytes *in vitro*. *J Clin Invest* **64:**1415–1422, 1979
6. Gleich GJ et al: Identification of a major basic protein in guinea pig eosinophil granules. *J Exp Med* **137:**1459–1471, 1973
7. Butterworth AE et al: Damage to schistosomula of *Schistosoma mansoni* induced directly by eosinophil major basic protein. *J Immunol* **122:**221–229, 1979
8. Gleich GJ et al: Cytotoxic properties of the eosinophil major basic protein. *J Immunol* **123:**2925–2927, 1979
9. Wassom DI et al: Elevated serum levels of the eosinophil granule major basic protein in patients with eosinophilia. *J Clin Invest* **67:**651–661, 1981
10. Chusid MJ et al: The hypereosinophilic syndrome: analysis of 14 cases with review of the literature. *Medicine (Baltimore)* **54:**1–27, 1975
11. Parillo JE et al: The cardiovascular manifestations of the hypereosinophilic syndrome: prospective study of 26 patients with review of the literature. *Am J Med* **67:**572–582, 1979
12. Kazmierowski JA et al: Dermatologic manifestations of the hypereosinophilic syndrome. *Arch Dermatol* **114:**531–535, 1978
13. Parillo JA et al: Immunologic reactivity in the hypereosinophilic syndrome. *J Allergy Clin Immunol* **64:**113–121, 1979
14. Seiler G et al: The role of specific eosinophil granules in eosinophil-induced experimental encephalitis. *Neurology* **19:**478–488, 1969
15. Durack DT et al: Neurotoxicity of human eosinophils. *Proc Natl Acad Sci USA* **76:**1443–1447, 1979
16. Parillo JE et al: Therapy of hypereosinophilic syndrome. *Ann Intern Med* **89:**167–172, 1978
17. Parillo JE, Fauci AS: Human eosinophils: purification and cytotoxic capability of eosinophils from patients with the hypereosinophilic syndrome. *Blood* **51:**457–473, 1978
18. Shulman LE: Diffuse fasciitis with hypergammaglobulinemia and eosinophilia: a new syndrome? *J Rheumatol* **1(Suppl 1):**82, 1974
19. Shulman E: Diffuse fasciitis with eosinophilia: a new syndrome? *Trans Assoc Am Physicians* **88:**70–86, 1975
20. Moore TL, Zuckner J: Eosinophilic fasciitis. *Semin Arthritis Rheum* **9:**228–234, 1980
21. Barnes L et al: Eosinophilic fasciitis. *Am J Pathol* **96:**493–507, 1979
22. Michet GJ et al: Eosinophil fasciitis: report of 15 cases. *Mayo Clin Proc* **56:**27–34, 1981
23. Wells GC: Recurrent granulomatous dermatitis with eosinophilia. *Trans St Johns Hosp Dermatol Soc* **57:**46–56, 1971
24. Wells GC, Smith N: Eosinophilic cellulitis. *Br J Dermatol* **100:**101–110, 1979
25. Spigel GT, Winkelman RK: Well's syndrome: recurrent granulomatous dermatitis with eosinophilia. *Arch Dermatol* **115:**611–613, 1979
26. Churg J, Strauss L: Allergic granulomatosis, allergic angiitis, and periarteritis nodosa. *Am J Pathol* **27:**277–301, 1951
27. Kimura T et al: Unusual granulation combined with hyperplastic change of lymphatic tissue. *Trans Soc Pathol Jap* **37:**179, 1948
28. Kawada A et al: Eosinophilic lymphofolliculosis of the skin (Kimura's disease). *Jpn J Dermatol* **76:**61–72, 1966
29. Wells GC, Whimster IW: Subcutaneous angio-lymphoid hyperplasia with eosinophilia. *Br J Dermatol* **81:**1–15, 1969
30. Wilson-Jones E, Bleehen S: Inflammatory angiomatous nodules with abnormal blood vessels occurring about the ears and scalp (atypical or pseudopyogenic granuloma). *Br J Dermatol* **81:**804–815, 1969
31. Ofuji S et al: Eosinophilic pustular folliculitis. *Acta Derm Venereol (Stockh)* **50:**195–203, 1970
32. Ishibashi A et al: Eosinophilic pustular folliculitis (Ofuji). *Dermatologica* **149:**240–247, 1974
33. Holst R: Eosinophilic pustular folliculitis: report of a European case. *Br J Dermatol* **95:**661–664, 1976

ERYTHEMA ELEVATUM
DIUTINUM

Stephen I. Katz

Definition

Erythema elevatum diutinum is a rare chronic skin disease characterized by red, purple, and yellowish papules, plaques, and nodules that are usually distributed acrally and symmetrically over extensor surfaces. It is characterized histologically by a leukocytoclastic vasculitis.

Historical Aspects

In 1894, Radcliffe-Crocker and Williams [1] described a 6-year-old patient with persistent pink and purple nodules over the hands, elbows, knees, and buttocks and reviewed the small number of clinically similar cases reported by Hutchinson [2] and Bury [3]. As the group of patients could be collectively characterized as having red, raised lesions with a strong tendency toward persistence of lesions rather than to involution, they suggested the descriptive term *erythema elevatum diutinum*. In that report, Radcliffe-Crocker and Williams distinguished the Bury type of erythema elevatum diutinum, occurring in young females with a family history of gout or "rheumatism," from the Hutchinson type, occurring in elderly gouty males. Radcliffe-Crocker and Williams felt that the two types of erythema elevatum diutinum might be phases of one disease; however, any distinction between these two types has for decades been abandoned. Although for many years cases of erythema elevatum diutinum were confused with what was later described by Radcliffe-Crocker to be granuloma annulare [4], it was Della-Favera [5], Weidman and Besancon [6], and Haber [7] who clearly differentiated these two diseases histopathologically. In the 1930s, extracellular cholesterosis [8] was introduced as a new entity but it cannot be distinguished from erythema elevatum diutinum [9,10] and should not be separated nosologically.

Etiology and Pathophysiology

Although the cause of erythema elevatum diutinum is unknown, the finding of C1q binding activity in the sera of some patients, the exacerbation of disease with spontaneous streptococcal infections or with streptokinase-streptodornase skin tests, the Arthus-like histology of all spontaneous and streptokinase-streptodornase–induced lesions, and the positive 4-hr streptokinase-streptodornase skin test reactivity in many patients suggests an immune complex etiology for this disease. It may be, as Jensen and Esquenazi [11] have proposed from animal studies, that chemoattraction occurs as a direct result of an immune reaction taking place between the chemotactic stimulus and the surface of the responding cell. In the case of erythema elevatum diutinum, the neutrophil surface would have to be coated with a substance that binds bacterial cell products (streptokinase-streptodornase or perhaps others), and the resultant immune complex reaction results in the movement of these neutrophils to the site of antigenic deposition. The impaired neutrophil chemotaxis observed in two patients could be explained by deactivation of

neutrophil responsiveness by circulating chemotactic factor as has been described for other chemotactic factors [12]. Another testable hypothesis would be that these patients lack a chemotactic factor inhibitor which is a basic, homeostatic, controlling influence [13]. Dapsone, which is effective in erythema elevatum diutinum, may stimulate production of this inhibitor which, in turn, shuts off the pathologic process.

Clinical Features and Course of Disease

Erythema elevatum diutinum is most frequently seen in adults but may occur at any age [14]. The lesions are multiple and often progress from papules to plaques or nodules. Coalescence of lesions may result in gyrate or irregular forms. The early lesions are often pink or yellowish and may later become red or purple. Early lesions are soft and may be tender while older lesions may become doughy or hard.

The distribution of lesions is highly characteristic. They are usually distributed symmetrically on the extensor surfaces and have a striking predilection for the skin overlying joints, especially on the hands, elbows, and knees (Figs. 1 to 3), although lesions may cover large areas of skin

Fig. 2. Erythema elevatum diutinum. Nodular, scaling, and crusted lesions on elbows and wrists. Papular lesions on forearms.

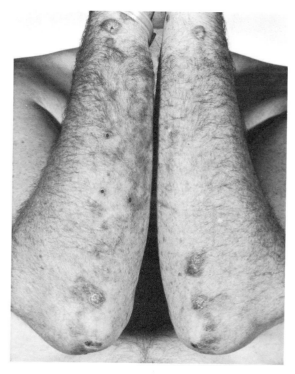

Fig. 1. Erythema elevatum diutinum. Nodular lesions on dorsa of hands and on wrists. Each lesion had been present for several years.

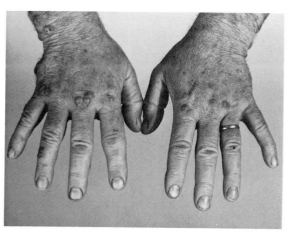

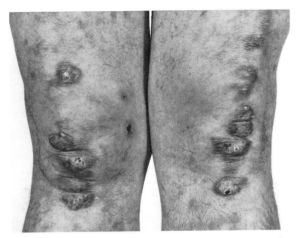

Fig. 3. Erythema elevatum diutinum. Nodular, crusted, and scaling lesions on knees.

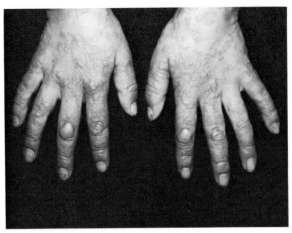

Fig. 4. Erythema elevatum diutinum. Papules, nodules, and plaques on dorsa of hands.

(Figs. 4 and 5). They also have a predilection for the buttocks (Fig. 6) and for the skin overlying the Achilles tendon. The face and ears may be affected but the trunk is generally spared, as are the mucous membranes. Lesions may be round or oval and the surface is usually smooth with the occasional presence of scale. They are usually freely movable from the underlying tissues. Petechia or purpura is sometimes seen in early lesions (especially after discontinuation of dapsone therapy). Bulla formation or hemorrhagic crusting with ulceration may also be seen, especially in very edematous lesions. Some old nodules or plaques may become fibrotic and may resemble xanthomas. Occasionally lesions involve spontaneously and often leave atrophic wrinkled hyper- or hypopigmented areas with loss of underlying collagen.

Symptoms vary, the lesions being totally asymptomatic in some and very painful in others. The lesions are sometimes characterized as aching or

Fig. 5. Erythema elevatum diutinum. Numerous papules and plaques on thighs and legs with nodular lesions on knees.

Fig. 6. Erythema elevatum diutinum. Papules and nodules on buttocks and thighs.

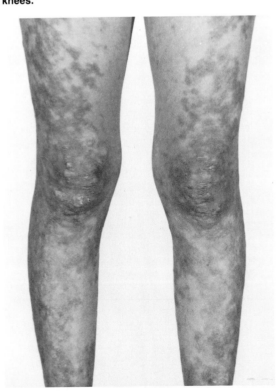

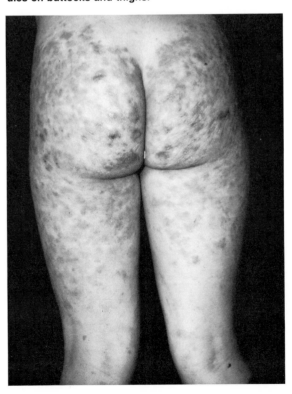

burning. Often there is an associated systemic abnormality, the most common of which is arthralgia of varying severity [7]. More recent studies have described patients with a long history of recurrent pharyngeal and sinopulmonary infections, most commonly streptococcal [14].

The course of the disease is highly variable. Although Haber [7] stated that the disease "is essentially chronic and progresses, in most cases, over a period of 5 to 10 years, to eventual resolution," there are few well-documented instances of spontaneous long-term resolution. Follow-up of five patients reported in 1977 [14] has shown that each of the individuals has persisting disease which has varied from 11 to 28 years. There are periods of waxing and waning; some patients have only one or two lesions or crops of new lesions every 2 to 3 weeks and others have new lesions once every month or two. Streptococcal infections have been reported to exacerbate the disease [14]. Changes in temperature, and especially cold weather, have also been said to aggravate existing lesions or be associated with the eruption of new lesions.

Fig. 7. Erythema elevatum diutinum. Biopsy of lesion showing myriads of neutrophils in vessel wall and strewn throughout the dermis. × 188.

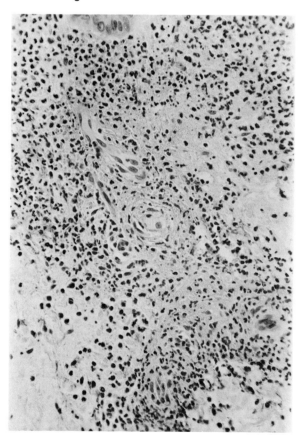

Histopathology

Erythema elevatum diutinum was one of the first skin diseases to be designated to be a form of necrotizing vasculitis. Weidman and Besancon [6] felt that the vasculitis with prominent neutrophils along with the marked hyalinization of vessel walls were the outstanding features of this disease, which they clearly differentiated from granuloma annulare. Indeed, histologically the lesions are highly characteristic and easily differentiated from the other clinical considerations but may be difficult to differentiate from other types of leukocytoclastic vasculitis. Most small, upper, and mid dermal blood vessels show endothelial swelling as well as a significant number of neutrophils and their fragments in and around their walls (Figs. 7 and 8). Fibrinoid degeneration, referred to as *toxic hyalin* of the vessel walls, is usually present (Fig. 8). An admixture of lymphocytes and a smaller number of eosinophils may be seen perivascularly. Neutrophils and their fragments are also commonly strewn throughout the upper and mid dermis and may be seen in large numbers between collagen bundles. There may be an unaffected zone of collagen just beneath the epidermis as in granuloma faciale (Fig. 9). On the other hand, the epidermis may be affected as a result of the dermal infiltrate and edema and may show varying degrees of injury from slight acanthosis to frank necrosis. Older lesions may show a fibrotic replacement of the dermis accompanied by capillary proliferation (Fig. 10). Even when the dermis appears to be totally replaced by these changes, one can often find small foci of the leukocytoclastic vasculitis cited above. In the older lesions there may also be varying amounts of extracellular cholesterol deposits. This

Fig. 8. Erythema elevatum diutinum. High-power view of Fig. 7 showing endothelial swelling, fibrinoid necrosis of the vessel wall ("toxic hyalin"), and neutrophilic fragments in vessel wall. × 405.

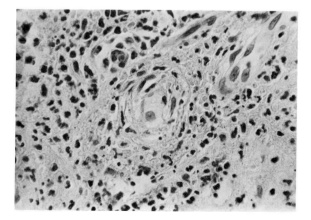

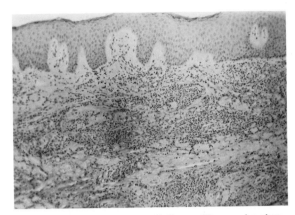

Fig. 9. Erythema elevatum diutinum. Biopsy showing leukocytoclastic vasculitis with neutrophils strewn throughout the dermis and unaffected zone of collagen just beneath the epidermis. ×96.

is especially the case in lesions that have a yellowish xanthomatous appearance clinically. This particular histologic variant of erythema elevatum diutinum, which was formerly called *extracellular cholesterosis* [8], is unassociated with disturbances of lipid metabolism. It probably occurs as a result of the heavily damaged tissue with extracellular and intracellular deposits consisting of cholesterol esters [9,10]. None of the histologic findings cited is pathognomonic for erythema elevatum diutinum, although the constellation of histologic findings in both recently erupted and older lesions of erythema elevatum diutinum may serve to distinguish this entity from other forms of leukocytoclastic vasculitis.

Laboratory Findings

Most patients have elevated erythrocyte sedimentation rates. In addition, in most patients tested, there are markedly positive 4- and 24-hr skin test reactions to intradermally injected streptokinase-streptodornase, extracellularly elaborated products of Lancefield group C strains of streptococci [14,15]. When biopsied at 4 or 6 hr after the skin test, reactions show most of the histologic features of leukocytoclastic vasculitis. In addition to the markedly positive skin test reactions, many patients develop satellite lesions peripheral to the skin test reactions (Fig. 11). These lesions also show the histopathologic features of erythema elevatum diutinum.

There have been several patients reported who have IgA (mainly) or IgG monoclonal gammopathies or even myeloma [14,16–20]. Though the concurrence of these two diseases may be coin-

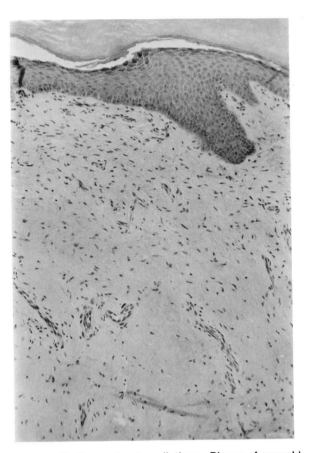

Fig. 10. Erythema elevatum diutinum. Biopsy of very old lesion showing homogenization and fibrocytic replacement of the dermis and capillary proliferation. ×96.

cidental, elevated levels of IgA in other patients with erythema elevatum diutinum [10,15,21–23] and the rarity of both erythema elevatum diutinum and IgA monoclonal gammopathy would suggest that this association may be more than chance. In addition, C1q binding activity (indicative of IgG- or IgM-containing circulating immune complexes) has been identified in the sera of three of five patients [14]. Defective neutrophil chemotaxis has been detected in two patients [14].

Direct immunofluorescence or immunoperoxidase studies of lesional skin of patients with erythema elevatum diutinum occasionally reveal immunoglobulin and complement deposition in and around blood vessels [15,20,24]. Our extensive immunofluorescent studies of early, spontaneous lesions and streptokinase-streptodornase skin test were not helpful [14]. The small admixture of eosinophils in the infiltrates obviated any critical attempts to identify true immunoglobulin or complement deposition in lesional skin. Eosinophils are fluorophilic and their granules take up any fluoresceinated antibody as well as free fluorescein

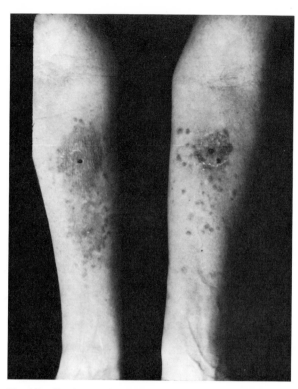

Fig. 11.   Erythema elevatum diutinum. Skin test reaction 72 hr after intradermal injection of 0.1 mL of a 40/10 concentration of streptokinase-streptodornase. Note satellite lesions.

in the concentration range used for conjugated reagents (10^{-6} to 10^{-8} M). Ultrastructural studies have not demonstrated any amorphous electron-dense deposits (thought to be immune complexes) in or around blood vessel walls (our unpublished data). Furthermore, intradermal histamine was not followed by skin lesions or any identifiable immunoglobulin or complement deposition in two patients tested [14].

Differential Diagnosis

Although there was, for many years, confusion between erythema elevatum diutinum and granuloma annulare, there is now little difficulty in differentiating the two clinically and histologically. Recurrent febrile neutrophilic dermatosis of Sweet [25], characterized by painful red plaques accompanied by fever and neutrophilic leukocytosis, can usually be distinguished from erythema elevatum diutinum by the distribution and character of lesions. Also, although Sweet's syndrome is characterized histologically by the presence of a dense neutrophilic infiltrate, which may be diffuse or, at times, perivascular, there is no leukocytoclastic

vasculitis. Xanthomas can easily be distinguished histologically, as can multicentric reticulohistiocytosis. There is occasional difficulty in differentiating erythema elevatum diutinum from granuloma faciale histologically (not clinically); however, the latter lesion usually shows far less vascular involvement, more eosinophilia, and regular sparing of the overlying epidermis. As stated above, extracellular cholesterosis of Urbach [8] should be regarded as a variant of erythema elevatum diutinum. Other forms of leukocytoclastic vasculitis may be very difficult to distinguish from erythema elevatum diutinum, especially histologically: The distribution, character, and chronicity of individual lesions is highly suggestive of erythema elevatum diutinum.

Treatment

Case reports [15,21,23,26,27] and a study of a series of patients [14] have indicated the regularity with which dramatic response is obtained when dapsone or sulfapyridine is given to patients with erythema elevatum diutinum. The prompt recurrence of skin lesions and systemic symptoms following sulfone withdrawal is evidence of the suppressive but not curative effect of sulfones in this disease (Fig. 12). It seems that the disease exacerbations are more severe with each subsequent withdrawal of medication. A few prior case reports have stated that dapsone is not effective in treating erythema elevatum diutinum [15,28]. Dosage, however, varies considerably and is probably crucial [14]. In addition to its beneficial effect in erythema elevatum diutinum, dapsone therapy is occasionally beneficial in other forms of leukocytoclastic vasculitis. Recently, niacinamide has been reported to suppress effectively erythema elevatum diutinum [29]. Systemic corticosteroids are not effective.

The mechanism(s) of action of sulfones in alleviating the signs and symptoms of erythema elevatum diutinum is not known. Many hypotheses have been offered for its dramatic effect in the treatment of dermatitis herpetiformis, another inflammatory disease in which neutrophils are the predominant infiltrating cells. Provost and Tomasi [30] have postulated and presented data in support of the interference of dapsone with complement deposition in dermatitis herpetiformis. Thompson and Souhami [31] have suggested that dapsone inhibits the hemorrhagic component of Arthus' reactions in guinea pigs, and Millikan and Conway [32] have proposed that dapsone interferes with

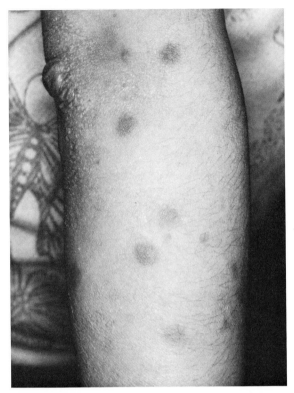

Fig. 12. Erythema elevatum diutinum. Red painful vasculitic nodules on arm erupting 12 hr after cessation of dapsone therapy.

patients. Dapsone undoubtedly acts at the very end stage of the pathologic process because of its rapidity of action, the prompt recurrence of reactivity after its withdrawal, and the marked decrease in the severity of streptokinase-streptodornase skin test reactions after institution of treatment. An understanding of the exact mechanism(s) of action of dapsone would contribute to the understanding of the pathophysiology of erythema elevatum diutinum and many of the other neutrophilic dermatoses.

Conclusion

Salient features of erythema elevatum diutinum that serve to distinguish it from other forms of leukocytoclastic vasculitis include the symmetry of erythematous lesions, the persistence of lesions, their distribution (mainly localized to extensor aspects, especially over joints), their evolution into fibrotic nodules with only tiny foci of vasculitis, the exquisite sensitivity of the patients to skin testing with streptokinase and streptodornase [14], and the dramatic response of the disease to sulfone or sulfapyridine therapy, with rapid resolution of existing skin lesions, cessation of new lesion formation, and diminution of systemic symptoms. Lesions and systemic complaints recur within 12 to 48 hr of discontinuing therapy. Although the precise cause is unknown, an immune complex etiology is suggested.

activation of the alternative complement pathway. Our extensive human and animal studies have not substantiated any of these claims [33]. Specifically, C3 may be detected in the normal-appearing skin of dermatitis herpetiformis patients after they have been kept free of lesions for 2 to 8 weeks by taking sulfone or sulfapyridine therapy. Our human studies are in keeping with those of Seah et al. [34] in this regard and with those in vitro data reported by Schifferli and Russell-Jones [35]. Also when Diasone, a water-soluble sulfone, is given to Hartley strain or C4-deficient guinea pigs in a dose of 150 mg/kg per day, there is no effect on the active or reverse passive Arthus' reaction or on the Forssman's reaction [33]. It is interesting that many diseases in which dapsone is most effective are those in which neutrophilic infiltrates are prominent [36]. Various investigators have shown that dapsone inhibits lysosomal enzyme activity [37,38] and interferes with the myeloperoxidase-H_2O_2-halide-mediated cytotoxic system in polymorphonuclear leukocytes [39]. Although these findings may account for the effect of the drug on neutrophils or on their lysosomal enzymes at the site of injury, they probably do not account for the lack of influx of neutrophils into the dermis in treated

References

1. Radcliffe-Crocker H, Williams C: Erythema elevatum diutinum. *Br J Dermatol* **6**:1–9, 1894
2. Hutchinson J: On two remarkable cases of symmetrical purple congestion of the skin in patches, with induration. *Br J Dermatol* **1**:10–15, 1888
3. Bury JS: A case of erythema with remarkable nodular thickening and induration of the skin associated with intermittent albuminuria. *Illus Med News* **3**:145–149, 1889
4. Radcliffe-Crocker H: Granuloma annulare. *Br J Dermatol* **14**:1–9, 1902
5. Della-Favera GB: Erythema elevatum diutinum and granuloma annulare. *Dermatol Z* **17**:541–558, 1910
6. Weidman FD, Besancon JH: Erythema elevatum diutinum: role of streptococci, and relationship to other rheumatic dermatoses. *Arch Dermatol Syphilol* **20**:593–620, 1929
7. Haber H: Erythema elevatum diutinum. *Br J Dermatol* **67**:121–145, 1955
8. Urbach E et al: Extrazelluläre Cholesterinose. *Arch Dermatol Syphilol (Berlin)* **166**:243–272, 1932
9. Laymon CW: Extracellular cholesterolosis. *Arch Dermatol Syphilol* **35**:269–284, 1937
10. Herzberg JJ: Die extracelluläre Cholesterinose (Kerl-Ur-

bach), eine Variante des Erythema elevatum diutinum. *Arch Klin Exp Dermatol* **205:**477–496, 1958

11. Jensen JA, Esquenazi V: Chemotactic stimulation by cell surface immune reactions. *Nature* **256:**213–215, 1975

12. Ward PA, Becker EL: The deactivation of rabbit neutrophils by chemotactic factor and the nature of the activatable esterase. *J Exp Med* **127:**693–703, 1968

13. Till A, Ward PA: Two distinct chemotactic factor inactivators in human serum. *J Immunol* **114:**843–848, 1975

14. Katz SI et al: Erythema elevatum diutinum—skin and systemic manifestations, immunologic studies, and successful treatment with dapsone. *Medicine (Baltimore)* **56:**443–455, 1977

15. Cream JJ et al: Erythema elevatum diutinum: an unusual reaction to streptococcal antigen and response to dapsone. *Br J Dermatol* **84:**393–399, 1971

16. Duperrat B, Rappaport MM: Erythema elevatum diutinum associé a un myélome plasmocytaire diffus. *Bull Soc Fr Dermatol Syphiligr* **66:**6–8, 1959

17. Archimandritis AJ et al: Erythema elevatum diutinum and IgA myeloma: an interesting association. *Br Med J* **2:**613–614, 1977

18. Kövary PM et al: Paraproteinemia in erythema elevatum diutinum. *Arch Dermatol Res* **260:**153–158, 1977

19. Sams WM Jr et al: Necrotizing vasculitis associated with lethal reticuloendothelial diseases. *Br J Dermatol* **80:**555–560, 1968

20. Jones RR et al: Erythema elevatum diutinum with IgA paraproteinemia. *Br J Dermatol* **105(Suppl 19):**41–42, 1980

21. Abdel-Aziz AHM, Robertson DEH: Erythema elevatum diutinum: immunoglobulin, bacterial skin tests and response to dapsone. *Cutis* **12:**549–553, 1973

22. Mraz JP, Newcomer VD: Erythema elevatum diutinum: presentation of a case and evaluation of laboratory and immunological status. *Arch Dermatol* **96:**235–246, 1967

23. Vollum DI: Erythema elevatum diutinum: vesicular lesions and sulphone response. *Br J Dermatol* **80:**178–183, 1968

24. Wolff HH et al: Erythema elevatum diutinum. *Arch Dermatol Res* **261:**17–26, 1978

25. Sweet RD: Acute febrile neutrophilic dermatosis. *Br J Dermatol* **76:**349–356, 1964

26. Fort S, Rodman OG: Erythema elevatum diutinum: a review and report of a case. *Arch Dermatol* **113:**819–822, 1977

27. Kalkoff KW: Zur Behandlung des Erythema elevatum diutinum mit 3-Sulfanilamido-6-methoxypyridazin (Lederkyn). *Dermatol Wochenschr* **142:**788–800, 1960

28. Lugt LVD: Erythema elevatum et diutinum. *Dermatologica* **119:**65–71, 1959

29. Kohler IK, Lorincz AL: Erythema elevatum diutinum treated with niacinamide and tetracycline. *Arch Dermatol* **116:**693–695, 1980

30. Provost TT, Tomasi TB: Evidence for the activation of complement via the alternate pathway in skin diseases. II. Dermatitis herpetiformis. *Clin Immunol Immunopathol* **3:**178–186, 1974

31. Thompson DM, Souhami R: Suppression of the Arthus reaction in the guinea pig by dapsone (Abstr). *Proc R Soc Med* **68:**273, 1975

32. Millikan LE, Conway FR: Effect of drugs on the Pillemer pathway—dapsone (Abstr). *J Invest Dermatol* **62:**541, 1974

33. Katz SI et al: Effect of sulfones on complement deposition in dermatitis herpetiformis and on complement-mediated guinea pig reactions. *J Invest Dermatol* **67:**688–692, 1976

34. Seah PP et al: Complement in the skin of patients with dermatitis herpetiformis. *Br J Dermatol* **89(Suppl 9):**12, 1973

35. Schifferli JA, Russel-Jones R: Dapsone and complement. *Lancet* **2:**368–369, 1981

36. Lang PG Jr: Sulfones and sulfonamides in dermatology today. *J Am Acad Dermatol* **1:**479–492, 1979

37. Barranco VP: Inhibition of lysosomal enzymes by dapsone. *Arch Dermatol* **110:**563–566, 1974

38. Mier PD, Van Den Hurk JJMA: Inhibition of lysosomal enzymes by dapsone. *Br J Dermatol* **93:**471–472, 1975

39. Stendahl O et al: The inhibition of polymorphonuclear leukocyte cytotoxicity by dapsone: a possible mechanism in the treatment of dermatitis herpetiformis. *J Clin Invest* **62:**214–220, 1978

GRAFT-VERSUS-HOST DISEASE

Evan R. Farmer

Antoinette F. Hood

Graft-versus-host disease (GVHD) is a clinical syndrome characterized by cutaneous changes, diarrhea, and liver dysfunction. GVHD is seen most commonly as a sequela of bone marrow transplantation, which increasingly is used in the treatment of aplastic anemia [1], acute leukemia [2,3], and some immunodeficiency disorders [4]. Bone marrow transplantation uniquely differs from transplantation of other organs because the transfused marrow contains proliferating immunologically competent cells. With successful engraftment there is replacement of the host marrow by immunocompetent donor cells capable of reacting against the "foreign" tissue antigens of the host (Fig. 1). The term *graft-versus-host reaction* (GVHR) refers to the inflammatory reaction mounted by the donor cells against a specific host organ—skin, liver, or gastrointestinal tract. Graft-versus-host disease is a clinical syndrome composed of the sum of these reactions in an individual patient. Therefore, the patient has GVHD, while the skin or liver or intestinal tract has a GVHR. Associated with high morbidity and mortality, GVHD represents the major impediment to the success of the bone marrow transplantation procedure.

Graft-versus-host disease is not limited to patients with marrow transplants but may also occur in (1) the immunosuppressed patient receiving leukocyte-rich blood transfusions [5–7] and (2) the immunodeficient fetus through maternal-fetal transfer of leukocytes [8,9].

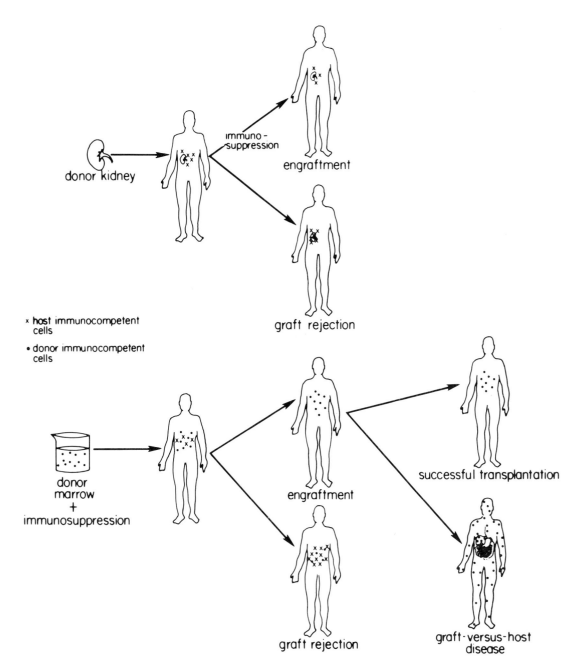

× host immunocompetent
cells

• donor immunocompetent
cells

Fig. 1. This schematic diagram contrasts the sequence of events in kidney transplantation vs. bone marrow transplantation in which the major difference is the presence of donor immunocompetent cells in the marrow graft and their ability to cause graft-versus-host disease.

Incidence

The incidence of GVHD following successful engraftment with allogeneic (transplant between non-identical individuals) marrow varies from 58 to 80 percent [2,10,11]. These figures include a spectrum of disease from the mild to the severe. Although the severity of disease which develops is not absolutely predictable, it appears to be related to

(1) the histocompatibility match between donor and recipient and (2) the preparatory regimen used [10].

The incidence of GVHD developing in syngeneic (transplant between identical twins) marrow transplant patients is quite low. Disease that does occur is of short duration, tends to be limited to the skin, and resolves spontaneously [12–14].

The incidence of GVHD following blood transfusions in immunosuppressed patients or as the result of maternal-fetal transfer in immunodeficiency disease is unknown but probably quite low.

Pathogenesis

In the 1966 Harvey lecture, Billingham stated the conditions for a graft to be able to mount a GVHR [15]. These conditions were as follows:

1. The graft *must* contain immunologically competent cells.
2. The host must possess important transplantation isoantigens that are lacking in the graft donor, so that the host appears foreign to it and is therefore capable of stimulating it antigenically.
3. The host itself must be incapable of mounting an effective immunologic reaction against the graft, at least for sufficient time for the latter to manifest its immunologic capabilities—i.e., *the graft must have some security of tenure.*

Over the subsequent 15 years these principles have generally held true, but with modification of condition 2. We now know that changes of a GVHR may also occur in syngeneic marrow transplants who possess identical transplantation isoantigens [12–14]. The GVHR that occurs in these patients is similar to the GVHR that occurs in allogeneic transplants except that it is usually much less severe [12–14].

It is important to understand the techniques that are currently employed in marrow transplantation. The actual regimen used in the various transplant centers may vary somewhat, but the underlying rationale is the same [16].

As previously outlined, one of the earliest theories of the pathogenesis of GVHD was advanced by Billingham, which stated that the donor immunocompetent cells were reacting to transplantation isoantigens in the recipient tissues that were lacking in the graft and thus appeared foreign to it [15]. All tissues should therefore be at risk to develop a GVHR; this has not been the case as GVHRs in humans seem to develop specifically in the skin, gastrointestinal tract, liver, lungs, and lymphoid tissue, but not in the nervous system, bone, or endocrine system.

Streilein in 1971 [17], in an effort to resolve this dilemma, postulated that the immunologic target in GVHD was the host lymphocyte. The destruction of the skin, gastrointestinal tract, etc., could therefore be explained by the "innocent bystander" effect as the immunocompetent cells were attacking the residual host's lymphocytes.

GVHD would possibly limit its own progression by the elimination of the host lymphocytes.

By the mid to late 1970s, it was clear that GVHD was not a single disorder but actually composed of two separate phases, acute and chronic, each having different clinical manifestations and probably a different pathogenesis. Acute GVHD is now thought to be due to the attack of donor immunocompetent T lymphocytes (thymus-derived) and null lymphocytes against host histocompatibility antigens. The null lymphocytes may attack antigens that are common to both the donor and recipient and are termed *autocytotoxic* lymphocytes. This phenomenon can best be demonstrated by the development of acute GVHD in syngeneic transplants. The appearance in the peripheral blood of suppressor lymphocytes (T lymphocytes) that modulate the null lymphocytes may account for the cessation of acute GVHD [18,19]. This theory differs from that of Streilein in that (1) the target tissue is not limited to a specific cell type and (2) the attacking immunocompetent cells may attack cells with similar antigens.

Chronic GVHD that occurs after a period of engraftment seems to be produced by cells that differentiate within the host. The composition of these cells is unknown. The suppressor cells that seem to be modulating the acute GVHD may also be found in patients with chronic GVHD, but these cells do not seem to play a defined role in either establishing or subduing the process. These suppressor cells, however, probably do play a role in the development of the late immunoincompetence and susceptibility to microbial infections that are characteristic of chronic GVHD [18,20,21].

Clinical Manifestations

Clinically distinguishable acute and chronic forms of GVHD have been described. The acute phase may evolve directly into the chronic phase or the two reactions may occur independently of each other (see Table 1).

Acute Graft-versus-Host Disease

Acute GVHD usually develops 10 to 40 days after marrow transplantation. The earliest symptom of the cutaneous GVHR is mild pruritus which may be localized or generalized. Patients also often complain of discomfort or pain when pressure is exerted on their palms or soles. The first recognizable visible skin change in acute cutaneous

Table 1   Clinical-pathologic correlation of cutaneous graft-versus-host reaction

Clinical lesion	Histopathology	Electron microscopy	Immunofluorescence
Acute			
	Basal vacuolization may be observed several days before a clinically detectable eruption		
Discrete but subtle erythematous macular or papular lesions on upper trunk and feet	Focal vacuolization of the basal cell layer and dyskeratosis of individual keratinocytes; mild perivenular mononuclear cell infiltrate	Dyskeratotic cells show loss of desmosomes, aggregation of tonofilaments and cytoplasmic organelles with apoptosis; close contact with lymphocytes occasionally observed	Occasional dermal-epidermal junction deposition of granular IgM, IgG, and C3
Confluent areas of macular or papular erythema which become generalized (erythroderma)	Increased vacuolization and dyskeratosis; vacuoles may coalesce to form small subepidermal clefts; endothelial cell swelling; perivascular mononuclear cell infiltrate		
Bullae, most prominent over pressure or trauma sites	Subepidermal blister formation; roof of blister composed of epidermis with numerous dyskeratotic cells; variable perivascular mononuclear cell infiltrate		
Chronic			
Violaceous lichenoid papules on distal extremities	Compact hyperkeratosis, hypergranulosis, mild irregular acanthosis, moderate basal vacuolization and dyskeratosis; mild perivascular mononuclear cell infiltrate; melanin incontinence	Epidermal changes similar to those in the acute phase	
Confluent areas of dermal sclerosis with overlying scale involving trunk, buttocks, hips, and thighs; hair loss and anhidrosis common	Hyperkeratosis, epidermal atrophy or acanthosis, rare dyskeratosis, mild perivascular mononuclear cell infiltrate, melanin incontinence, loss of hair follicles, entrapment of sweat glands, dense dermal sclerosis; occasional perieccrine plasma cell infiltrate		Dermal-epidermal junction deposition of IgM in globular or linear pattern

GVHR is a subtle, blanchable, erythematous, macular or papular eruption which initially appears on the upper trunk, neck, hands (Fig. 2), and feet, especially the palms and soles. Concurrently there may be mild edema and a violaceous hue imparted to the skin over the pinna and periungual areas. If the reaction is controlled at this point, there is gradual diminution of the erythema, desquamation, and subsequent appearance of postinflammatory hyperpigmentation. If the eruption progresses, small individual lesions coalesce to form large areas of confluent erythema; occasionally the eruption becomes generalized. Blister formation may accompany the more severe and widespread erythematous eruption. The blisters are most promi-

nent on the palms and soles and over pressure or trauma sites. A positive Nikolsky's sign can be elicited in skin adjacent to the blisters. The bullae are initially filled with clear fluid but may become hemorrhagic. When the blisters rupture, the underlying dermis is exposed, indicating the subepidermal location of the lesion. The occurrence of widespread erythema with blister formation has been described as the toxic-epidermal-necrolysis-like (TEN-like) form of acute cutaneous GVHR [22]. The mortality associated with TEN-like GVHR is high. Individuals who do survive heal without scarring but develop postinflammatory hyperpigmentation at sites of involvement. A grading system has been developed that is helpful in

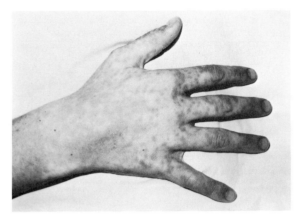

Fig. 2. Acute cutaneous graft-versus-host reaction. This discrete and confluent erythematous maculopapular eruption developed 30 days after an allogeneic marrow transplant.

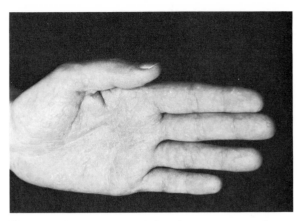

Fig. 3. Lichenoid phase of chronic cutaneous graft-versus-host reaction. The palmar surface of the hand and fingers show numerous violaceous, shiny, flat-topped papules resembling lichen planus.

management of patients with acute cutaneous GVHR (Table 2) [23].

In addition to involving the skin, acute GVHRs may occur simultaneously or independently in the liver [24], intestinal tract [24], and bronchial mucosa [25]. The degree of involvement in any one organ and the number of target organs involved with GVHRs is quite variable. Liver involvement is manifested by nausea, vomiting, right upper quadrant pain and tenderness, and abnormal liver function tests, particularly elevations of serum glutamic oxaloacetic transaminase (SGOT) and bilirubin. Involvement of the intestinal tract is manifested by nausea, vomiting, cramping abdominal pain, and watery diarrhea. Diarrhea may be quite severe and fluid loss may approach that seen in cholera. Pulmonary involvement is clinically characterized by a dry nonproductive cough and subsequent development of pneumonia [25]. Fever may accompany a GVHR involving any of the organ systems.

Chronic Graft-versus-Host Disease

Chronic GVHD, which occurs months to years after marrow transplantation, may or may not be preceded by acute GVHD. The skin and the liver are the organs primarily involved in chronic GVHRs.

Lichenoid Graft-versus-Host Reaction. In many patients the cutaneous disease is manifested initially by the appearance of violaceous lichenoid papules. These lesions, which are seen most commonly on the distal extremities, especially the palms (Fig. 3) and soles, may become generalized. The violaceous papules closely resemble the lesions of lichen planus; however, their margins are less distinct and less angulated than classic lichen planus lesions. The eruption, which may be accompanied by mild pruritus, resolves, leaving a macular hyperpigmentation. Periareolar erythema and scattered macular hypopigmentation (vitiligo) are also seen in association with the lichen-planus-like lesions.

Sclerodermoid Graft-versus-Host Reaction. A second type of cutaneous lesion observed in chronic GVHR is characterized by sclerosis. Individual morphea-like lesions, ranging in size from 1 to 10 cm, may coalesce to form large confluent areas of sclerosis. The skin markings disappear, and there is a firm indurated feel on palpation. There may be significant discomfort, loss of mobility, and even joint contractures. Recurrent, often persistent pyoderma with (ecthyma-like) ulcer formation is common. Skin appendages are affected; hair loss and diminished sweating are observed. Sicca membranes have been reported [26]. In contrast to the lichenoid lesions, the sclerodermoid lesions are located more centrally, with prominent involvement of skin on the trunk, buttocks, hips, and thighs. Particularly severe sclerosis is often seen in areas of previous inflammation, especially following a herpes zoster infection.

Table 2   Clinical grading of acute cutaneous graft-versus-host reaction

Grade	Clinical lesions
1	Erythematous maculopapuler eruption involving less than 25% of the body surface
2	Erythematous maculopapuler rash involving 25–50% of the body surface
3	Erythroderma
4	Bulla formation

Source: Adapted from Glucksberg et al [23].

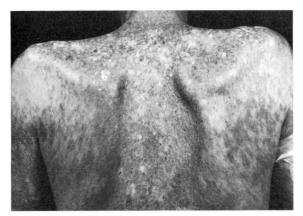

Fig. 4.   Sclerodermoid phase of chronic cutaneous graft-versus-host reaction. Fourteen months after an allogeneic marrow transplant this patient demonstrated sclerodermoid plaques and areas of poikiloderma-like changes consisting of dyspigmentation, atrophy, and scaling.

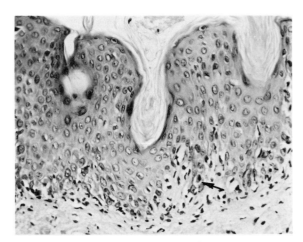

Fig. 5.   Acute cutaneous graft-versus-host reaction. The epidermis demonstrates mild spongiosis, exocytosis of lymphocytes, dyskeratotic keratinocytes (*arrow*), and vacuolar alteration of the basal cell layer. In the papillary dermis is a mild lymphocytic infiltrate tending to aggregate at the dermal-epidermal junction. (H & E, ×310).

Poikiloderma-like changes frequently develop during the sclerodermoid phase and consist of dyspigmentation, telangiectasia, scaling, and atrophy (Fig. 4). These changes may be generalized but are especially noted on the face and trunk.

We have observed spontaneous resolution of the sclerotic phase of chronic GVHR in several patients. Over a 1- to 2-year period their skin became appreciably softer, ulcers healed, contractures improved, and the ability to sweat returned.

Pathology

Since 1977 skin biopsies have been routinely obtained at weekly intervals on all patients undergoing bone marrow transplantation at our institution. Consequently we have been able to follow the histopathologic evolution of cutaneous GVHR in considerable detail.

Acute Graft-versus-Host Reaction

One to two days preceding a clinically detectable eruption, histopathologic abnormalities may be observed. The earliest alteration consists of focal vacuolar change in the basement membrane zone of the epidermis and hair follicle epithelium. Vacuolar changes may also occur as sequelae of the chemotherapy or x-irradiation given in preparation for transplantation; however, if these changes are due to an ongoing GVHR, an inflammatory infiltrate will be seen in the papillary and upper reticular dermis. This infiltrate, which is quantitatively quite variable, is composed predominantly

of mononuclear cells with an occasional eosinophil. Although the cells are primarily distributed around vessels of the superficial venular plexus, exocytosis of individual cells into the epidermis commonly occurs (Fig. 5). As the reaction progresses, the vacuolar changes become more pronounced, intercellular edema is observed, and there is loss of polarity of epidermal cells in the lower epidermis. Individual dyskeratotic cells appear in the basal cell layer and lower stratum malpighii. These distinctive cells with homogeneous bright eosinophilic cytoplasm, small pyknotic nuclei, and surrounding clear halo or lacunae have been termed ''mummified'' cells [24]. Occasionally mononuclear cells may be seen in close apposition to the dyskeratotic cells, the so-called satellite lymphocytes [27]. In severe acute GVHR the vacuoles coalesce to form subepidermal clefts, microvesicles, and even bullae. Necrotic epidermis may slough, leaving exposed dermis. Lerner and coworkers devised a grading system based on the degree of epidermal alteration to quantify the histologic changes in cutaneous GVHR [28] (Table 3). Additional epidermal changes that may be due to GVHR, chemotherapy, or irradiation include compact laminated orthohyperkeratosis, epidermal atrophy with flattening of the rete ridges, and unevenly distributed melanin granules within keratinocytes.

In association with the perivenular mononuclear cell infiltrate there is marked endothelial cell swelling and narrowing of the vascular lumina. Dermal hemorrhage is common and may be due either to thrombocytopenia or incompetent vessel walls.

Table 3 Histopathologic grading system for acute cutaneous graft-versus-host reaction

Grade	Histopathologic features
0	Normal epidermis or epidermal changes of other cutaneous disorders
1	Focal or diffuse vacuolar alteration of the basal cell layer
2	Dyskeratotic squamous cells in epidermis and/or hair follicle epithelium
3	Subepidermal cleft or microvesicle formation
4	Complete separation of epidermis from the dermis

Note: In grades 1–4 there is usually a superficial perivascular infiltrate of mononuclear cells with exocytosis of these cells into the lower half of the epidermis.
Source: Adapted from Lerner et al [28].

Leukocytoclastic vasculitis is not seen as a feature of cutaneous GVHR. Melanin granules, free and within melanophages, are often present in the papillary dermis.

As acute GVHR resolves, the basal vacuolar changes diminish, the dyskeratotic cells move upward to be shed with the stratum corneum, the perivascular inflammatory infiltrate decreases, and endothelial cell swelling subsides. Dermal scarring and loss of elastic tissue do not occur unless there has been a superimposed pyoderma, viral infection, or other traumatic event.

Histopathologic changes similar to acute cutaneous GVHR occurring in patients receiving allogeneic bone marrow transplants have also been reported in patients receiving syngeneic bone marrow transplants [12] or autologous (stored marrow reinfused into the same individual) bone marrow transplants. These changes, which usually are mild and transient, consist of vacuolar alteration of the basal cell layer, dyskeratosis, and a scant superficial perivenular lymphocytic infiltrate. None of the cases reported has developed clinically or histologically severe acute cutaneous GVHR or evolved to chronic cutaneous GVHR.

Extracutaneous Graft-versus-Host Reaction

Acute GVHRs occurring in organs other than the skin show mild-to-severe epithelial cell necrosis associated with a predominantly mononuclear cell infiltrate. Biopsies taken from mildly to moderately involved intestines show necrotic epithelial cells, crypt abscess formation, and a mixed inflammatory infiltrate composed of lymphocytes, plasma cells, and occasional eosinophils [24,28,29]. Biopsies from florid lesions show complete denudation of the mucosal surface [24,28,29]. In hepatic GVHR there is a lymphocytic infiltration of the portal triad with necrosis of the bile duct epithelium,

hepatocytes, and Kupffer cells [24,28]. Lesional biopsies from patients with pulmonary GVHR demonstrate a lymphocytic bronchitis with lymphocyte-associated necrosis of the bronchial mucosa and the submucosal glands [25].

Chronic Graft-versus-Host Reaction

Surveillance skin biopsies obtained during the interval between acute and chronic GVHR show no significant recognizable abnormalities. As with acute cutaneous GVHR, vacuolar changes along the basement membrane zone are observed in biopsies taken several days before the clinically apparent lesions in chronic cutaneous GVHR.

Lichenoid Graft-versus-Host Reaction. Examination of biopsies from well-developed lichenoid lesions show hyperkeratosis (which is generally orthokeratotic), hypergranulosis, moderate irregular acanthosis, and moderate vacuolar changes in the basal cell layer (Fig. 6). Individual eosinophilic dyskeratotic keratinocytes with or without nuclei are present in the basal layer and lower stratum malpighii. These cells are for the most part histologically indistinguishable from the dyskeratotic, "mummified" epidermal cells described in acute cutaneous GVHR and from dyskeratotic cells or colloid bodies described in lichen planus. The follicular epithelium shows changes similar to those observed in the epidermis.

Fig. 6. Lichenoid phase of chronic cutaneous graft-versus-host reaction. The epidermis demonstrates hyperkeratosis, hypergranulosis, irregular acanthosis, mild spongiosis, exocytosis of lymphocytes, vacuolar alteration, and squamatization of the basal cell layer. In the papillary dermis is a bandlike infiltrate consisting of lymphocytes, mononuclear cells, and melanophages. (H & E, ×125).

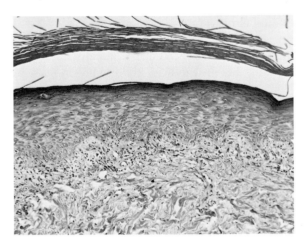

In the papillary and upper reticular dermis there is a mild perivascular infiltrate composed of lymphocytes, mononuclear cells, melanophages, and rarely a few plasma cells or eosinophils. Inflammatory cells occasionally are seen in the epidermis.

Lichenoid GVHR can be histologically distinguished from lichen planus only by its scant, predominantly perivenular infiltrate; the epidermal changes in the two diseases are identical. Interestingly, patients treated in the mid-1970s had more intense dermal infiltrates associated with this phase of GVHR. The current findings may reflect either better histocompatibility matching between recipient and donor or better methods of therapy.

Sclerodermoid Graft-versus-Host Reaction. Biopsy specimens from sclerodermoid lesions exhibit a thickened reticular dermis composed of hypertrophic, densely packed, brightly eosinophilic collagen bundles (Fig. 7). In many cases, the normal distinction between the papillary and reticular dermis is lost and the papillary dermis is entirely replaced by thick sclerotic collagen fibers. Hair follicles disappear; eccrine glands lose their surrounding fat and become "entrapped" in dense collagen. Arrector pili muscles and eccrine ducts are relatively spared until late in the course. A variable perivascular and periadnexal mononuclear cell infiltrate is present. This infiltrate is composed of lymphocytes, mononuclear cells, and occasional plasma cells and melanophages. An inflammatory infiltrate is not observed along the dermal-subcutaneous junction. The overlying epidermis shows hyperkeratosis, keratotic plugging, hypergranulosis, irregular acanthosis or epidermal atrophy, occasional dyskeratotic cells, and diminished melanin in the basal cell layer. Except for the epidermal changes and the lack of infiltrate at the dermal-subcutaneous junction, the histologic changes observed in the sclerodermoid lesions of chronic GVHR are quite similar to changes present in the lesions of progressive systemic scleroderma and morphea.

Extracutaneous Chronic Graft-versus-Host Reaction. The minor salivary glands demonstrate the histologic features of Sjögren's syndrome, initially consisting of a patchy and periductal infiltrate composed of lymphocytes and plasma cells [30,31]. These inflammatory cells may also be found within the duct walls and glandular acini. Fibrosis subsequently develops, resulting in dilatation of the ducts and destruction and loss of the acini with replacement by the fibrous tissue. Sialomucin normally present within the acini and ducts is markedly reduced in advanced cases.

The gastrointestinal tract in general shows a focal process consisting of an inflammatory cell infiltrate with subsequent development of submucosal fibrosis. Most of the changes have been seen in the esophagus, small bowel, and colon with little alteration being noted in the stomach. The esophagus may show ulceration of the mucosa with vacuolar changes in the basal cell layer and a submucosal infiltrate composed of lymphocytes and plasma cells [31]. Mucosal and submucosal fibrosis subsequently develops [31,32]. Both the large and small intestines show similar inflammatory cell infiltrates and fibrosis, but with predominant involvement in the small bowel [31,32].

Biopsy and autopsy specimens of the liver show a variety of changes. Initially there is a mixed inflammatory cell infiltrate in the portal zones consisting predominantly of lymphocytes but with an admixture of plasma cells, histiocytes, eosinophils, and neutrophils. Portal fibrosis develops with destruction of the bile ducts and leads to atresia. Occasional individual cell necrosis of the ductal epithelium may be seen [31]. In the peri-

Fig. 7. Sclerodermoid phase of chronic cutaneous graft-versus-host reaction. The epidermis shows mild compact hyperkeratosis and keratotic plugging. There is hyalinization of the collagen throughout the dermis with loss of the appendageal structures. (H & E, ×90).

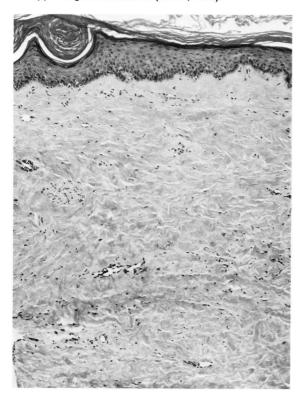

portal region the hepatocytes may be normal [32] or show piecemeal necrosis [31].

Autopsy specimens of pulmonary tissue have shown a lymphoplasmacytic bronchitis with destruction of the submucosal glands, resembling the changes seen in the minor salivary glands [31]. Interstitial infiltrates are present consisting of lymphocytes and plasma cells, but no fibrosis [32] or blood vessel changes that are seen in pulmonary scleroderma have been demonstrated [31].

Lymph node specimens have demonstrated a focal to diffuse decrease in the number of lymphocytes with an increase in the number of plasma cells [31,32]. The germinal centers are usually poorly formed to absent, being replaced by a hyalinized eosinophilic material [31].

Muscle specimens have demonstrated a polymyositis with interstitial perivascular infiltrates composed of lymphocytes and plasma cells and with fibrosis and atrophy of myofibers. Occasionally extensive necrotizing plasmacytic polymyositis has also been seen [31].

Electron Microscopy

The first electron microscopic descriptions of acute cutaneous GVHR were reported by Woodruff and his colleagues in 1971 [27]. They examined the mucous membranes and external epithelia of rhesus monkeys who received allogeneic marrow transplantation and reported three types of epidermal alterations. The first change consisted of desmosomal lysis, loss of cellular cohesion between individual keratinocytes, acantholysis, and suprabasal lacuna formation. In the second type of change, injured keratinocytes, which were often in direct contact with lymphocytes, exhibited alterations of the endoplasmic reticulum and mitochondria and the formation of autolytic vacuoles. The third change was characterized by encasement of individual keratinocytes by lymphocytes. Subsequently there was disruption of the tonofilaments and compaction of the cytoplasm. These cells corresponded to the dyskeratotic cells with satellite lymphocytes observed with the light microscope. The authors concluded that the acantholysis, autophagocytosis, and dyskeratosis of epidermal cells were due to the invading "aggressor" lymphocytes.

Electron microscopic examination of the dyskeratotic cells seen in humans with acute cutaneous GVHR demonstrated dense aggregation of tonofilaments and cytoplasmic organelles and loss of desmosomes [5,33,34]. Some of these degenerating or dyskeratotic cells appeared to be phagocytized by neighboring keratinocytes [5], a process

also known as apoptosis [35]. Direct contact of lymphocytes with degenerating keratinocytes has been observed by some authors [33,34] but not by others [5].

Immunofluorescent Microscopy

There have been conflicting reports regarding the presence or absence of immunoglobulin and complement deposition in cutaneous GVHR. In patients with acute GVHR Tsoi et al. [36] demonstrated granular IgM deposition at the dermal-epidermal (D-E) junction in 39 percent and C3 deposition in 75 percent of the cases. Ullman and coworkers examined one patient with acute cutaneous GVHR and reported granular, diffuse, and bandlike C3 deposition at the D-E junction in addition to granular deposition of IgG, IgM, and C3 in the vessel walls [37]. Saurat et al. examined 17 patients with GVHR and were unable to demonstrate either immunoglobulin or complement deposition [38]. At the Johns Hopkins Medical Institutions, 22 patients with acute cutaneous GVHR were examined with multiple sequential specimens per patient for immunoglobulin and complement deposition [39]. Complement (C3) deposition was observed along the D-E junction in 41 percent of our patients; immunoglobulin deposition was uniformly absent. The deposition of C3 did not correlate with either clinical or histologic disease activity. Eight patients who never clinically developed GVHD demonstrated C3 deposition in the skin, which implies some nonspecificity to this finding.

Therefore, while deposition of C3 and IgM has been reported in a few patients with acute cutaneous GVHR, it is not a consistent finding and it is difficult to attribute an important role to these immunoreactants in the pathogenesis of the disease. Examination of skin biopsies from patients with chronic GVHR reveals more consistent findings. IgM was seen deposited along the D-E junction in a globular pattern analogous to lichen planus [38] or in a linear fashion [36,39]. Whether the deposition of immunoreactants is playing a role in the pathogenesis of the disorder or is merely an epiphenomenon is not known at this time.

Differential Diagnosis

Acute Cutaneous Graft-versus-Host Reaction

An erythematous maculopapular eruption that develops within the first $2\frac{1}{2}$ months after successful marrow transplantation often poses a major diagnostic dilemma. The differential diagnosis includes GVHR, drug reaction, and viral exanthem. Concurrent evidence of GVHRs involving the liver or gastrointestinal tract makes the diagnosis of cutaneous GVHR more likely. In the absence of these findings, however, other parameters must be evaluated and used in establishing the diagnosis. Periungual erythema, auricular erythema, and pressure-induced pain on the palms and soles are features that favor the diagnosis of GVHR. In acute cutaneous GVHR, lesions tend to appear on the distal extremities and spread centrifugally in contrast to a drug reaction, which often appears first on the thorax and then involves the extremities. The presence of purpura is not an integral feature of cutaneous GVHR. Pruritus is variable in GVHR and has not been a helpful feature in the differential diagnosis. A skin biopsy is helpful if it shows the characteristic features of GVHR. If the initial skin biopsy does not support the diagnosis of acute cutaneous GVHR, and shows only nonspecific or minimal abnormalities, then additional biopsies may be necessary to establish the diagnosis. This is required only in the absence of other organ involvement with acute GVHRs. A therapeutic trial with low-dose prednisone has been useful in differentiating a drug reaction from cutaneous GVHR since drug eruptions respond to much lower doses (1 mg/kg per day) of corticosteroids than are required to suppress GVHR. Differentiation of GVHR from a viral exanthem may be extremely difficult unless the characteristic GVHR periungual and auricular erythema or palm and sole pain are present. Some cases require observation over time before the diagnosis can be established.

A few patients with severe acute GVHR develop a blistering eruption with a positive Nikolsky's sign. Clinically these patients have the appearance of toxic epidermal necrolysis (TEN). All our cases have had concurrent evidence of GVHR involving the liver or gastrointestinal tract, allowing us to differentiate this eruption from drug-induced TEN. A skin biopsy will support the diagnosis of acute GVHR and allow differentiation from the other, more common blistering disorders.

Chronic Cutaneous Graft-versus-Host Reaction

Chronic GVHR presents changes in the skin that mimic lichen planus, lichenoid drug reaction, scleroderma, and poikiloderma. The lichen planus-like lesions of chronic GVHR are not as sharply angulated as are the lesions of idiopathic lichen planus; the characteristic nail and mucous membrane lesions of lichen planus have not been described in GVHR. The sclerodermoid lesions and poikiloderma-like lesions appear identical to their respective idiopathic counterparts. The diagnosis is therefore established by the development of these lesions at least 3 to 6 months following successful marrow transplantation. The oral and ocular mucous membranes may develop lesions that are identical clinically and histologically with Sjögren syndrome.

Treatment

Therapy in bone marrow transplantation is directed toward (1) prevention of GVHD and (2) treatment of disease when it occurs. Theoretically, GVHD will not occur if the donor and the recipient are a perfect histocompatible match, i.e., HLA-identical and mixed lymphocyte culture nonreactive. This ideal transplantation does occur between identical twins. Since GVHD may develop with transplants from well-matched individuals and rarely with transplants from identical twins [12], there must be other factors as yet undiscovered that play a role in the development of GVHD.

Prevention of the development of GVHD has been attempted by two techniques: (1) chemotherapy from the time of transplantation and (2) modification of the marrow prior to infusion into the recipient. Currently, methotrexate is being used following bone marrow transplantation in an attempt to prevent or modulate the disease. More recent studies have demonstrated significant prevention of GVHD with regular administration of cyclosporin-A. Removal of the cells thought to be responsible for the development of GVHD from the marrow prior to infusion has been attempted by fractionation and in vitro treatment with antithymocyte antibodies. X-irradiation of peripheral white blood cells that are transfused during periods of aplasia is routinely used.

Once the disease is established, administration of high-dose corticosteroid with or without adjunctive agents such as methotrexate or azathioprine is effective. High-dose methotrexate with citrovorum factor rescue has been used in some refractory cases. Cyclosporin-A has been reported to be of some benefit for established disease, particularly acute cutaneous GVHR [40]. Antithymocyte globulin has been used as a direct attack on the cells thought to be responsible for the disease [41]. In general, we have found that the earlier therapy is begun, at the first sign of the disease, the better is the outcome. The combination of corticosteroids and azathioprine provides some control of the chronic phases of the disease.

Good nursing care is of paramount importance for the physical and psychologic well-being of these patients. Hyperalimentation, protective isolation, antibiotics, and physical therapy may be needed following transplantation.

With regard to specific skin care, good cutaneous hygiene with mild soap followed by lubrication seems to give the most symptomatic relief. Topical corticosteroids, in our experience, have not been helpful during either the acute or chronic phases of cutaneous GVHR. Systemic antihistamines provide only partial relief for the pruritus associated with either the acute or chronic phases. For the rare TEN-like phase of acute cutaneous GVHR, treatment analogous to a burn patient with aseptic techniques, saline compresses, antibiotics, and careful handling of the patient provides some help.

Following discharge from the hospital, we advise avoidance of excessive sunlight exposure and routine use of topical sunscreen agents. Although the status of sunlight as a factor in triggering GVHD has not been definitely determined, we have seen patients whose disease seemed to be precipitated by a sunburn.

Course and Prognosis

Acute Graft-versus-Host Disease

The natural history of acute or chronic GVHD can be predicted by the severity of the clinical manifestations. In acute GVHD mild abnormalities of the skin, gastrointestinal tract, or liver may spontaneously resolve without therapy. Moderate to severe GVHD is always treated aggressively and the natural history of the disease is modified by the regimen used. The patient is consequently subjected to many additional side effects of the therapy, the most serious complication being an increased susceptibility to infection. Patients with severe acute GVHD frequently develop localized or disseminated bacterial, fungal, or viral infections. The most common viral agents are cytomegalovirus, herpes simplex, and varicella-zoster virus.

Progressive interstitial pneumonitis is a common cause of death. Many of the infective organisms enter through the respiratory tract; however, breaks in the integrity of the skin (fissures and ulcerations) and bowel mucosa are other portals of entry.

Survival, once acute GVHD has developed, appears to be related to the severity of the disease. Acute GVHR is the primary or associated cause of death in 17 to 73 percent of bone marrow transplantation patients [2,3,10,11]. Survival is improving as we have become more adept at recognizing and treating early disease and dealing with the complications associated with aggressive immunosuppression.

Chronic Graft-versus-Host Disease

Patients with chronic cutaneous GVHR are compromised by limitation of motion secondary to tight (taut) skin and joint contractures. They often develop cutaneous bacterial infections, especially with *Staphylococcus aureus,* and chronic ulcerations which heal slowly.

Chronic GVHD may spontaneously resolve. One patient developed a moderately severe lichenoid phase which evolved into the sclerodermoid form of GVHR. Except for routine prophylactic methotrexate administered during the first 100 days posttransplantation, he was not being treated with immunosuppressive agents. Two years after the onset of cutaneous disease, the GVHR began to resolve spontaneously. This sclerodermoid phase, including joint contractures, resolved in a cephalad to caudad progression, leaving only residual postinflammatory hyperpigmentation. Early in the course of his disease he had required mechanical dilation of a strictured esophagus; his difficulty in swallowing resolved as his skin disease cleared. We have observed the resolution of the sclerotic phase of chronic GVHR in several other patients. Over a 1- to 2-year period their skin becomes appreciably softer, ulcers heal, contractures improve, and ability to sweat returns. Persistent xerosis and hyperpigmentation are common sequelae.

References

1. Storb R et al: Marrow transplantation in thirty "untransfused" patients with severe aplastic anemia. *Ann Intern Med* **92:**30–36, 1980
2. Blume KG et al: Bone marrow ablation and allogeneic marrow transplantation in acute leukemia. *N Engl J Med* **302:**1041–1046, 1980
3. Bortin MM, Rimm AA: Bone marrow transplantation for acute myeloblastic leukemia. *JAMA* **240:**1245–1252, 1978
4. Bortin MM, Rimm AA: Severe combined immunodeficiency disease: characterization of the disease and results of transplantation. *JAMA* **238:**591–600, 1977
5. De Dobbeleer GD et al: Graft vs. host reaction: an ultrastructural study. *Arch Dermatol* **111:**1597–1602, 1975
6. Ford JM et al: Fatal graft-versus-host disease following transfusion of granulocytes from normal donors. *Lancet* **2:**1167–1169, 1976
7. Rosen RC et al: Acute leukemia and granulocyte transfusion: fatal graft-versus-host reaction following transfusion

of cells obtained from normal donors. *J Pediatr* **93**:268–270, 1978

8. Grogan TM et al: Graft-versus-host reaction (GVHR): a case report suggesting GVHR occurred as a result of maternofetal cell transfer. *Arch Pathol* **99**:330–334, 1975

9. Morhenn VB, Maibach HI: Graft vs. host reaction in a newborn. *Acta Derm Venereol (Stockh)* **54**:133–136, 1974

10. Tutschka PJ et al: Preparative regimens for marrow transplantation in acute leukemia and aplastic anemia. *Am J Pediatr Hematol Oncol* **2**:363–370, 1980

11. Thomas ED et al: One hundred patients with acute leukemia treated by chemotherapy, total body irradiation, and allogeneic marrow transplantation. *Blood* **49**:511–533, 1974

12. Rappeport J et al: Acute graft-versus-host disease in recipients of bone marrow transplants from identical twin donors. *Lancet* **2**:717–720, 1979

13. Barnes DWH, Loutiti JF: Acute GVH disease in recipients of bone marrow from identical twin donors. *Lancet* **2**:905, 1979

14. Gluckman E et al: Graft-versus-host disease in recipients of syngeneic bone marrow. *Lancet* **1**:253–254, 1980

15. Billingham RE: The biology of graft-versus-host reactions. *Harvey Lect* **62**:21–78, 1966–1967

16. Buckner CD et al: Human marrow transplantation—current status, in *Progress in Hematology VIII*. Edited by EB Brown. Grune & Stratton, New York, 1973, pp. 299–324

17. Streilein JW: A common pathogenesis for the lesions of graft-versus-host disease. *Transplant Proc* **3**:418–421, 1971

18. Parkman R et al: Human graft-versus-host disease. *J Invest Dermatol* **74**:276–279, 1980

19. Reinherz EL et al: Aberrations of suppressor T cells in human graft-versus-host disease. *N Engl J Med* **300**:1061–1073, 1979

20. Tsoi MS et al: Nonspecific suppressor cells in patients with chronic graft-versus-host disease after marrow grafting. *J Immunol* **123**:1970–1976, 1979

21. Santos GW et al: Bone marrow transplantation—present status. *Transplant Proc* **11**:182–187, 1979

22. Peck GL et al: Toxic epidermal necrolysis in a patient with graft-versus-host reaction. *Arch Dermatol* **105**:561–569, 1972

23. Glucksberg H et al: Clinical manifestations of graft-versus-host disease in human recipients of marrow from HL-A-matched sibling donors. *Transplantation* **18**:295–304, 1974

24. Slavin RE, Santos GW: The graft versus host reaction in man after bone marrow transplantation: pathology, pathogenesis, clinical features and implication. *Clin Immunol Immunopathol* **1**:472–498, 1973

25. Beschorner WE et al: Lymphocytic bronchitis associated with graft-versus-host disease in recipients of bone-marrow transplants. *N Engl J Med* **299**:1030–1036, 1978

26. Lawley TJ et al: Scleroderma, Sjögren-like syndrome, and chronic graft-versus-host disease. *Ann Intern Med* **87**:707–709, 1977

27. Woodruff JM et al: Early secondary disease in the rhesus monkey. II. Electron microscopy of changes in mucous membranes and external epithelia as demonstrated in the tongue and lip. *Lab Invest* **27**:85–98, 1972

28. Lerner KG et al: Histopathology of graft-versus-host reaction (GVHR) in human recipients of marrow from HL-A-matched sibling donors. *Transplant Proc* **6**:367–371, 1974

29. Sale GE et al: Gastrointestinal graft-versus-host disease in man: a clinicopathologic study of the rectal biopsy. *Am J Surg Pathol* **3**:291–299, 1979

30. Gratwhol AA: Sjögren-type syndrome after allogeneic bone-marrow transplantation. *Ann Intern Med* **87**:703–706, 1977

31. Shulman HM: Chronic graft-versus-host syndrome in man: a long-term clinicopathologic study of 20 Seattle patients. *Am J Med* **69**:204–217, 1980

32. Graze PR, Gale RP: Chronic graft-versus-host disease: a syndrome of disordered immunity. *Am J Med* **66**:611–620, 1979

33. Grogan TM et al: Graft-versus-host reaction. *Arch Dermatol* **113**:806–812, 1977

34. Gallucci BB et al: The ultrastructure of the human epidermis in chronic graft-versus-host disease. *Am J Pathol* **95**:643–654, 1979

35. Weedon D et al: Apoptosis: its nature and implications for dermatopathology. *Am J Dermatopathol* **1**:133–144, 1979

36. Tsoi MS et al: Deposition of IgM and complement at the dermoepidermal junction in acute and chronic cutaneous graft-versus-host disease in man. *J Immunol* **120**:1485–1492, 1978

37. Ullman S et al: Immunoglobulins and complement in skin in graft-versus-host disease. *Ann Intern Med* **85**:205, 1976

38. Saurat JH et al: Skin antibodies in bone marrow transplanted patients. *Clin Exp Dermatol* **1**:377–384, 1976

39. Farmer ER et al: Cutaneous graft-versus-host reactions: a prospective sequential immunopathologic study in man. *Clin Res* **27**:241A, 1979

40. Powles RL et al: Cyclosporin A for the treatment of graft-versus-host disease in man. *Lancet* **2**:1327–1331, 1978

41. Storb R et al: Treatment of established human graft-versus-host disease by antithymocyte globulin. *Blood* **44**:57–75, 1974

ACUTE FEBRILE NEUTROPHILIC DERMATOSIS (SWEET'S SYNDROME)

Herbert Hönigsmann

Klaus Wolff

Definition

Acute febrile neutrophilic dermatosis is an uncommon, recurrent, fairly dramatic skin disease characterized by painful plaque-forming inflammatory papules and associated with fever, arthralgia, and peripheral leukocytosis.

Historical Aspects

In 1964 Sweet [1] described a distinct hitherto unrecognized condition for which he employed the descriptive term *acute febrile neutrophilic dermatosis*. More than 100 cases have since been reported [2], and this may indicate that the disease is not a new condition, but rather was lumped in the past with other dermatoses such as erythema multiforme or erythema nodosum.

Incidence

The disease has a worldwide distribution and there is no racial predilection [3,4]. There is a striking preponderance of the female sex. The ratio of females to males was 15:1 in Sweet's report [2] and 18:1 in another large series [3]; all of our own patients have been women. Most of the reported patients have been in their mid-thirties to mid-fifties, but on rare occasions the condition may affect younger people. The youngest patient recognized was a 3-month-old Japanese girl [5].

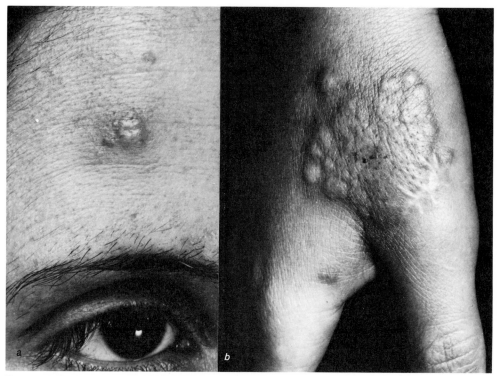

Fig. 1. Acute febrile neutrophilic dermatosis. Typical lesions consisting of coalescing, plaque-forming papules. (*a*) Lesion on the forehead. (*b*) Lesion on the dorsum of the right hand exhibiting the "relief of a mountain range" feature. *[From [7], with permission.]*

Etiology

There is no known cause of acute febrile neutrophilic dermatosis. In the majority of the patients a febrile upper respiratory tract infection, tonsillitis, or influenza-like illness precedes the skin lesions by 1 to 3 weeks [6]. However, there is no conclusive evidence for a causative role of bacterial or, more specifically, streptococcal infection. Fever and peripheral leukocytosis suggest a septic process, but antibiotics do not influence the course of the disease. Massive tissue leukocytosis strongly implies a pathogenic role of leukotactic mechanisms [7], but so far no studies have been performed on complement and its components, on the function of leukocytes and their response to chemotactic stimuli, and on circulating immune complexes in this syndrome. The clinical appearance, course, and histopathology, which reveals some morphologic features of vascular alteration, indicate that Sweet's syndrome may represent a form of hypersensitivity reaction [7]. The favorable response to systemic corticosteroids is consistent with this concept.

Clinical Features

The typical skin lesions are red or bluish-red papules or nodules which show a strong tendency to coalesce and to form irregular, sharply bordered plaques (Fig. 1). Such lesions have been compared to a "relief of a mountain range" [6] (Fig. 1*b*). The pronounced inflammatory edema is often responsible for a transparent, vesicle-like appearance of the lesions despite the fact that they are solid upon palpation [2,7] (Fig. 2). This phenomenon has been described as an "illusion of vesiculation" [1]. In later stages the tops of the papules may occasionally become studded with tiny pustules and central clearing may lead to annular or arcuate patterns. The lesions are tender and often painful and tend to enlarge over a period of days or weeks and eventually resolve without scarring after weeks or months. The eruption may present with a single or with multiple lesions, characteristically in an asymmetric distribution. Most commonly, the face, neck, and upper extremities are involved, but lesions also develop on the lower limbs. Widespread or even generalized forms have

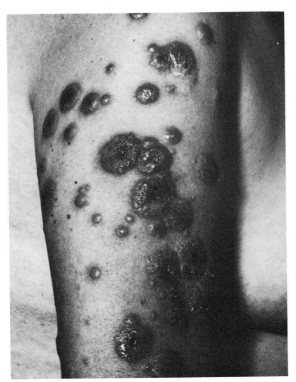

Fig. 2. Acute febrile neutrophilic dermatosis. Multiple, confluent papules and plaques which, at first sight, give the illusion of vesiculation, but are solid upon palpation. *[From [11], with permission.]*

been reported, but lesions on the trunk are uncommon. About half of the patients experience recurrences, often in previously involved sites.

The systemic symptoms that characteristically accompany the skin eruption are fever and leukocytosis and the patients often appear dramatically ill. However, it has been recognized that not all cases of acute febrile neutrophilic dermatoses express the whole spectrum of symptoms [8], and Sweet's syndrome may therefore not always be acute nor always febrile and may lack leukocytosis [7,9]. A period of feverish state may precede the skin disease by several days or sometimes by several weeks and may be present throughout the entire course. Additional symptoms that may occur to varying degrees are headache, arthralgia, and general malaise. Inconsistent findings are conjunctivitis or episcleritis [2], but these have been noted in over 60 percent of patients in one large series [3]. Excepting one single observation (personal communication, R. Travers to R. D. Sweet, see [2]), mucosal lesions are not a feature of the syndrome.

Laboratory Findings

An elevated red blood cell sedimentation rate and peripheral leukocytosis with neutrophilia are the most consistent laboratory findings. White blood cell counts range from 10,000 to 20,000, but, as pointed out above, quite a number of patients do not exhibit leukocytosis, which originally had been thought to represent an integral symptom.

Pathology

The most prominent histopathologic features are edema of the papillary body (Fig. 3) and a dense infiltrate of leukocytes in the lower dermis [6]. The infiltrate may be diffuse or perivascular consisting predominantly of neutrophils with occasional eosinophils and some lymphoid cells. Perivascular foci of leukocytoclasia are quite common and, at low magnification, may suggest vasculitis [7,10] (Fig. 4). However, except for a slight dilatation of the small blood vessels there are no signs of vascular damage. Usually, the epidermis is normal. Spongiosis and exocytosis have been reported in some cases and rarely there may be a subcorneal pustule (Fig. 3).

Electron microscopy does not reveal endothelial cell damage, but rather signs of metabolic activation as indicated by the abundance of endoplasmic reticulum, mitochondria, and multiple Golgi areas [7] (Fig. 5). The vessels are separated from the cellular infiltrate by a relatively broad electron lucent zone occupied by multiple concentrically arranged basal laminae and a finely fibrillar and

Fig. 3. Acute febrile neutrophilic dermatosis. Massive edema of the papillary body with polymorphs scattered throughout the upper dermis. In the center of the lesion there is focal spongiosis and formation of a subcorneal pustule. × 150.

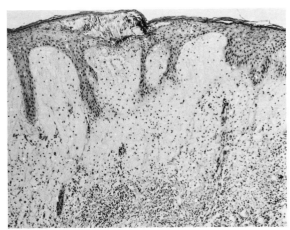

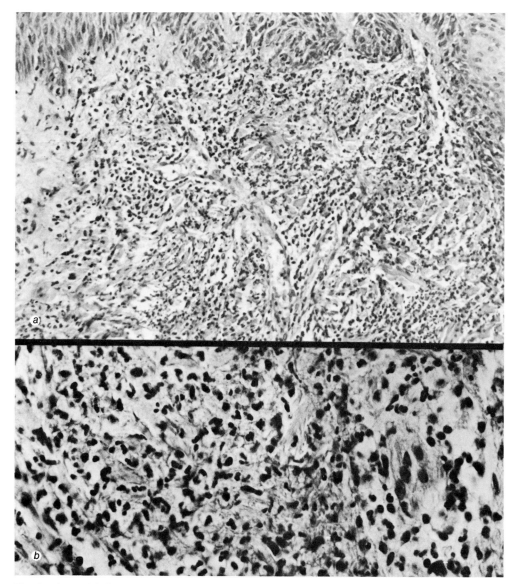

Fig. 4. Acute febrile neutrophilic dermatosis. (*a*) Dense inflammatory infiltrate in the upper and mid dermis predominantly composed of polymorphonuclear leukocytes. ×250. *[From [7], with permission.]* (*b*) Higher magnification shows thickening of the vessel walls and perivascular foci of leukocytoclasia. ×600. *[From [11], with permission.]*

vesicular material consisting of plasma constituents and cell debris, which may also be found in the vascular lumen (Fig. 5). Such findings are consistent with endothelial repair and regeneration after previous endothelial damage.

Immunofluorescence

In three patients investigated by us so far, direct immunofluorescence of lesional skin was noncontributory. In one case, deposits of IgG, IgM, and fibrin were found diffusely distributed in a perivascular arrangement, but this may only represent

a nonspecific inflammatory exudate [11]. Investigations of very early lesions have not been performed so far; possibly, immune complexes or immunoglobulin deposits do exist in early lesions of Sweet's syndrome but escape detection because they are degraded rapidly. This would be analogous to the situation in immune complex vasculitis.

Associated Diseases

There have been several isolated reports of Sweet's syndrome and associated diseases of questionable pathogenic relevance, such as ulcerative colitis

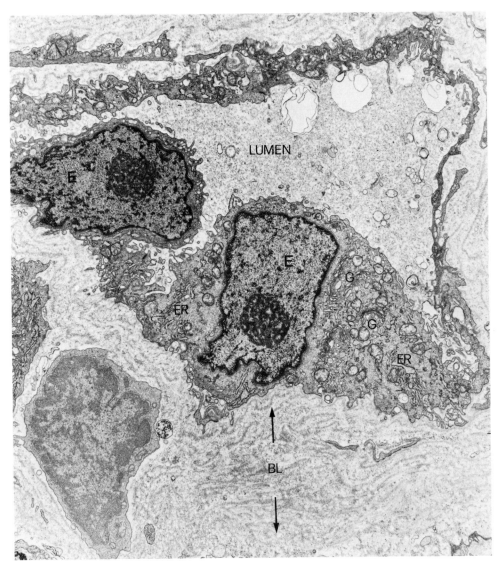

Fig. 5. Acute febrile neutrophilic dermatosis. Endothelial cells (E) exhibit signs of metabolic activation as indicated by the abundance of endoplasmic reticulum (ER), multiple Golgi areas (G), and numerous mitochondria. Vesicles and cellular debris in the lumen may indicate previous cellular damage, and multiple concentric basal laminae (BL) suggest repeated vascular damage and regeneration. Original magnification ×25,000. *[From [7], with permission.]*

[1], benign monoclonal gammopathy [12], transient myeloid proliferation [13], and various malignant tumors [9,10,14]. More importantly, there is an increasing number of reports on patients with acute myeloid leukemia and associated Sweet's syndrome [9,15–20]. In the majority of the cases reported so far, the skin lesions preceded the diagnosis of leukemia by several months or even years. Thus, thorough hematologic follow-up of patients with Sweet's syndrome is recommended. However, in view of the small number (10 cases) with associated leukemic disease it would be premature to consider Sweet's syndrome a paraneoplastic condition [11,19].

Diagnosis and Differential Diagnosis

Early Sweet's syndrome may clinically resemble erythema multiforme, but the asymmetrical distribution pattern, the absence of oral and genital mucosal involvement, and the pronounced tenderness of the lesions should alert the physician to consider Sweet's syndrome. After a few days the distinctive coalescing, irregular, and marginated plaques can easily be separated from the target-like lesions of erythema multiforme and the typical histopathology will permit the correct diagnosis [2,6]. Differential diagnosis also includes erythema nodosum, which is primarily a nodular, deep-seated eruption most commonly occurring on the lower legs, which are only occasionally, but never exclusively, involved in Sweets syndrome. The histological finding of septal panniculitis will clearly rule out acute febrile neutrophilic dermatosis. Solitary lesions may clinically mimic herpes simplex (Fig. 1a) because of their peculiar transparent, pseudovesicular appearance, but palpation will reveal their solid consistency.

Individual plaques may be suggestive of erythema elevatum diutinum, but this disease is characterized, histologically, by leukocytoclastic vasculitis, and its course is definitively chronic. Pyoderma gangrenosum will not give rise to confusion because of its characteristic ulceration. A disease that shows a very similar histopathologic picture with pronounced tissue neutrophilia and leukocytoclasia without signs of vasculitis is bowel-bypass syndrome [21], but its clinical presentation is quite different.

Treatment

Despite the fact that the systemic symptoms, fever, and leucocytosis suggest a septic process, there is no response to antibiotics. Prompt relief of cutaneous and systemic symptoms is obtained by systemic corticosteroids in doses of 30 to 60 mg prednisolone daily, which are tapered to 10 mg within 2 or 3 weeks. In some patients prolonged treatment with lower doses (10 to 20 mg on alternate days) for 2 or 3 months may be necessary to suppress recurrences. Recently a dramatic response to oral potassium iodide (900 mg daily for 2 weeks) has been reported in a group of Japanese patients [22].

Course and Prognosis

Acute febrile neutrophilic dermatosis is a benign condition. The pathogenic significance of associated malignant diseases remains to be clarified. Without treatment the eruption may persist for weeks or even several months and then involute without leaving scars. Recurrences have to be expected in approximately 50 percent of the patients at various time intervals after therapy-induced or spontaneous remission.

References

1. Sweet RD: An acute febrile neutrophilic dermatosis. *Br J Dermatol* **76**:349–356, 1964
2. Sweet RD: Acute febrile neutrophilic dermatosis—1978. *Br J Dermatol* **100**:93–99, 1979
3. Gunawardena DA et al: The clinical spectrums of Sweet's syndrome (acute febrile neutrophilic dermatosis)—a report of eighteen cases. *Br J Dermatol* **92**:363–373, 1975
4. Sanchez de Paz F: Tesis doctoral, La Facultad de Medicina de la Universidad Complutense de Madrid, 1977
5. Itami S, Nishioka K: Sweet's syndrome in infancy. *Br J Dermatol* **103**:449–451, 1980
6. Crow KD et al: Acute febrile neutrophilic dermatosis. Sweet's syndrome. *Dermatologica* **139**:123–134, 1969
7. Hönigsmann H, Wolff K: Acute febrile neutrophilic dermatosis (Sweet's syndrome), in *Major Problems in Dermatology*, vol 10, *Vasculitis*. Edited by K Wolff, RK Winkelmann; consulting editor, A Rook. Lloyd-Luke, London, 1980, pp 307–316
8. Sweet RD: Further observations in acute febrile neutrophilic dermatosis. *Br J Dermatol* **80**:800–805, 1968
9. Matta M et al: Sweet's syndrome: systemic association. *Cutis* **12**:561–565, 1973
10. Shapiro L et al: Sweet's syndrome (acute febrile neutrophilic dermatosis). *Arch Dermatol* **103**:81–84, 1971
11. Hönigsmann H et al: Akute febrile neutrophile Dermatose. *Wien Klin Wochenschr* **91**:842–847, 1979
12. Holst R, Mobacken H: Acute febrile neutrophilic dermatosis (Sweet's syndrome). *Acta Derm Venereol (Stockh)* **51**:63–66, 1971
13. Dymock RB et al: Acute febrile neutrophilic dermatosis (Sweet's syndrome) with myeloid proliferation. *Australas J Dermatol* **19**:24–27, 1978
14. Greer KW et al: Acute febrile neutrophilic dermatosis (Sweet's syndrome). *Arch Dermatol* **111**:1461–1463, 1975
15. Klock JC, Oken R: Febrile neutrophilic dermatosis in acute myelogenous leukemia. *Cancer* **37**:922–927, 1976
16. Pirard C, Dellancy A: Syndrome de Sweet et leucémie myéloide aigue. *Ann Dermatol Venereol (Paris)* **104**:160–161, 1977
17. Raimer SS, Duncan C: Febrile neutrophilic dermatosis in acute myelogenous leukemia. *Arch Dermatol* **114**:413–414, 1978
18. Goodfellow A, Calvert H: Sweet's syndrome and acute myeloid leukaemia. *Lancet* **2**:478–479, 1979
19. Burton JL: Sweet's syndrome, pyoderma gangrenosum and acute leukemia. *Br J Dermatol* **102**:239, 1980
20. Spector JI et al: Sweet's syndrome. Association with acute leukemia. *JAMA* **244**:1131–1132, 1980
21. Ely PH: The bowel bypass syndrome: a response to bacterial peptidoglycans. *J Am Acad Dermatol* **2**:473–487, 1980
22. Horio T et al: Treatment of acute febrile neutrophilic dermatosis (Sweet's syndrome) with potassium iodide. *Dermatologica* **160**:341–347, 1980

HERITABLE MELANIN DEFICIENCY SYNDROMES
Diagnosis and Prophylactic Treatment with Sun-Protective Agents

Thomas B. Fitzpatrick

Madhu A. Pathak

Franz Greiter

David B. Mosher

John A. Parrish

Melanin pigmentation of human skin can be described in two categories: the first, constitutive or intrinsic skin color, and the second, facultative or inducible skin color [1]. *Constitutive skin color* designates the genetically determined levels of cutaneous melanin pigmentation in accordance with the genetic programs of the cells in the absence of direct or indirect influences (e.g., solar radiation, hormones, or other environmental factors). *Facultative skin color* characterizes the increase in melanin pigmentation above the constitutive level and arises from the complex interplay of solar radiation and certain pituitary hormones upon the genetically endowed melanogenesis of the individual. The facultative skin color change brought about by solar radiation is commonly referred to as *suntan*.

1. Constitutive Melanin Pigmentation. The melanin pigmentary system of the human skin is based on two cell types: dendritic melanocytes and nondendritic keratinocytes. The melanocytes synthesize specialized organelles called *melanosomes* within which the pigment melanin is synthesized and contained. Melanosomes are transferred to the keratinocytes and transported by these cells to the epidermal surface or stratum corneum. The production and the transfer of these chromoprotein-carrying organelles, the melanosomes, is a complex process involving the structural and functional organization of both melanocytes and keratinocytes. This functional unit, consisting of one melanocyte and approximately 36 keratinocytes, is known as the *epidermal melanin unit*. The functional activity of the multicellular epidermal melanin unit, rather than the melanocyte alone, is the focal point for the determination of skin color. This unique symbiotic relationship results in a uniform and wide distribution of pigment granules throughout the entire epidermis, although the melanocyte population of the epidermis is no more than 10 to 25 percent of the population of the keratinizing basal cells. The structural basis of normal melanin pigmentation of mammalian skin depends on the following factors: (1) the formation of pigment granules, the melanosomes; (2) the melanization of melanosomes, involving the synthesis of the enzyme *tyrosinase* and the enzymatic oxidation of tyrosine into melanin; (3) the movement of the melanosomes from the protoplasmic mass, the perikaryon, into the dendrites of the melanocytes; (4) the transfer of these melanosomes into the keratinizing epidermal cells, the keratinocytes; (5) the incorporation of melanosomes by these cells either as single discrete particles or as *melanosome complexes;* (6) the degradation of the melanosomes within keratinocytes; and (7) the rate of exfoliation of keratinocytes (see Fig. 3).

2. Facultative Melanin Pigmentation: Action of Light. Solar radiation markedly influences skin color. Increased melanin pigmentation that occurs after exposure of human skin to sunlight or to ultraviolet (UV) radiation from artificial sources is familiarly known as *tanning*. Tanning of the skin involves two distinct photobiologic processes: (1) immediate tanning (IT), sometimes referred to as immediate pigment darkening (IPD) reaction, and (2) delayed tanning (DT). The biophysical, biochemical, and ultrastructural bases of these two processes will be reviewed briefly, with special emphasis

on the effects of UV radiation on *(a)* changes in the number of melanocytes, *(b)* synthesis of melanosomes, i.e., the number of melanosomes and their size, *(c)* melanization of melanosomes, and *(d)* the transfer of melanosomes to keratinocytes and concomitant changes in keratinocytes concerning *(e)* the number of melanosomes transferred, and *(f)* the distribution pattern of melanosomes within the keratinocytes.

Melanogenesis and Melanin Pigmentation: Biologic Basis of Heritable Deficiency Syndromes and Dermatoheliosis

Biologic Basis [2]

The Epidermal Melanin Unit. The epidermal melanin unit is a functional and structural unit comprised of a specialized, dendritic, pigment-producing exocrine gland, the *melanocyte,* that sits on the basal lamina and projects its dendrites into the keratinocytes (Fig. 1). In a three-dimensional image, there is 1 melanocyte to 36 keratinocytes. The melanocyte is derived from the neural crest and is part of a family of cells comprising the *melanocyte system* located (in addition to the epidermis) in the hair bulb, the uveal tract, the retinal pigment epithelium, and the stria vascularis of the inner ear. Variations in skin color are predominantly due to the content of specialized chromophoric subcellular organelles, the *melanosomes,* which are the secretory product of the exocrine melanocytes and which are transferred to keratinocytes. The content of melanin in melanosomes is determined by the level within the melanosome of active tyrosinase, an aerobic oxi-

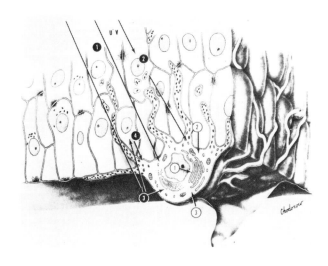

Fig. 1. Epidermal melanin unit illustrating the possible pathways of intrinsic and environmental (UVR) influences on melanocytes. *Intrinsic* (black numbers on white background): (1) genome of melanocytes, (2) keratinocyte influences, and (3) dermal influences. *Environmental* (UVR) (white numbers on black background): (1) UVR influences melanocyte directly, (2) UVR stimulates keratinocyte to influence melanocyte, (3) UVR stimulates dermis to influence melanocyte directly or (4) indirectly by action on keratinocytes.

dase, containing copper as a prosthetic group which catalyzes the oxidation of the precursor, tyrosine, to the insoluble high-molecular-weight polymer melanin (Fig. 2). The level of skin color in humans is not determined by changes in the number of melanocytes but by the *functional activity* of these cells: to produce and transfer melanosomes to the cluster of keratinocytes in the epidermal melanin unit (Fig. 3). Defects in this scheme can lead to decreased or increased pigmentation by blocks at various steps. For example, if no, or a reduced amount of, melanin is deposited on the melanosome because of an inactive tyrosinase, melanin pigmentation is reduced or absent (human oculocutaneous albinism). If melanosomes are synthesized but not transferred to keratinocytes, there will be a dilution of skin and hair pigmentation even though melanocytes are full of pigmented melanosomes.

Components of the Melanin Pigmentary System.

MELANOCYTES. The number of melanocytes varies from region to region but does not vary with differences in skin color. The highest number is on the head/neck and genitalia (1900 to 2300 per square millimeter), and one-half this number on the trunk and extremities (890 to 1200 per square millimeter). Melanocytes undergo occasional mitotic division to maintain their population.

MELANOSOMES. The melanosome is the site of melanin synthesis in the melanocyte. Melanosomes are 0.4 by 0.7 μm in size with an ellipsoidal shape and an *internal structure* comprised of internal membranous filaments. The melanization varies and is classified into four stages—I, II, III, IV—determined by the degree of melanization. These characteristics (size, shape, and melanization) are regulated by transcription and translation of information coded by "pigmentary genes."

Fig. 2. Biosynthesis of eumelanin and phaeomelanin. [Modified from Prota [3].]

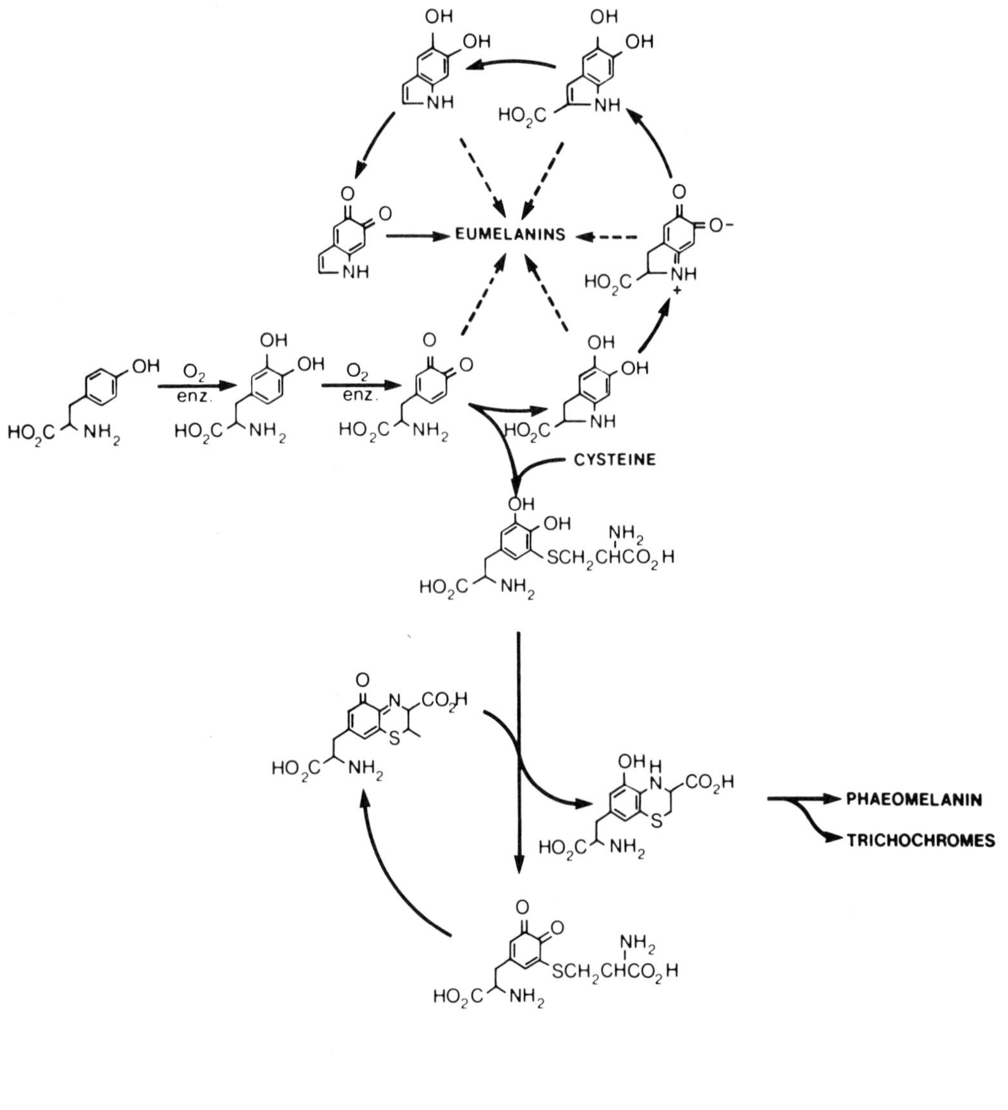

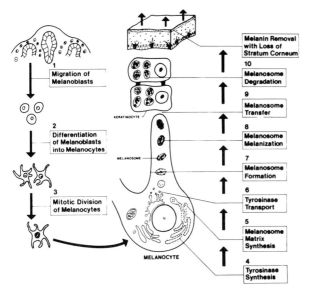

Fig. 3. Morphologic and metabolic pathway of epidermal melanin pigmentation.

The melanosomal attributes are specified by nucleotide sequences within DNA; the level (gene transcription or translation) is not yet known. It is now known that vesiculoglobular bodies (VGB), 400 Å in diameter, are present in normal melanosomes. The role of the VGB in the ontogeny of the melanosome is not known; some believe it transfers tyrosinase. Melanosomes in pigmented hair and in black skin are larger, approximately 1.0 μm in length. In these melanocytes of the pigmented hair bulb and in black skin, the melanosomes transferred to keratinocytes remain as discrete organelles (nonaggregated) in contrast to white skin, in which the melanosomes become aggregated—two or more particles within membrane-limited vesicles. These membrane-limited, melanosome-containing organelles resemble the membrane-limited, melanosome-containing organelles within macrophages which have been identified as phagolysosomes (secondary lysosomes). The aggregated melanosomes undergo gradual degradation into small electron-dense particles.

TYROSINASE. The majority of investigators believe that tyrosinase is the single enzyme that catalyzes the oxidation of tyrosine to dopa and dopa to dopaquinone. Three different molecular forms (isoenzymes) have been designated T1, T2, and T3. T1 and T2 are the soluble forms, while T3 is the bound enzyme. Most (90 percent) of the tyrosinase in human melanoma cells is T3. Serum tyrosinase has been recently detected in patients with metastatic melanoma and metastatic breast carcinoma. The purification of tyrosinase has not yet been achieved; this is eagerly awaited because it would then be possible to develop a radioimmunoassay for tyrosinase in serum and in tissue.

MELANIN. Mammalian melanins are all derived from tyrosine but are so complex and insoluble that they must be defined on the basis of their color, origin, and chemical properties (Fig. 2). Melanins that are brown-black are intractably insoluble nitrogenous pigments and are termed *eumelanins;* they consist of heteropolymers, mainly 5,6-dihydroxyindole [3]. Melanins that range in color from light yellow to red are called *phaeomelanins,* and, while also derived from tyrosine, they are formed by the interaction of cysteine and glutathione with dopaquinone (Fig. 2). Phaeomelanins have *been found only in hair* and in some human melanomas. These complex sulfur-containing macromolecules, the phaeomelanins, are soluble in dilute alkali and have been shown to be formed by benzothiazole, 1,4-benzothiazine, and tetrahydroisoquinoline systems. In addition there is another group of phaeomelanins that are called *trichochromes.* The trichochromes are the most precisely defined of all the melanins and are characterized by a pH-dependent chromophore consisting of two conjugated 1,4-benzothiazine units derived from cysteinyldopa.

Recently it has been proposed that the eumelanin and phaeomelanin pathways are always intermeshed. In other words, in most mammals and humans, the phenotypic color reflects the relative mixtures of the two metabolic pathways: eumelanin and phaeomelanin. For example, the sulfur content of eumelanin is 6 compared to 10 percent for phaeomelanin. Eumelanins are remarkable in some of their special properties. The stability of melanin is evidenced by its presence in the ink sacs of fossilized squid about 180 million years old. Heating melanin to 600°C does not alter it. Melanins are not biodegradable. Melanins contain intrinsic free radicals and can absorb radicals, e.g., free radicals produced by exposure of tissue to light. Melanin absorbs light strongly throughout the UV and visible electromagnetic spectrum; there is a strong featureless absorption increasing toward the shorter wavelengths. Melanin is thought to be an amorphous semiconductor in which photon-phonon coupling, by way of excited electronic states of the melanin, plays a role. Melanin binds drugs probably through charge-transfer complexes in which the drug donates electrons and melanin acts as an electron acceptor. Metals (including those with a high content of zinc) are bound to melanin by virtue of their capacity to act as a cation-exchange material.

Control of Melanogenesis and Melanin Pigmentation

Ultraviolet-Induced Melanin Pigmentary Response in Skin [4].

IMMEDIATE TANNING REACTION. This can best be seen in pigmented individuals or in the previously tanned areas of fair-skinned individuals. IT can be induced by both long-wave UV (315 to 400 nm) and visible light (400 to 700 nm). UVA (315 to 400 nm) radiation is more effective in induction of IT than is visible light. UVB radiation, the sunburn-producing spectrum, does not stimulate IT as effectively as does UVA radiation. This selective induction of IT by UVA is related to the depth of penetration and absorption of this radiation at the dermal-epidermal junction. The skin begins to be hyperpigmented with 5 to 10 min of midday summer sun exposure and can be maximally pigmented with 1 hr of irradiation. The hyperpigmentation fades rapidly within 30 to 60 min; thereafter the color usually fades gradually, so that after 3 to 4 hr the irradiated areas are barely hyperpigmented. Sometimes, however, after prolonged sun exposure, 90 to 120 min, skin may remain hyperpigmented for as long as 36 to 48 hr, after which time newly synthesized melanin [new melanogenesis or delayed tanning (DT)] begins to hyperpigment the skin.

DELAYED TANNING REACTION AND HYPERPIGMENTATION OF THE SKIN (TABLE 1). Delayed tanning is a process which involves the production, transfer, distribution, and, to a limited extent, degradation of melanosomes. The degree of melanin pigmentation that occurs following exposure of human skin to solar radiation varies to a certain extent with the total dose of solar radiation received, but more importantly it is regulated by the genetically controlled functional capacity of the epidermal melanin unit of the individual. Genes control the structure of the melanosomes, the level of tyrosinase activity, the polymerization process of the indolequinone and other intermediates, and the development of the dendrites that transfer the melanosomes to keratinocytes. Solar radiation or UV radiation from artificial sources influences the genetically controlled normal melanin pigmentation (facultative color) of the skin in one or more of the following ways: (1) an increase in the number of functional melanocytes (dopa-positive) as a result of proliferation of melanocytes and also possibly the activation of the dormant or resting melanocytes; (2) hypertrophy of the melanocytes and increased arborization (branching) of the dendrites of melanocytes; (3) augmentation of melanosome synthesis manifested by an increase in the number of melanosomes both in the melanocytes and in malpighian cells (keratinocytes); (4) an increase in tyrosinase activity due principally to the synthesis of new tyrosinase in the proliferating melanocytes; (5) an increase in the transfer of melanosomes from melanocytes to keratinocytes as the result of increased turnover of keratinocytes; (6) an increase in the size of melanosomes and also an increase in the size of the melanosome complex.

ACTION SPECTRUM FOR MELANOGENESIS. Wavelengths shorter than 320 nm, which cause sunburn (erythema), are considered to stimulate melanogenesis or delayed tanning most effectively. The generally held concept of the initiation of melanogenesis only by UVB should be modified; longwave UV radiation (UVA) must be included in the melanogenic spectrum. It must be stressed, however, that if one were to estimate the quantum efficiency for melanogenesis by UVB and UVA, it would be apparent that UVB is more efficient in the induction of melanogenesis than is UVA. It requires approximately a minimum of 50 to 100 mJ/cm^2 to stimulate melanogenesis by UVB, whereas a minimum of 10 to 12 J/cm^2 of UVA is required to stimulate melanogenesis. Visible radiation (400 to 700 nm) and infrared radiation ($\lambda > 750$ nm) are extremely weak in the induction or stimulation of melanogenesis. A single exposure in the range of 25 to 30 J/cm^2 of visible light will not stimulate melanogenesis.

Hormonal Control. Melanin pigmentation is the process that occurs in the epidermal melanin unit by which melanized melanosomes are produced in melanocytes *and* transferred to keratinocytes. In addition to UV radiation, which enhances the melanin pigmentation by an as yet unknown mechanism, the polypeptide hormones of the anterior pituitary gland stimulate pigmentation. These polypeptide hormones are produced by cleavage of larger peptides. These polypeptides, called originally *melanocyte-stimulating hormones* (MSH), are of two types, *alpha MSH* and *beta MSH*; alpha MSH is a single polypeptide of 13 amino acid residues, identical in sequence to the terminal portion of ACTH; ACTH has one-fortieth the pigmentation effect of alpha MSH. Beta MSH (human) has 22 amino acids. Although the precise mechanism of action of MSH in human beings has not yet been established, there is some considerable understanding of the mode of action of MSH in mammalian melanocytes, especially in the mouse. The sequence of events is as follows. Melanocytes

Table 1 Light and ultrastructural changes in epidermal melanin unit in the delayed tanning reaction after repeated exposures to UVB, UVA, or UVA plus oral 8-methoxypsoralen (8-MOP)

Nature of observations	Nonexposed skin	Exposed skin after UVB, UVA, or UVA plus oral 8-MOP
Macroscopic:		
Degree of visual pigmentation		Increased with UVB + +; UVA + + +; UVA plus 8-MOP + + + +
Onset of visual pigmentation		UVA within 36–43 hr; UVB within 24–72 hr; UVA + 8-MOP within 96–120 hr
Light microscopic:		
Melanin granules	Barely visible in fair whites but easily visible in blacks and Mongoloids	Increased in all Skin Types; most with UVA + 8-MOP
Number of melanocytes	About 700–950/mm² in unexposed skin and 1000–1300/mm² in habitually exposed skin; no racial differences in population density	Increased 2–3 times within 7–10 days; most remarkable increase in UVA + 8-MOP
Perikaryon of melanocytes	Small	Markedly enlarged
Dendrites of melanocytes	Poorly developed	Prominent and marked arborization
Dopa reaction (tyrosinase)	Weak	Strong; UVA + 8-MOP > UVA; UVA ≥ UVB
Tyrosine reaction (tyrosinase)	Barely detectable or absent	Increased and easily detectable in all races
Electron microscopic		
In melanocytes:		
Number of melanosomes	Few	Markedly increased
Melanization of melanosomes	Predominantly unmelanized in fair skin (stages I–III); melanizing forms (stages III–IV) in dark skin	Melanized melanosomes (stages III and IV) notably increased. In UVA and UVA + 8-MOP most of the melanosomes are fully melanized; in UVB melanosomes are in various stages of melanization.
Size of melanosomes	Small (400–500 nm in long axis) in whites; large in blacks (500–700 nm in long axis)	Some increased; some are 700–800 nm, even in whites.
Distribution of melanosomes	Perinuclear and rarely in dendrites	Variable (diffused in perikaryon and dendrites); more prominent in dendrites particularly with UVA or UVA + 8-MOP
10-nm (100 Å) filaments	Dense, perinuclear aggregation	Diffusely scattered in perikaryon and dendrites
Golgi apparatus	Poorly developed	Well developed, marked increase in size and number
Rough endoplasmic reticulum	Poorly developed	Well developed
Microtubules	Perinuclear	Perinuclear and in dendrites
In keratinocytes:		
Distribution pattern of melanosomes	Aggregated (melanosome complexes) in whites, nonaggregated in blacks and Australoids, and mixed (aggregated and single) in Mongoloids	Slightly altered (more single and aggregated melanosomes) in whites and Mongoloids; in blacks nonaggregated form
Ratio of nonaggregated vs. aggregated	Predominantly aggregated in whites; nonaggregated in blacks	Increased ratio of nonaggregated form, particularly with UVA + 8-MOP
Autophagic vacuoles in melanocytes and keratinocytes	Absent or very rare	Usually seen in UVB and UVA + 8-MOP treated skin
Lipid droplets	Absent or very rare	Usually seen in UVB and UVA + 8-MOP treated skin

possess a unique membrane-bound receptor molecule that is present in the late S and G_2 phase of the cell cycle. This receptor interacts with alpha MSH, and this induces the formation of adenylate cyclase, which, in turn, leads to the formation of cyclic AMP. The increase in cyclic AMP leads to increased tyrosinase synthesis, and pari passu, increase in melanin formation. Recent studies [5] using mouse melanoma cells in culture suggest the following hypothesis: cyclic AMP activates a protein kinase which, in turn, inactivates an inhibitor of tyrosinase, through a phosphorylation reaction.

Increased cyclic AMP levels are correlated with increased tyrosinase, increased pigmentation, cessation of cell division, and outgrowth of dendritic processes of the melanocyte.

The Epidermal Melanin Density Filter: Nature's Shielding Skin Pigment Layer (Fig. 4)

In humans, active epidermal melanin units (melanocytes producing and transferring melanosomes) provide a front line of defense against UV and visible radiation. In the eye, melanocytes occur in abundance in the uveal tract and in the retinal pigment epithelium and protect the eye from UVA and visible radiation, inasmuch as UVB is filtered by the cornea. Melanized epidermis (both constitutive and facultative epidermal pigmentation) is a cloak that shields the epidermis and dermis by reducing the transmission of damaging UVB and UVA radiant energy (Fig. 4). While the stratum corneum is the same thickness in white and black skin, black skin has more cell layers and more melanin [6,7]. Also, approximately 5 times less UVB and UVA reach the dermis of blacks as compared with Caucasians, with transmission differences in the stratum corneum not being very significant and absorption by the epidermis (containing melanosomes) being more marked in the black [8]; in Caucasian skin the stratum corneum is the major site of UV radiation filtration. A sun protection factor (SPF, see definition below) increasing from 3 to 30 was observed with increasing degrees of pigmentation in a study by Olson et al [9]. Protection by a UVA-induced pigmentation is 2:3 against broadband UV radiation [10], while 7 days of four 8-methoxypsoralen-UVA treatments per day provides a protection of 4:7 [11].

Despite this paucity of quantitative studies on the role of melanin in protection against UV radiation, there is general acceptance of the protective effects of epidermal melanin against the damaging effects of UV radiation. Blacks and Type IV and V Caucasians are far less susceptible to acute and chronic actinic damage, and there is a reciprocal relationship between solar elastosis and skin color. Sun-induced nonmelanoma skin cancer on the exposed areas of the face and upper extremities is very rare in blacks living in areas with high UVB flux; on the other hand, black albinos living in these same areas (Africa) are very susceptible to skin cancer and develop solar keratoses and skin cancer in childhood.

Skin Color and Sun-reactive Skin Types in White Skin

The 2 billion *nonwhite* world population has a very low incidence of melanoma (less than 0.9 per 100,000) compared to an average incidence of 4.5 per 100,000 in whites (25.0 per 100,000 in Australia) and very few nonmelanoma skin cancers (basal cell and squamous cell carcinomas). Also, non-

Fig. 4. Comparison of epidermal melanin density filter to a camera.

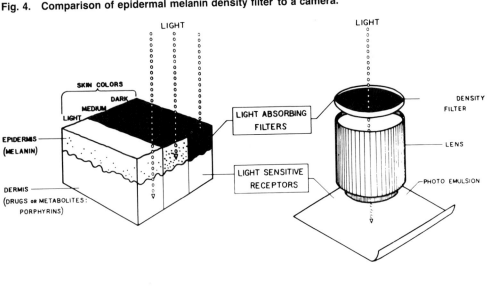

white persons have virtually no dermatoheliosis (for definition, see below). These susceptible white people (living in northern Europe, the United Kingdom, North America, South Africa, and Australia) have *white* skin (e.g., in the unexposed areas of the buttocks) while the 500 million people living in the Middle East, although classified as "white," have constitutively a *tan* (i.e., in the unexposed and exposed skin) not white skin. The fact is that even the susceptible white people (with white unexposed skin) are not all alike in their reactions to sun exposure or in their potential risk for developing sun-induced skin disorders.

There are two concerns about the effects of sun exposure on the skin of healthy individuals. The first is the development of delayed erythema or acute sunburn reaction, and the second is the potential long-term risk of repeated UV radiation exposure, namely dermatoheliosis ("aging") and malignant tumors of the skin. There is considerable human variability in the tendency to develop these changes. This variability is based in large part on the inherent epidermal melanin content of skin not habitually exposed to sunlight (constitutive skin color) and on the genetic capacity of the skin to darken or tan in response to UV irradiation (facultative skin color, or tan). A careful history of the reaction of each patient to sun exposure—tendency to sunburn and capacity to tan—enables the physician to categorize patients with white unexposed skin by *Skin Types* and thereby to be able to estimate the relative risk of the development of the acute and chronic changes related to UV radiation exposure.

There is a special high-risk normal white-skinned population who have poor tolerance to sunlight (Skin Type I). These are most often light-skinned people with red or blond hair, blue eyes, and freckles (ephelides). Identification of this subgroup who are genetically inadequately protected from sunlight signals a group of people who must use additional protective measures. Heavily tanned, swarthy-skinned (Skin Type IV) people have little or no sunburn response to sun exposure except to develop an "immediate" tan; often these people have only occasional and limited need for ancillary sun protection.

How do we identify the white population at high risk for the development of sun-induced skin changes, including skin cancer? A simple working classification has been proposed [12] (Table 2) that is based, not on the phenotype (i.e., hair and eye color), but on what patients tell us about their responses to an *initial* sun exposure—three *minimum erythema doses* (MEDs), or about 1 hr in

Table 2 Working classification of sun-reactive skin types

Skin Type*	Erythema and tanning reactions† to first exposure in summer to 3 minimum erythema doses (MED) (MED = 15–30 min of noon sun)
I	Always burn, never tan
II	Usually burn, tan less than average (with difficulty)
III	Sometimes mild burn, tan about average
IV	Rarely burn, tan more than average (with ease)

* Type I and Type II persons all have pale skin color and often but not always have blue eyes, red scalp hair, and may or may not have freckling; however, some persons with dark brown hair and blue or green eyes have Type I and Type II sun reactions.
† At ages 12 to 40 years
Source: From Fitzpatrick [12].

northern latitudes in the summer. If we ask two questions about their responses to three MED exposures—"How much painful sunburn do you have after 24 hours?" "How much tan will you develop in a week?"—there are two groups of the white population with a clear-cut answer. One group will reply: "A painful burn at 24 hours and no tan at 7 days." This is Type I sun-reactive skin type; they may have dark hair and brown eyes! Another group will respond: "No burn at 24 hours and a dark tan at 7 days." This group is called Skin Type IV. A subgroup of Skin Type I will answer: "A painful burn at 24 hours (the same as Skin Type I response) and a light tan at 7 days"; this group is Skin Type II. A subgroup of Skin Type IV will testify to "a slightly tender burn at 24 hours and a good tan at 7 days"; this is Skin Type III and is the largest group. Types I and II are at high risk for sun-induced skin damage; Type IV persons have a low risk for sun-induced skin damage; Type III persons are at moderate risk, but persons in this group often have a history of repeated and prolonged sun exposure—often deliberately to obtain a cosmetic tan!

Of the three factors affecting melanin pigmentation in humans—genes, UV radiation, and hormones—only genes and the UV radiation in sunlight are major determinants of pigmentation in the normal population. Genes determine *constitutive pigmentation;* UV radiation and hormones determine *facultative pigmentation.* Genes set the level of tyrosinase production and determine the rate of synthesis and the number and size of melanosomes within the melanocyte itself, and they also control the manner of melanosome degradation in keratinocytes. After three MEDs of sun exposure, persons with Skin Types I and II develop few or very few melanized melanosomes, and these melanosomes, in fact, are rapidly degraded in keratinocytes so that a melanin filter never develops in the stratum corneum and the epidermis is virtually devoid of melanin. In Type IV skin, after three MEDs there is a high level of tyrosinase and a large number of heavily melanized melanosomes; the whole epidermis contains myriads of UV filtering melanin particles. The Type IV skin in response to sun exposure creates a "density filter" that absorbs UVB and thus prevents damage to the nucleus by photons. To prepare Types I and II for sun exposure, we need to encourage the use of an effective sunscreen to substitute for their inherent congenital deficiency of the melanin density filter that is present in normal white persons with Skin Types III and IV. Like some other heritable metabolic defects, melanin deficiency cannot be corrected by replacing melanin, but by preventing the damage with chemical preparations that have the same function as melanin.

Heritable Syndromes with Congenital Diffuse Hypomelanosis of the Skin

Certain persons are genetically predisposed to the development of severe sunburn and dermatoheliosis because of congenital deficiency of preformed epidermal melanin (constitutive melanin pigmentation) and their limited capacity to develop protective melanin pigmentation (facultative melanin pigmentation) following exposure to sunlight.

Three heritable syndromes in humans with poor tolerance to sunlight are all characterized by varying degrees of reduction or total absence of both constitutive melanin pigmentation (skin color in covered areas of the body) and facultative melanin pigmentation (tanning following exposure to UV radiation) (see Table 3).

Oculocutaneous Albinism, Recessive (OCAR) [13]

OCAR is the most easily recognizable of these three syndromes primarily because of the ocular findings, especially the decrease in visual acuity which is a major disabling feature of OCAR. Some of these persons can, however, develop tanning (especially some black albinos) and most albinos are able to increase their tolerance to sunlight by gradual progressive exposure to sun, which increases the protection by an increase in the thickness of the stratum corneum. Nevertheless, the majority of persons with OCAR living near the equator or in northern latitudes who are careless about sun protection will develop marked dermatoheliosis and nonmelanoma skin cancers, particularly squamous cell carcinomas.

Oculocutaneous Albinoidism, Dominant (OCAD) [14]

This autosomal dominant syndrome has been only rarely reported but is far more common than is realized as families have not been recognized. Patients with OCAD do not have visual impairment (i.e., decrease in visual acuity) and only rarely have nystagmus but they all have iris translucency and absence of the macular reflex, as in OCAR. The hair color is blond or light brown or red. They have slightly more capacity to tan (Type II) than persons with OCAR.

Cutaneous Albinoidism, Hereditary Pattern Not Defined

These patients might be considered to have "normal" skin with Skin Type I. There is no visual impairment or iris translucency. The hair color is blond, light brown, or red; the phenotypic expression of hair and eye color may be deceptive as these patients may, in fact, have dark hair and pigmented irides. Freckling is common in persons with cutaneous albinoidism, especially those with red hair. Cutaneous albinoidism is the characteristic "Celtic" phenotype and is, therefore, seen most frequently in the following ethnic groups: Bretons, Cornish, Irish, Scottish, and Welsh. Most

Table 3 Heritable syndromes with congenital diffuse hypomelanosis of the skin

	Skin*	Eye
Oculocutaneous albinism (autosomal recessive)	Decrease or absence of epidermal melanin	Decreased visual acuity Iris translucency Nystagmus
Oculocutaneous albinoidism (autosomal dominant)	Decrease or absence of epidermal melanin	Iris translucency Nystagmus (rare)
Cutaneous albinoidism† (hereditary pattern not established)	Decrease or absence of epidermal melanin	No eye abnormalities

* Skin of covered areas is white; in exposed areas some tanning is possible in all three syndromes, including oculocutaneous albinism, tyrosine-positive type.
† This is presently known as Skin Type I.

ethnologists do not accept the Celtic-speaking peoples as a racial entity. Nevertheless, a large proportion of Celtic peoples have the phenotype of skin, hair, and eye color that is here called *cutaneous albinoidism*. These persons are at high risk for dermatoheliosis and skin cancer.

Cutaneous albinoidism is a term that replaces the so-called Skin Type I; persons with this disorder are not considered to be "normal" but are examples of a heritable melanin deficiency syndrome and need to be educated regarding sun exposure and sun protection at an early age.

The Relationship of Skin Color to Sun-induced Skin Damage (Skin Cancer and Dermatoheliosis) (Table 4)

Whiteness is, ironically, an inferior quality of human skin. If the skin can be considered as humans' "oldest clothes" (as John Donne said), then translucent, hairless, white skin is an ineffective shield as it is an easy target for the repetitive, lifetime exposures of damaging UV radiation. These repeated insults can ultimately result in skin cancer and, in addition, to a syndrome we have called *dermatoheliosis*.

Dermatoheliosis describes the effects of repeated exposures to the sun of normal skin. These effects occur following the first exposures in early life and are cumulative and irreversible. The magnitude and variety of the effects depend on the natural defense mechanisms and on whether or not susceptible persons use effective topical sun-protective agents throughout life. The dermatoheliosis syndrome is a polymorphic response to sun exposure of various components of the skin: (1) the *vascular system* of the dermis, with acute, transient, mediator-induced vasodilatation (sunburn erythema) or permanent dilatation of vessels (telangiectasia); (2) the *keratinocytes* of the epidermis, leading to localized atypical keratinocytic hyperplasia (solar keratosis) (Fig. 5); (3) the *melanocytes* of the epidermis, leading to macular pigmented lesions with sharply irregular borders and variegated brown color (freckles) and to isolated smooth-bordered, uniformly brown macules (solar lentigo); and (4) the *connective tissue components* of the dermis, collagen, and elastic tissue, leading to wrinkling, roughening, and yellowing of the skin.

Dermatoheliosis, which is analogous to pneumoconiosis, is a preventable environmental hazard that can potentially affect the health of approxi-

Table 4 Relationship of dermatoheliosis and skin cancer to solar ultraviolet radiation (UVR) and to natural defense mechanisms

$$\text{Dermatoheliosis and skin cancer} = \frac{\text{UVR intensity (I)} \times \text{duration: total life dose of sun exposure (D)}}{\text{Natural defense mechanisms (NDM)}}$$

Dermatoheliosis and skin cancer
  Single exposure (15–35 min, or 50 mJ UVB)
    Sunburn (erythema)
    Delayed tanning (melanogenesis)
  Multiple exposures (years)
    Skin cancer
      Basal cell cancer
      Squamous cell cancer
      Malignant melanoma
    Dermatoheliosis
      Solar keratoses
      Solar lentigo
      "Aging" (wrinkling)
      Red, "weather-beaten" face (telangiectasia)

I = Ultraviolet intensity of sun (290–320 nm UVB) (320–400 nm UVA)
  Ozone (in the stratosphere) reduces UVB
  Latitude is inversely related to intensity
  Weather (clouds)
  Smog
  Sun's angular altitude (maximal at 1000–1400 hr)
  Altitude (4% increase/300 m)
  Surface reflectivity (snow, sand most reflective)

D = Duration (total life dose) of solar exposure (years)
  Age
  Sex
  Site
    Habitually exposed areas: face, ears, neck, backs of hands
    Relatively exposed areas: lower legs (in females), back, chest, arms
    Rarely exposed areas: breasts (in females), bathing trunk area, scalp
  Climate (cool temperatures increase exposure time)
  Behavioral patterns
    Occupation (outdoor vs. indoor)
    Leisure (outdoor vs. indoor)
    Type of recreation (outdoor vs. indoor)
    Clothing (seasonal variations)
    Intermittent intense exposures ("weekenders")

NDM = Natural defense mechanisms
  Ethnic variation
    Constitutive skin color (color of unexposed skin)
    Facultative skin color
      Sun-reactive Types I–IV (based on personal history of sunburning and tanning)
  DNA repair mechanisms, fully expressed in the genetic disease, xeroderma pigmentosum
  Immunologic surveillance

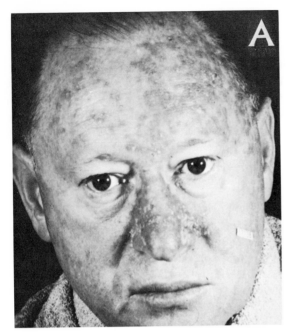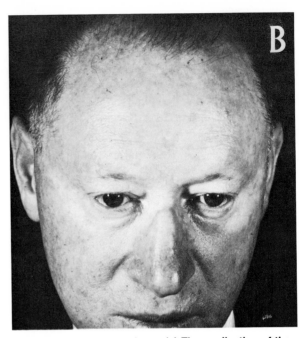

Fig. 5. Effect of topical application of 5% 5-fluorouracil in an oil-in-water emulsion-type base. (*a*) The application of the 5-fluorouracil has been limited to the skin of the left half of the forehead and the entire nose. Note the marked inflammatory reaction in the keratoses. Marked inflammation developed in areas of clinically normal-appearing skin, thereby indicating the presence of latent keratoses. (*b*) Photograph taken a few weeks after all the reaction had subsided; the skin of the face is free of keratoses and appears normal.

mately 25 percent of the population of the United States. Excessive exposure to the sun in normal white persons leads to acute and chronic dermatoheliosis. Persons at risk need to be identified at an early age and need to be made aware of the noxious long-term effects of the sun so they may protect themselves by (1) avoiding exposure during the peak flux of UVB in the middle hours of the day and (2) using substantive and effective topical sunscreens in a daily program of self-protection.

The relationship of skin cancer and the dermatoheliosis syndrome (sun-induced skin damage) to solar UV radiation is summarized in Table 4. In the table you will notice that the natural defense mechanisms against sun-induced skin damage include skin color (ethnic variation).

Prevention of Sunburn, Dermatoheliosis, and Skin Cancer with Topical Sunscreens

Individuals of Skin Types I and II are genetically predisposed to repeated sunburn and skin injury depending on (1) their congenital partial or total deficiency of melanin in the epidermis (constitutive melanin pigmentation) and (2) their genetic capacity to develop protective melanin pigmentation following exposure to the sun (facultative melanin pigmentation, or suntanning).

Inasmuch as it is not possible by topical or systemic agents to alter the constitutive or facultative pigmentation, these deficiency states must be managed by use of filtering chemical preparations (sunscreens). Sun-protective topical preparations contain light-absorbing chemical agents in suitable lotion or ointment vehicles. These formulations attenuate the deleterious responses of normal white skin to excessive exposures of UVB (290 to 320 nm) and UVA (320 to 400 nm) obtained during outdoor work, sports activities, or sunbathing (Table 5).

These mixtures of a UV-absorbing agent and a vehicle may be true solutions or dispersions of comparatively large particles. The vehicle may be nonvolatile, partly volatile, or completely volatile.

Most of the topical sunscreens available absorb UVB radiation, and more recently most sunscreens also absorb UVA radiation. The active agents are either PABA, PABA esters (glyceryl PABA, isoamyldimethyl PABA, octyldimethyl PABA), benzophenones (such as sulisobenzone, oxybenzone, dioxybenzone), ethylhexyl-*p*-methoxycinnamate, diethanolamine-*p*-methoxycinnamate, homomenthyl salicylates, or anthranilate. All compounds have different absorption spectra but only the benzophenones and anthranilates have significant absorption in the UVA range. The formulation bases used are alcohol or mild lotions or creams;

Table 5 Comparative efficacy (SPFs) of sunscreens under indoor and outdoor conditions

Indications and Skin Type	Trade name	Type of formula	Sun-protection factor	
			Indoor solar simulator	Outdoor sunlight
I and II	PreSun 15	Clear lotion	15	10
	Pabanol	Clear lotion	15	6–8
	Supershade 15	Milky lotion	20	9
	Eclipse 15	Milky lotion	15–18	9
	Tiscreen	Milky lotion	16–22	10
	MMM—What A Tan!	Milky lotion	15	12
	Piz Buin 8 (European)	Cream	22	13
	Clinique	Cream	15–19	7
III	Sundown	Milky lotion	8–10	4–6
	Blockout	Milky lotion	6–8	4–6
	UVAL	Milky lotion	10–14	3–4
IV	Sunguard	Milky lotion	6	4
	Sea & Ski	Milky lotion	8	3

From Pathak et al [15].

the vehicle in which the sunscreen chemical is incorporated can affect whether a sunscreen remains effective under the stress of prolonged sunbathing, sweating, and swimming. This property, known as "substantivity," varies considerably among the various sunscreen formulations that are available, some of which are retained on the skin and others of which easily wash off after sweating or swimming. For example, all sunscreens containing 5% PABA do not have equal sun protection factor values, or SPFs (ratio of amount of time one can spend in the sun with a sunscreen to time without to obtain minimal erythema doses—MEDs—or a mild sunburn reaction). Opaque formulations containing titanium dioxide, talc, or zinc oxide are physical sunscreens and act as reflectors for impinging radiation. They are useful for limited areas such as the nose, lips, or other very limited vulnerable areas.

The daily use of sunscreens by persons will depend on the acceptability of the preparation. An alcoholic lotion base is preferred by men but is disliked by children (because of stinging) and older women (because of drying the skin). For daily use, milky lotions are more acceptable to women and children but less acceptable to men; creams are preferred by older women and skiers.

Determination of the Sun-Protection Factor (SPF)

The erythema response is at present the most reasonable estimate of the acute deleterious effects of sunlight. It is the basis of the SPF by which sunscreens are now standardized for effectiveness in susceptible subjects. The SPF value is defined as the ratio of the amount of energy required to

produce a minimum erythema dose (MED) through a sunscreen product film applied topically to the amount of energy required to produce the same MED without any treatment. The use of a "protection factor" as a means of standardization of topical sun-protective agents is regarded as a means of comparison of various formulations with regard to their effectiveness. The SPF may range from 2 (minimal protection) to 22 (maximum protection).

Until the last few years, the assessment of sunscreens has been relatively haphazard and not properly standardized. New technology has made available suitable UV sources that simulate sunlight exposure, and this new technology now needs to be utilized for the development and standardization of the UV radiation sources to be used in the laboratory for evaluating new formulations. Evaluations of actual usage conditions of sun-protective agents in human volunteers can be performed in field trials or under standardized conditions with environmental chambers, treadmills, immersion, etc., to determine the effects of sweating and swimming.

Sunscreen Usage

Indications for Usage. There are many indications for sunscreen usage. People who burn readily and tan poorly or not at all (Skin Types I and II) are more susceptible to the acute (sunburn reaction) and chronic (wrinkling, actinic damage, and skin cancers, including melanoma) solar damage to the skin. Habitual sunscreen usage in these people is thought to block enough UV radiation to decrease significantly the risk of acute skin changes and dermatoheliosis. These changes are attributed to sunburn spectrum (UVB) UV radiation. The need for sunscreen usage is dependent upon degree of sensitivity to UV radiation, season of year, and geographic location. UVB is most intense north of the equator in the months around the summer equinox and least so in late December.

The deleterious effects of sun exposure are cumulative and irreversible. Even Skin Type III persons can develop skin cancer and dermatoheliosis depending on the total lifetime exposures. They should always use prophylactic sunscreens if there is prolonged or excessive sunlight exposure, especially on the face and chest in males and females and the lower legs in females as these are the sites of origin of sun-induced skin cancer (epithelial cancers and malignant melanomas).

Methods of Usage. Persons with Skin Types I and II should *never* sunbathe and should adopt a program of daily application of effective sunscreens (SPF 15) as a habit and from an early age—in much the same manner as daily brushing of the teeth is adopted to prevent dental caries.

Most topical sunscreen formulations are most effective if applied 1 hr before sun exposure. All sunscreens should be reapplied after swimming or sweating. People who are most susceptible to sunburn reactions must be most careful to protect themselves during peak UVB hours extending from 11:00 a.m. to 2:00 p.m. and can usually be more casual about exposure before 9:00 a.m. and after 4:00 p.m. For those who are particularly susceptible to sunburn (Skin Types I and II) daily application of sunscreen from mid-April to October in the northern United States should provide protection from incidental brief and unplanned prolonged sun exposure. Those who wish to acquire some natural tan should apply their sunscreen after one-half hour of unprotected sun exposure.

Selection of Type of Sunscreen. The question of which sunscreen formulation is best for which patient is complex. The sun blocker must be selected with attention to the patient Skin Type, previous history of photosensitivity and clinical diagnosis, history of allergies, and desire to have an alcohol-, gel-, or cream-based preparation.

Patients with very fair skin who normally burn after sun exposure (Skin Types I and II) may be able to tolerate 3 or more hours of prolonged passive sunbathing with the most effective sunscreens (SPF 15). One who tans moderately but requires an hour for mild sunburn may be adequately protected with sunscreens with an SPF of 6. A patient who tans deeply (Skin Type IV) and

never sunburns rarely needs a sunscreen. Since Skin Typing is only an approximation of relative susceptibility of the individual to sunlight, conservative selection of a product with high SPF (6 or more) is probably desirable. Many patients object that sunscreens prevent tanning; it is true that sunscreens do prevent or minimize the tanning reaction, but most permit appreciable suntan, albeit at a slower pace. Maximum tan in sunscreen-protected skin can be achieved by repeated exposures. None of the sunscreens augment the delayed tanning reaction. The tan is generally as cosmetically acceptable as one obtained without sunscreen usage. For those patients who tan moderately (Skin Type III), after the tan is established a sunscreen with a lower SPF may be selected for regular use.

Which of the Sunscreen Products is Best?

There has been a gratifying response of the Food and Drug Administration (FDA) and pharmaceutical industry to the repeated pleas of the academic community to standardize sunscreens. Unfortunately the original concept of the SPF by Greiter et al. [16] has been maligned by an SPF "race" in the industry. Entrepreneurial pharmaceutical companies have marketed preparations claiming an SPF of 26 or more. At present there is no regulatory control of such practices and the experimental data (under either laboratory or field conditions) establishing the claims is not published in refereed medical journals—except by a very few companies. For the present, therefore, preparations from these latter companies should be selected for use.

Adverse Reactions to Topical Sunscreen Preparations

Contact dermatitis occasionally develops from use of PABA, certain PABA esters, benzophenones, and cinnamates. Glyceryl PABA seems to be the most common cause of allergic contact dermatoses from sunscreens; cross-reactivity may occur to PABA, benzocaine, procaine, *p*-phenylenediamine, and sulfanilamide. A photocontact dermatitis has been described with isoamyldimethyl PABA. That PABA cross-reactivity may include sulfanilamide and thiazides (Diuril, Hydrodiuril, etc.) makes this potential reaction of some medical significance. Sensitivity to octyldimethyl PABA alone has not been reported to date. Contact reactions may also occur with the benzophenones, though this seems uncommon. Recent information suggests photocontact sensitivity to some sunscreen formulations may be due to 6-methylcoumarin, not to the actual sunscreening chemical agent. Some formulations contain parabens and lanolin, not uncommon contact sensitizers.

PABA may stain clothing yellow, especially after sun exposure. Users must guard against the notion that sunscreens prevent or block all light; casual use of sunscreens is also usually associated with periodic and sometimes severe sunburn reactions.

Future Development of New Sunscreens

Future development of new sunscreens should follow these guidelines:

1. Neutral skin-protecting bases, which retain the neutral conditions of the skin as far as possible.
2. Restriction of active ingredients (i.e., UV radiation filters) to an absolutely necessary minimum.
3. Sunscreens should include agents that absorb both UVB and UVA.

If the SPF is to become a valuable guide to the development and the evaluation of different sunscreening agents, the methods of SPF determination need to be clearly defined and used on an international basis. The use of the SPF as a publicity stunt is an example of how a useful index can be exploited by short-sighted, publicity-minded manufacturers.

Some Common Myths Regarding Sun Exposure

1. *Suntan preparations increase tan.* Sunscreen agents should not be confused with dyes or oils which comprise many of the common so-called suntan lotions or quick tan lotions. There is no commercially available lotion that enhances the delayed tanning reaction. Mineral oils, emollients, baby oils, etc., lubricate and even change the optical properties of the skin but do not protect from sunburn or promote suntan. Dye-containing agents give a rapidly developing yellow-brown-orange hue to the skin; this offers no sun protection, is washed away within a few days, and has quite variable patient acceptability.

2. *Remaining in the shade will prevent sunburn.* Even though a person may remain out of direct sunlight and in the shade on a bright, clear day, reflected and scattered sunlight can still cause an erythema response, in about twice the time required in direct sunlight. For the same reason a hat is inadequate protection for the face.

3. *It is difficult to get sunburned on a cloudy day.* On a bright, hazy, cloudy day, it is possible to receive 70 to 80 percent of the amount of UV radiation that is present on a bright clear day. In addition to the direct solar radiation, considerable scattered radiation from the sky will be striking the skin surface. The risk of overexposure is also increased because the clouds filter the infrared radiation that normally causes the sensation of heat that may be the only danger signal a patient experiences.

4. *Other myths concern sunburn responses related to altitude and to reflected radiation from water, sand, snow, and ground.* Each 1000-ft increment of altitude adds 4 percent of the erythema-producing UV spectrum so that the intensity of sunlight is 20 percent greater at 5000 ft than at sea level. *Water is a very poor reflector* and reflects no more than 5 percent of the UV radiation. Sand is about one-quarter as reflective as is the sky; hence a person sitting under an umbrella on the sand can be burned by both indirect radiation from the sky (skylight) and reflection from the sand. Fresh snow also functions as a very effective reflector.

References

1. Quevedo WC Jr et al: Light and skin color, in *Sunlight and Man: Normal and Abnormal Photobiologic Responses.* Edited by MA Pathak et al; TB Fitzpatrick, consulting editor. Univ of Tokyo Press, Tokyo, 1974, pp 165–194
2. Fitzpatrick TB et al: Biochemistry and physiology of melanin pigmentation, in *Biochemistry and Physiology of Skin.* Edited by LA Goldsmith. Oxford, New York, in press
3. Prota G: Recent advances in the chemistry of melanogenesis in mammals. *J Invest Dermatol* **75:**122–127, 1980
4. Pathak MA et al: Sunlight and melanin pigmentation, in *Photochemical and Photobiological Reviews*, vol 1. Edited by KC Smith. Plenum, New York, 1976, pp 211–239
5. Lerner AB et al: Action of melanocyte-stimulating hormone on pigment cells, in *Proceedings of the Cold Spring Harbor Conference on Cell Proliferation.* Edited by GH Sato. Cold Spring Harbor Conferences on Cell Proliferation, Hormones and Cell Culture, book A, vol 6, 1979, 979 pp
6. Thomson ML: Relative efficiency of pigment and horny layer thickness in protecting the skin of Europeans and Africans against solar ultraviolet radiation. *J Physiol (Lond)* **127:**236–246, 1955
7. Weigand DA et al: Cell layers and density of Negro and Caucasian stratum corneum. *J Invest Dermatol* **62:**563–568, 1971

8. Kaidbey KH et al: Photoprotection by melanin—a comparison of black and Caucasian skin. *J Am Acad Dermatol* **1**:249–260, 1979

9. Olson RL et al: Skin color, melanin and erythema. *Arch Dermatol* **108**:541–544, 1973

10. Kaidbey KH, Kligman AM: Sunburn protection by long-wave ultraviolet-induced pigmentation. *Arch Dermatol* **114**:46–48, 1978

11. Gschnait F et al: Photoprotective effect of a psoralen-UVA induced tan. *Arch Dermatol Res* **263**:181–188, 1978

12. Fitzpatrick TB: Soleil et peau. *Journal de Medicine Esthétique* **2(7)**:33–34, 1975

13. Witkop CJ Jr et al: Albinism, in *Metabolic Basis of Inherited Disease,* 4th ed. Edited by JB Stanbury et al. McGraw-Hill, New York, 1978, pp 283–316

14. Fitzpatrick TB et al: Dominant oculocutaneous albinism. *Br J Dermatol* **91**:23, 1974

15. Pathak MA et al: Topical and systemic approaches of protection of human skin against harmful effects of solar radiation, in *The Science of Photomedicine.* Edited by JD Regan, JA Parrish. Plenum, New York/London, in press

16. Greiter F et al: History of sunscreens and the rationale for their use, in *Principles of Cosmetics for the Dermatologist.* Mosby, St Louis, in press

URTICARIA AND
ANGIOEDEMA

Susan Bromberg Schneider

John P. Atkinson

Urticaria and angioedema are common medical problems, readily recognized by classical historical features and physical examination. One out of five people will, at least once in their lifetime, have one or more episodes of urticaria or angioedema.

Urticaria is the inimitable itchy, pink-red, discomforting affliction better known as "the hives." It usually occurs as diffusely distributed, erythematous, variably sized wheals often with serpiginous borders and a central pallor. Onset is rapid (within minutes) and duration transient (disappears within 24 hr or sooner). Its heralding feature is pruritus. The lesions characteristically blanch with pressure, consistent with the presence of dilated vessels.

Angioedema presents as areas of "swelling," larger than urticaria, occurring more often singly but sometimes as multiple lesions. It is usually without much erythema. The onset is subacute, evolving within hours and resolving within hours to days. The lesions are usually not pruritic but rather are described by patients as stinging, burning, or tingling. Angioedema may occur anywhere on the body, including the face, limbs, trunk, palms, soles, genitalia, and mucosal surfaces. The most common sites are the face and extremities. Gastrointestinal symptoms such as colic, nausea, vomiting, and diarrhea are seen with visceral (mucosal) involvement. Laryngeal angioedema with hoarseness, stridor, dyspnea, and airway obstruction can also occur. This is certainly the most serious and only life-threatening feature of the disease. Airway involvement is fortunately uncommon in acute urticaria and angioedema and rare in all forms of chronic urticaria and angioedema except hereditary angioedema. In some patients lesions known as "giant hives" have features of both urticaria and angioedema in that they are pruritic and erythematous but involve the deeper dermis.

Urticaria and angioedema share a similar appearance by light microscopy. The histologic picture is that of interstitial edema, manifested by separation of collagen bundles and dilatation of cutaneous vessels and lymphatics. These abnormalities are detected in the upper dermis in urticaria and in the deep dermis and subcutaneous tissue in angioedema. A paucity of inflammatory cells—neutrophils, mononuclear cells, or eosinophils—is the rule. In clinical practice, urticaria is more frequently biopsied than angioedema, because the latter is often located on the face where one is hesitant to leave a scar. Furthermore, it is difficult to obtain sufficiently deep tissue to localize the pathology with a usual punch biopsy. A significant proportion of pathologic reports in both urticaria and angioedema return with descriptions such as "normal skin" or "no pathologic diagnosis." Immunofluorescence is routinely negative for IgG, IgM, C3, or C4. If positive, one should consider urticarial vasculitis.

Urticaria and angioedema may occur singly or in association with one another. In a series of 554 cases reported by Champion and Roberts [1], 40 percent of patients had urticaria alone, 11 percent had angioedema alone, and the majority (49 percent) had a combination of urticaria and angioedema, with urticaria as the predominant clinical lesion in the combined group. Although these entities are seen in conjunction with one another, they are not to be considered synonomous. They are, in fact, as discussed above, reasonably well distinguished (see Table 1) by their gross appearance, rapidity of onset, duration, histologic location, and the discomfort they cause to the patient.

An arbitrary distinction is made in the literature with regard to acute and chronic forms of urticaria and angioedema. "Acute" disease has been defined as signs and symptoms of less than 6 weeks duration. Chronic illness is described, depending on the author, as daily or intermittent disease for greater than 6 weeks to greater than 6 months.

Attempts to characterize acute vs. chronic disease by their clinical features has led to several generalizations. Demographically "acute disease" exhibits no age predominance and affects males as frequently as females. Some authors suggest an increased frequency of atopy in the population with acute disease, although this increase is probably modest. The course of acute disease is that of an isolated, nonrecurrent event, or that of a self-limited series of many events. In contrast, chronic urticaria and angioedema, occurring as infrequently as one or two attacks per year, or as frequently as several attacks per day, is seen more commonly in females in the third or fourth decade of life. There is no correlation with an atopic history. In most physicians' experience, over 80 percent of cases are idiopathic, with a natural history of approximately 50 percent being in remission by 6 months, 70 percent in remission by 1 year, and 90 percent in remission by 5 years. The resolution of nonidiopathic disease depends in large part upon the recognition of its etiology and institution of the appropriate treatment of the causative factor.

Several excellent reviews of the pathogenesis, etiology, and therapy of urticaria and angioedema have been published in recent years [1–12]. The discussion that follows is largely based on these reviews as well as the authors' personal experience with patients seen at the National Institutes of Health (NIH) and the Washington University School of Medicine. Our intent is to emphasize a con-

Table 1 A comparison of urticaria and angioedema

	Urticaria	Angioedema
Onset	Acute as lesions appear rapidly (within minutes)	Subacute as lesions evolve slowly (within hours)
Symptoms	Pruritus Erythema prominent	Stinging or burning, or tingling sensation at eventual site of swelling; erythema usually not prominent
Duration	Hours	Hours to days
Histopathology	Dilatation of blood vessels Tissue edema ± Perivascular infiltrate	Dilatation of blood vessels Tissue edema ± Perivascular infiltrate
Location	Dermis	Deep dermis and subcutaneous tissue

servative commonsense approach to the diagnostic evaluation of urticaria and angioedema and to present a therapeutic scheme that we have found successful in the treatment of patients.

Pathophysiology: Mediators, Modulators, and Their Mechanisms of Release

Sir Thomas Lewis' classic experiment with urticaria produced by stroking the skin provides the basis for the modern theory of mediator involvement in the pathophysiology of urticaria and angioedema. In his study, a tourniquet placed about the involved limb of a patient with urticaria (providing what he termed "circulatory arrest") prevented the natural course and resolution of the lesions. With subsequent removal of the tourniquet, the swelling eventually reversed and the skin changes returned to normal [13]. Lewis concluded that vasoactive mediators concentrated by occlusion and then dispersed by tourniquet release were responsible for the lesions.

Logical candidates for such mediators are those with rapid and limited action. Lysozymes, terminal complement components, and other vasoactive substances that wield irreversible injury with cell death and necrosis are not reasonable considerations. Lesions of urticaria and angioedema are transient, with sparse inflammation and no necrosis. Thus, mediators with reversible actions such as histamine, arachidonic acid metabolites, bradykinin, serotonin, and C3 and C5 fragments become the rational "possibles."

Much work has been devoted to the identification of mediators and elucidation of their function in the pathophysiology of urticaria and angioedema. A variety of chemically diverse substances have been noted to exert vasoactive effects in animal models and humans. These are thought to assume either primary, incitatory roles in the initiation of urticaria and angioedema or modulatory functions, enhancing already initiated events. This network of interacting substances is not well defined. A list of vasoactive substances thus far identified in humans and a description of their actions by intradermal injection follows (Table 2).

Histamine

The intradermal injection of histamine, with its resultant wheal and flare, has become the experimental prototype of urticaria. Histamine, stored intracellularly in the granules within tissue mast cells adjacent to vessels and within circulating

Table 2   Intradermal injection of vasoactive substances

Substance	Results of intradermal injection		
	Erythema	Edema	Pruritus
Histamine	+	+	+
Bradykinin*	+	+	−
Serotonin†	+	±	−
PGE₁‡	+	+	−
PGE₂‡			
Acetylcholine§	+	±	−
C3a¶	+	+	+
C5a¶			

* Bradykinin, as potent a vasodilator as histamine, causes stinging pain rather than pruritus on injection.
† Response to intradermal serotonin is basically vasodilatory, with the appearance of erythema.
‡ Prostaglandins of the E series produce vasodilatory responses in humans in concentrations higher than physiologic. It is felt that, in nonexperimental conditions at physiologic concentrations, PGE₁ and PGE₂ potentiate the effect of other vasoactive substances, e.g., histamine and bradykinin.
§ Acetylcholine is a mediator of the cholinergic nervous system. As such, it exerts a vasodilatory effect on intradermal injection with resultant erythema with or without edema. It may also modulate mediator release from the mast cell.
¶ The anaphylatoxins cause erythema, edema, and pruritus through histamine release.

basophils, is the only vasoactive substance directly causing pruritus. Lewis' classic triple response, produced by stroking the skin and reproduced by histamine "pricked into the skin," well mimics the observed events of urticaria [13]: (1) dilation of capillaries and venules with subsequent erythema; (2) increase in vascular permeability with edema and wheal formation; and (3) local axon reflex, with dilatation of surrounding arterioles, and flare.

Serotonin

Serotonin is not contained within human mast cells but is found in high concentration within platelets. Its release may be produced by platelet-activating factor, a mediator derived from mast cells. Serotonin probably amplifies the response initiated with mast cell degranulation. Intradermal injection results in erythema without a wheal or pruritus.

Acetylcholine

Intradermal injection of acetylcholine results in vasodilatation and sometimes edema. It increases the tone of the vascular bed and can enhance mediator release from mast cells.

Kinin-Generating System

Bradykinin, an end product of one of the three Hageman factor-dependent pathways, is as potent a vasodilator as histamine. Intradermal injection results in increased capillary permeability and a sensation of "burning" or "stinging" pain, rather than pruritus.

Arachidonic Acid Metabolites of the Cyclooxygenase and Lipoxygenase Pathways

PGE_1 or PGE_2, injected intradermally in high concentration, produces a wheal-and-flare response as well as pain. An increase in serum histamine results in an increase of serum concentrations of the E series of prostaglandins, thereby potentiating histamine's effect. Slow-reacting substance of anaphylaxis (SRS-A) (recently shown to be of the family of molecules derived from the lipoxygenase pathway of arachidonic metabolism [14]) causes an increase in vascular permeability and contraction of smooth muscle. A large number of additional lipoxygenase metabolites are presently under investigation in regard to their potential role in mediating allergic events.

Complement

Activation of the classical and alternative complement cascades leads to production of two important vasoactive components, C3a and C5a. Injected intradermally, these potent degranulators of mast cells cause histamine release. The histamine in turn produces erythema, edema, and pruritus. C5a is also an important chemotactic factor.

Other Chemoattractants

Eosinophilic chemotactic factor of anaphylaxis (ECF-A), a chemotactant for eosinophils, and kallikrein, a chemotactant for neutrophils, mononuclear cells, and basophils, may contribute to the generation of the inflammatory response.

The vasoactive mediators are released by mechanisms categorized as immunologic and nonimmunologic.

Immunologic stimuli to mediator release include type I, type II, and type III mechanisms. Type I reactions, the classic immediate hypersensitivity reactions, are IgE-mediated. Examples of such reactions include the hypersensitivity response to pollens, certain drugs, foods, or insect stings. When a patient encounters antigen to which he or she is sensitive, either by the oral, inhaled, intravenous, intramuscular, or topical route, antigen combines with IgE bound to IgE receptors on mast cells. The antigen cross-links receptors to

induce mast cell degranulation, resulting in the release of histamine and other mediators.

Type II reactions are cytotoxic in nature, mediated by IgG or IgM. Antibody combines with the antigen on the cell surface and then activates complement. A clinical example of a type II immune mechanism is the classic ABO incompatibility transfusion reaction.

Type III reactions are IgG-, IgM-, or IgA-mediated. Circulating antigen-antibody complexes may deposit in target tissue, activate the complement cascade, and through C3a and C5a production induce mast cell content release. Examples of such reactions include serum sickness and immune complex-mediated collagen vascular diseases.

The nonimmunologic stimuli to mediator release will be fully discussed in the section entitled *Etiology*. Certain physical factors, pharmacologic agents, and genetic abnormalities can lead to the release of vasoactive substances by nonimmunologic means. For example, light, heat, pressure, and cold appear to directly affect mast cell degranulation. Genetically controlled deficiencies of inactivators of the inflammatory response permit uncontrolled and prolonged mediator responses. Furthermore, modulators of mediator release and actions exist that usually do not reproducibly incite, but may enhance, the release of mediators. These include alcohol, stress, emotion, exercise, and hormonal variation.

A schematic representation of factors that may incite or modulate mediator release is presented in Fig. 1. A biochemical sequence of events, initiated by antigen cross-linking IgE receptors on basophils and mast cells, leads to release of preformed mediators such as histamine from granules. Membrane potential changes, alterations in cyclic nucleotide concentrations, ionic fluxes, including sodium and calcium uptake, synthesis of arachidonic acid metabolites, and probably as yet undefined events occur within seconds of ligand-receptor interaction. The sequence of events, especially with regard to dependency of one event upon the next, is largely unknown. It is known that elevated intracellular cAMP levels decrease mediator release, and this is important for the therapeutic considerations to follow. β-Adrenergic agents bind to specific membrane receptors, thereby activating adenylate cyclase, the enzyme that synthesizes cAMP. Theophylline and related compounds inhibit phosphodiesterase, the enzyme that degrades cAMP. β Agonists and phosphodiesterase inhibitors not only alter mediator release but also modulate end-organ responsiveness. There is some evidence that serotonin and cholinergic agents

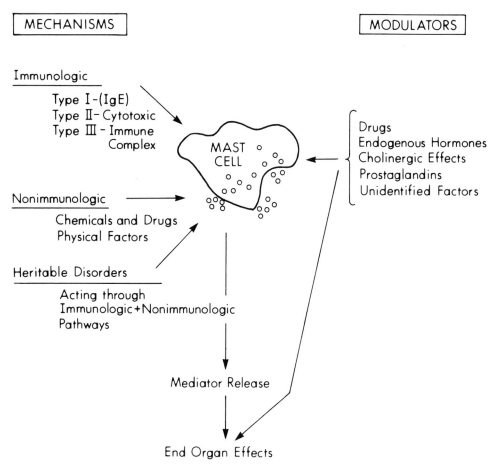

MECHANISMS

MODULATORS

Immunologic

Type I-(IgE)
Type II- Cytotoxic
Type III - Immune
    Complex

MAST CELL

Drugs
Endogenous Hormones
Cholinergic Effects
Prostaglandins
Unidentified Factors

Nonimmunologic

Chemicals and Drugs
Physical Factors

Heritable Disorders

Acting through
Immunologic+Nonimmunologic
Pathways

Mediator Release

End Organ Effects

Fig. 1. Scheme of pathophysiologic events. *(Adapted from Mathews [9].)*

can enhance mediator release by increasing intracellular cGMP concentrations. Antihistamines compete with released histamine for histamine receptors in vessel walls and other tissues.

Etiology (Table 3)

Drugs

Drugs are the most commonly identified cause of urticaria and angioedema. Exposure to pharmacologic agents may be by the oral, rectal, injected, topical, inhaled, or vaginal route. Temporal relationship of drug exposure to reaction ranges from minutes to hours to days, depending primarily upon the mechanism by which the drug produces its effect.

Drugs can elicit urticaria and angioedema by means of: (1) immediate (type I) IgE hypersensitivity, as seen with penicillin; (2) formation of antigen-antibody complexes (type III) with subsequent complement activation and histamine release, as seen with serum sickness type reactions

to drugs and foreign proteins; (3) direct mast cell degranulation and histamine release, as seen with nonspecific histamine releasers such as the opiate analgesics; (4) antibody-independent complement activation, as has been implicated in radiocontrast reactions; or (5) alteration of arachidonic acid

Table 3 Etiologic considerations in urticaria and angioedema

Drugs	Connective tissue disease
Blood products	Malignancy
Foods	Endocrinopathies
Aeroallergens/contactants	Urticaria pigmentosa
Infections/infestations	Systemic mastocytosis
Bites/stings	Genetic diseases
Physical agents	Hereditary angioedema
Cold	Carboxypeptidase deficiency
Cholinergic or heat	Familial cold
Pressure	Hereditary vibratory
Dermographia	Amyloidosis with deafness
Solar	and limb pain
Vibratory	Type VI solar urticaria—
Aquagenic	erythropoietic
Systemic diseases	protoporphyria
Serum sickness	Idiopathic disease

metabolism as seen with prostaglandin synthetase inhibitors such as aspirin.

A thorough history to search for possible drug exposure is essential in all cases of urticaria and angioedema. An account of the original sensitizing exposure to the drug may not be elicitable because of poor patient recall, unwitting exposure to trace amounts of drugs in foods or combination medicines, or the fact that not all drug reactions occur on a "previously sensitized" basis. While a complete account of prescribed medicines is usually obtainable, many patients fail to mention use of over-the-counter preparations such as cough drops, laxatives, cold remedies, or vitamins, or purposely avoid noting illicit drug intake. The physician must beware of such tendencies and make specific inquiries.

Many patients will be receiving more than one medicine at the time of onset of their urticaria and angioedema. This may make pinpointing a specific etiologic agent difficult. For example, a not uncommon consultative request of the allergist by medical and surgical specialists relates to "skin-testing" patients for one or more drug "allergies." It is unfortunate that a wide variety of skin tests for drugs does not exist and, for reasons to be discussed, will probably never be available. Reliable skin tests exist only for the assessment of immediate hypersensitivity and not for any of the other mechanisms by which drugs can cause reactions. They are available for only high-molecular-weight substances such as insulin or adrenocorticotropic hormone and for penicillin, with which extensive work in defining major and minor immunologic determinants has been performed [15].

Not only are skin tests not available for most drugs, but there are several limitations to the usefulness of skin tests for the diagnosis of drug reactions. First, as previously mentioned, they assess only one type of response to drug—IgE hypersensitivity. Second, false-positive reactions can occur. These are seen especially with drugs that are irritating on prick or intradermal injection, as well as with those like aspirin, dextrans, opium alkaloid, or polymyxin B, which can cause non-specific local histamine release on intradermal placement. Third, false-negative reactions may occur when the antigenic determinant to which the patient is allergic is a drug metabolite rather than the unprocessed drug tested, when the patient is on type I antihistamines, or when a recent drug reaction has occurred (since much of the antibody is already complexed to antigen).

A serologic test, the radioallergosorbent test (RAST), is available to measure IgE to a limited number of drugs [16]. In this assay, drug (antigen) is attached to insoluble carrier and incubated with the patient's serum. All antibody classes—IgG, IgM, IgA, IgD, IgE—directed against the drug are absorbed by the antigen-carrier complex. Serum is then removed and radiolabeled antihuman IgE is added. After washing, specific IgE antibody attached to insoluble carrier is measured by radiolabel uptake. Unlike skin tests, RASTs can be used at the time of acute drug reactions or while a patient is on antihistamines. Like the skin tests, the limitation of RAST is that, for reliable results, appropriate chemical determinants of the drug must be defined and used in testing. False negatives can occur if the wrong immunogenic determinants are used. Recent studies have also demonstrated a decrease in the sensitivity of RAST for IgE by interference of IgG blocking antibody [17]. Unlike skin tests, results to the RAST test are not immediately available.

In clinical practice, drugs most commonly causing urticaria and angioedema are: the penicillins; the sulfonamides; animal protein derivatives such as insulin, adrenocorticotropic hormone, thyroid extract, parathyroid hormone, and specific antisera; diuretics; aspirin and other nonsteroidal anti-inflammatory agents; opiate analgesics such as codeine, Demerol, and morphine; and radiocontrast materials.

An approach to the patient with suspected drug-induced urticaria and angioedema is outlined below:

1. *Identify the offending drug historically.* In the case of multiple-drug exposure, one can only statistically rank medicines as more likely or less likely to produce urticaria, realizing that any drug can potentially cause such reaction. Skin tests for drug IgE-mediated allergy, when available, are useful but cannot be used diagnostically to rule out an IgE-mediated event in the face of acute reaction, because of the complexing of antibody to drug already in the system. RAST testing requires days to weeks for results and suffers from a significant incidence of false negatives.

2. *Avoid usage of suspected drug or drugs.* Depending upon the mechanism, reintroduction may be accompanied by a more severe reaction than with initial use and should be avoided, if possible.

3. *Avoid use of structurally similar drugs.* Penicillin has multiple semisynthetic forms different only by the addition of a side chain to the 6-

aminopenicillenic acid nucleus. Cephalosporins are derivatives of 7-aminocephalosporanic acid and can cross-react with penicillins. Sulfonamides are similar to sulfonylureas, oral hypoglycemics, thiazides, furosemide diuretics, carbamic anhydrase inhibitors, and procaine-type local anesthetics. The aminoglycosides share cross-reactivity. Local anesthetics containing the *p*-aminophenol group, e.g., procaine and tetracaine, cross-react.

4. *Consider trace amounts of offending drug in foods.* Penicillin has been detected in trace quantities in milk and meat supplies, and there has even been an isolated report of a penicillin-like substance in a bottle of commercial soft drink [18]. It has been speculated that such presence in "occult sources" may account for the sensitizing of patients not knowingly exposed to the drug or for chronic urticaria and angioedema in very sensitive patients. However, in our experiences such highly sensitive individuals are uncommon and "trace antigen" in common foods and beverages is rarely the cause of chronic reactions.

Blood Products

Urticaria and angioedema due to blood or blood product transfusion can occur by several mechanisms. Except for cases of obvious "mismatch," it is often difficult to determine the exact etiologic agent of the urticaria to administered blood. Type II complement-mediated cytotoxic reactions, the classic hemolytic "transfusion reactions," are seen in cases of ABO incompatibility. Type I and type III reactions can occur to fresh frozen plasma, Factor 8, and cryoprecipitate. Reactions also may be directed to antigens "extrinsic" to blood or blood products, such as "contaminant" trace proteins or haptenic substances present in blood. Food antigen, drug or drug metabolites, or specific reaginic antibody of donor origin may elicit urticaria and angioedema in blood recipients.

Foods

Urticaria and angioedema can theoretically occur from virtually any food. The temporal relationship of food exposure to reaction ranges from minutes to hours. This wide range of reaction time may be a function of dose, degree of sensitivity, the fact that reaction can be directed to a product of enzymatic digestion rather than unaltered food protein, or the additive effect of other foods. The patient with a history of food reaction usually proves to have more than one food sensitivity.

The route of exposure to inciting food antigen is, as a rule, by ingestion, though inhalation or touch of such potent antigens as fish or peanut protein may precipitate systemic reactions in highly sensitive individuals.

Type I "allergic" reactions are seen most commonly with nuts, fish, seafood other than fish, eggs, berries, chocolates, and aliphatic aldehydes (present in odorous food such as garlic or as a combustion product of broiling or frying). Such immediate-hypersensitivity reactions usually occur within minutes of exposure and the causative agent is usually known or strongly suspected by the patient. Later IgE-mediated reactions, occurring within hours of exposure, have been observed with cereals, milk, eggs, potatoes, beef, pork, legumes, and oranges. Documentation of the precipitant is more difficult in such delayed reactions because of interim ingestion of other foods and the lack or obvious temporal "cause and effect" by history.

Foods effecting pharmacologic histamine release can cause urticaria and angioedema as a dose-related phenomenon in "normal" nonsensitive individuals. Such nonimmunologic intolerance is seen with ingestion of large quantities of certain foodstuffs such as strawberries, egg whites, or lobster and crayfish.

Nonobvious sources, the "hidden" natural and synthetic additives in foods, such as salicylates, benzoates, yeast, and azo dyes, have been implicated as the occult etiology in certain cases of urticaria and angioedema [19]. A limited number of remissions on restricted diets and anticandidal regimens in sensitive individuals has been reported.

An approach to the patient with food reaction as the cause of urticaria and angioedema is outlined below:

1. *Identify the offending food.* This is often difficult because of the ingestion of multiple foods and the occurrence of delayed reactions. However, the most serious reactions are the immediate IgE-mediated ones and the food involved is usually easily discerned. As with drug reactions, a careful history is necessary and can be supplemented by a diary account of diet and reactions. Patterns and temporal relationships of ingestions to reactions are sought.

Diagnostic aids for the determination of food allergy are meager. Skin tests to food antigens are associated with a significant incidence of false positives and false negatives. Futhermore, in exquisitely sensitive individuals, skin testing is a potentially dangerous procedure and may be complicated by anaphylaxis. RAST, a non-invasive alternative to skin testing, is available to a limited number of food antigens and again has false positives and false negatives [20]. Finally, diagnostic modalities in disrepute among allergists (e.g., leukocytotoxic food tests, sublingual food challenge, and others) in double-blind controlled studies reveal variable results from day to day, do not correlate with clinical sensitivity, and are unreliable [21]. They are not recommended.

2. *Avoid implicated foods.* The option of hyposensitization is not at this point available for foods.

3. *If the above measures are not effective in cases of chronic urticaria with daily or almost daily occurrences, elimination diet may be tried.* The menu in elimination diets consists of low allergenic food substances—rice, rice cereal, rice wafers, lamb, pears, spinach, celery, lettuce, salt, and cane or beet sugar. It is free of tartrazine (FD and C Number 5). It is devoid of foods with high salicylate or benzoate content, such as blueberries, loganberries, bananas, green peas, licorice, rhubarb, grapes, oranges, apples, wine, and beer. Yeast content is low.

Response to this restricted diet is assessed over a 7- to 14-day period. If resolution of urticaria is observed, additional foods are added, one at a time, every 2 to 3 days. If a reaction occurs to a newly added food, it is again removed to observe for resolution of urticaria. When and if it resolves, the same food is reintroduced to see whether urticaria recurs. The process of removal and reintroduction is repeated at least once. This is to ensure that the observed remissions and exacerbations indeed correlate with the removal and reintroduction of the food, rather than representing the natural waxing and waning course so characteristic of urticaria and angioedema.

It should be noted that the elimination diet is nutritionally deficient and should be attempted only on a short-term basis. Remissions of urticaria and angioedema on elimination diets are infrequently seen, in that food allergy is a rarely confirmed etiology of chronic disease.

Aeroallergens and Contactants

A history of seasonal exacerbations is helpful for the diagnosis of aeroallergen-induced urticaria and angioedema. Seasonal histories are characteristically seen with pollen sensitivities. The seasonal prevalence of pollens such as the grasses, trees, weeds, and seasonal molds varies with different geographic locations. In the St. Louis area, tree antigen predominates in the months of March and April, grasses in May and June, seasonal molds in the summer months and early fall, and weeds in the late summer through the first frost. A seasonal pattern is not seen with sensitivity to perennial antigens, such as house dust, feathers, perennial molds, and animal epithelium. In such instances, one must rely on situational accounts—such as urticaria "only when wearing one's down jacket," or urticaria "only since the new cat's arrival," or urticaria "only when working at the dog pound, and not on weekends at home." Notably, in aeroallergen-sensitive individuals, one often elicits a history of other allergic symptoms, such as rhinitis, asthma, or conjunctivitis. Although aeroallergens are common causes of allergic rhinitis and asthma, they are seldom implicated in urticaria and angioedema.

Contact urticaria can be seen to a wide variety of contactants [22] (see Table 4). Elimination schedules to everyday items such as mouthwash, toothpaste, shampoos, and certain fabrics may be attempted when suspicion of their involvement in urticaria exists.

Table 4 More common contactants in contact urticaria

Acrylic monomers	Horse dander
Alcohol	Horse serum
Algae and lichens	Laundry supplies
Aliphatic aldehydes	Lindane
Ammoniate of mercury	Menthol
Ammonium persulfate	Mouthwash
bleach	Nail polish
Arsphenamine	Neomycin
Arthropods	Nuts
Aspirin	Orange and lemon peel
Carrots	Penicillin
Cephalosporin	Perfumes
Chlorpromazine	Plants
Deodorant	Platinum salts
Dimethylsulfoxide	Pollen
Dyes	Potato
Egg white	Saliva from dogs
Emetine	and cats
Exotic woods	Shampoo
Facial and hand creams	Sheep wool
Fish, including cod	Silk
liver oil	Soaps
Flour	Sodium sulfide
Formaldehyde	Spices
Hair (cut)	Toothpaste
Hair sprays	

Source: Adapted from Fisher [22].

It is unnecessary and expensive to skin test all patients with chronic urticaria for immediate hypersensitivity (for aeroallergens) or delayed hypersensitivity (for contactants). Only when clinical suspicion and observed patterns warrant it should such testing be performed. Positive skin tests in the absence of clinical correlation are valueless.

The therapeutic approach to aeroallergen or contact-induced urticaria and angioedema is avoidance. Environmental manipulations such as a job change (particularly in industrial workers sensitive to pollutants or contactants) may be necessary. The efficacy of desensitization for urticaria has not been established.

Infections and Infestations

Case reports of the association of urticaria and angioedema with almost any type of infection are found in the literature. The mechanism by which infections effect urticaria is believed to be immunologic, by type I, or more likely, type III mediation. Urticaria has been seen concurrent with viral disease, bacterial infection, fungal disease, and parasitic infestation [23].

Urticaria may precede overt clinical manifestations of viral hepatitis and infectious mononucleosis. Approximately one-quarter of patients with viral hepatitis ("yellow urticaria") and 6 percent of patients with infectious mononucleosis exhibit urticaria as a part of their prodrome. In pediatric populations urticaria can be seen with the ubiquitous viral syndromes. The association of urticaria with specific viruses, such as Coxsackie and measles, has also been reported.

Bacterial infections have been linked to the development of urticaria and angioedema. Several anecdotal reports have cited resolution of urticaria with definitive therapy of dental abcesses, sinusitis, or intraabdominal infection. Though a search by history and physical examination for occult foci of infection should be undertaken, sophisticated and invasive diagnostic tests in the absence of appropriate history are not indicated.

In the past two decades several articles have dealt with *Candida* infection or yeast sensitivity as an etiologic factor in chronic urticaris [24]. Though some studies quote an incidence of yeast sensitivity as high as 20 percent in chronic urticaria patients, the actual frequency of yeast sensitivity as an etiologic agent to urticaria is probably much lower. Positive or negative skin tests for immediate hypersensitivity to yeast are not dependable predictors of patient response to anti-*Candida* regimen or low-yeast diets. Resolution of urticaria with use of oral Mycostatin or low-yeast diet has been seen in selected yeast-infected or yeast-sensitive patients with chronic disease.

Infestation with parasites is rare in the United States. Parasite infestations implicated in urticaria and angioedema include pinworm, ascariasis, schistosomiasis, echinococcosis, trichiniasis, fascioliasis, toxocaria, filariasis, strongyloidiasis, and ancylostomiasis. The presence of eosinophilia, elevated IgE, and appropriate systemic symptoms should alert the physician to pursue such a diagnosis. Not all patients with urticaria should be repetitively evaluated for ova and parasites, as this is an expensive and unnecessary procedure in the majority of cases.

Note that well-documented associations of infection with chronic urticaria and angioedema are infrequent.

Bites and Stings

Urticaria due to spiders, snakes, and insects can occur by immunologic mechanisms, such as previous sensitization seen with Hymenoptera sensitivity, or by nonimmunologic mechanisms, such as complement activation and mast cell degranulation seen with certain snake venoms.

The therapy of such urticaria is of course avoidance. High-risk Hymenoptera-sensitive patients are advised of such precautionary measures as avoidance of bright colors in personal clothing, refraining from use of perfumes, shunning outdoor picnics, and limiting yard work. Sensitive individuals should always carry, and be educated regarding the use of, epinephrine in emergencies. Commercial kits—the Anakit or Epipen—provide premeasured dosage vehicles for immediate administration of adrenalin. Desensitization to Hymenoptera venom is available for patients with severe reactions.

So-called papular urticaria is characterized by discrete pruritic lesions observed with insect bites. It is more long-lived than classic urticaria, and most frequently encountered in pediatric populations in the summer. The lesions are usually scattered on exposed parts, particularly the feet, arms, and legs. The duration of lesions rules out typical urticaria.

Physical Urticarias

The pathognomonic feature shared by the physical urticarias is their consistent reproducibility by their respective stimuli. Our knowledge of the in vivo mediators of urticaria and angioedema is in large part secondary to recent studies analyzing venous drainage from limbs of patients with physical urticarias. From these studies on experimentally induced lesions we know that histamine is released temporally in association with lesion development. Other mediators (serotonin, eosinophilic chemotactic factor of anaphylaxis, and arachidonic acid metabolites) have also been found in some of these patients with physical urticaria and probably interact with histamine in the production of the lesions [25].

Cold Urticaria and Angioedema. Cold urticaria is precipitated by temperature change rather than absolute temperatures. It becomes manifest with the rewarming of a cold-exposed part. There appears to be no age or sex predominance to the primary disease. Cold urticaria and angioedema may present focally with limited exposure or diffusely with extensive degrees of exposure. It may be associated with such systemic symptoms as nausea, vomiting, headache, tachycardia, and syncope. Mediators isolated with experimental cold challenge have included histamine and factors chemotactic to neutrophils and eosinophils [25,26].

As may be expected, a seasonal pattern is seen with cold urticaria. Commonly, symptoms are exacerbated in the winter. In the summer months, fatal cases of hypotension have been seen with total-body exposure during swimming. Patients may complain of swelling of the mouth, lips, tongue, and throat with ingestion of cold foods and beverages.

Cold urticaria and angioedema occurs as a primary disease entity or can be seen in association with other diseases, such as cryoglobulinemia, cryofibrinogenemia, paroxysmal hemoglobinemia of the Donath-Landsteiner type, or cold agglutinin syndrome. Also a familial form exists, either of an immediate type, occurring within 30 min of exposure and often associated with fever, chills, and arthralgias, or of a delayed type, occurring 9 to 18 hr after exposure and presenting as a localized and deep swelling.

The provocative test for cold urticaria is performed by placing an ice cube on the volar surface of the patient's forearm for 4 min and then observing for 10 min. A control test should be performed simultaneously on a nonaffected individual.

Periactin, 16 mg per day in four individual doses, is the preferred therapy for primary cold-induced urticaria. It is generally more effective for this disease than other type I antihistamines [27].

Cholinergic Urticaria. Cholinergic urticaria is mediated by the release of acetylcholine from the parasympathetic and/or sympathetic nervous systems. Stimuli to the liberation of acetylcholine include heat, exercise, sweating, anxiety, and other strong emotion. Vasoactive substances isolated in increased amounts from the systemic circulation after exercise challenge in patients with the disease include histamine and factors chemotactic to neutrophils and eosinophils [25,26].

Cholinergic urticaria appears as "punctate" lesions approximately 1 to 2 mm in diameter occurring locally or scattered over the upper trunk and limbs. It rarely involves the face. Wheals can be larger and may become confluent [28].

Provocative tests to cholinergic urticaria include: (1) the intradermal injection of 100 μL of methacholine (Mecholyl), with the production of a wheal and flare surrounded by smaller satellite lesions, (2) the application of warm water locally with the development of focal urticaria, and (3) a 10-min run in the doctor's office with the production of a generalized urticaria.

Evidence for the involvement of a neurogenic reflex in the pathophysiology of cholinergic urticaria is offered by a simple experiment. If a hand of a patient with the disease is placed in warm water, with a tourniquet distal to the immersed part, no urticaria or angioedema occurs. If the tourniquet is removed, urticaria and angioedema develop [2]. Further, unilateral cervical sympathetic blockage with procaine can prevent the appearance of induced urticaria on the blocked side [29]. One may conclude that a central perception of a temperature change takes place first, with a subsequent efferent reflex effecting the urticaria [8].

The most effective therapy of cholinergic urticaria is hydroxyzine (Atarax) at 100 to 200 mg/day in divided doses.

Pressure Urticaria and Angioedema. This type of urticaria and angioedema develops under points of pressure. Patients typically complain of involvement of the buttocks and back after a long trip, of the soles after a long walk, or of lesions beneath bra straps, belts, or other tight garments.

Onset may be immediate (within minutes of the stimulus) or delayed (several hours—4 to 6 hr mean and up to 24 hr). Systemic symptoms such as fever, chills, and nausea have been associated with the delayed variant. This delayed form can be a confusing entity unless the patient is specifically asked about the possibility. Histamine levels are elevated over experimentally induced blisters in the delayed form [25].

There are no standardized, reliable provocative tests for the diagnosis of pressure urticaria. One must rely on the history and location of the lesions. Repeated examination of a patient's lesions is helpful in arriving at the correct diagnosis, especially in this form of urticaria. In addition, patients will often relate an activity that reproducibly produces the swelling (such as squeezing a tennis ball), and the activity should be performed under observation.

Pressure urticaria and angioedema are usually poorly responsive to conventional antihistamines, but these should be tried as some patients respond. In some patients, relief has been achieved with theophylline preparations and/or low-dose systemic corticosteroids.

Dermographia. Dermographia literally means writing ("graphia") on the skin ("dermo"). Though it belongs in the classification of the physical urticarias, dermographia is not to be mistaken for pressure urticaria and angioedema, which is a response to sustained pressure.

In dermographia, stroking the skin results first in a white line of vasoconstriction, followed by pruritus, erythema, and swelling. This "wheal and flare" classically occurs immediately, and is resolved usually within 30 min. There is a rare form of dermographia which is seen 3 to 6 hr after a stimulus as linear red nodules. Lesions last from 24 to 48 hr and are burning and tender. Immediate dermographia may precede delayed lesions.

In approximately 50 percent of the population with dermographia the wheal and flare are mediated by IgE, as determined by Prausnitz-Küstner transfer. Dermographia is seen in 5 percent of the "normal" population and can be elicited in some patients with chronic idiopathic urticaria. A wheal-and-flare reaction is characteristically seen in stroking the lesions of urticaria pigmentosa and systemic mastocytosis (Darier's sign).

In most individuals dermographism is a curiosity only and rarely requires therapeutic intervention. If necessary, the therapy of choice for dermographism is the Type I antihistamines.

Solar Urticaria. Solar urticaria is uncommon. Though it can occur at any age, solar urticaria usually presents between the third and fourth decades of life. There is no increased incidence of atopy in these patients. Solar urticaria is characterized by the development of urticarial lesions in

Table 5 Solar urticaria

Type	Inciting wavelength, nm	Passive transfer	Therapy
I	280–320	+	p-Aminobenzoic acid
II	320–400	–	Benzophenones Titanium oxide Zinc oxide
III	400–500	–	Titanium oxide Zinc oxide
IV	400–500	+	Titanium oxide Zinc oxide
V	280–500	–	p-Aminobenzoic acid Titanium oxide Zinc oxide
VI	405	–	Oral β-carotene

light-exposed areas, usually within minutes of exposure [30]. These lesions are transient and disappear within hours. Aside from wheal-and-flare reactions, patients with large areas of exposure may suffer systemic symptoms, including shock. A delayed form of solar urticaria can occur, in which lesions develop 18 to 27 hr after light exposure. In such instances, the cause-and-effect relationship of light to disease signs and symptoms is not so evident.

There are six types of solar urticaria, distinguished by both the wavelength of light provoking the urticaria as well as the mechanism by which lesions are produced (Table 5).

Type I solar urticaria occurs at 280 to 320 nm of light. It can be passively transferred to other individuals and is therefore felt to be immunologically mediated. It is treated with topical 5% p-aminobenzoic acid, an effective screen for ultraviolet radiation between 280 and 320 nm. A 3-mm glass pane, which absorbs the inciting range of light, may serve as a protective shield.

Type II solar urticaria occurs at 320 to 400 nm. The mechanism by which the lesions are produced is unknown. It is treatable by sunscreens containing benzophenone compounds, titanium oxide, or zinc oxide. These are effective blockers to UVA radiation.

Type III solar urticaria, occurring at 400 to 500 nm, is treated with titanium or zinc oxide.

Type IV solar urticaria also occurs at 400 to 500 nm. Solar sensitivity of this type can be passively transferred, implying an immune mechanism. It is treated with titanium or zinc oxide.

The mechanism of type V solar urticaria, occurring at 280 to 500 nm, is unknown.

Type VI solar urticaria, better known as erythropoietic protoporphyria (EPP), is an inherited metabolic disorder. Urticaria, in fact, is a rare manifestation of EPP; more often there is simply an exaggerated sunburn (erythema, edema, etc.). The photosensitivity is induced by 405-nm radiation. Recent guinea-pig and human data have demonstrated complement activation with irradiation by 405-nm light in animals injected intraperitoneally with porphyrins and normal human serum containing uroporphyrin [31]. This suggests a role for complement activation in the pathogenesis of the cutaneous abnormality. Oral β-carotene, in doses of 180 mg daily, is useful in ameliorating but not completely abolishing the photosensitivity. The mechanism of action is unknown but it probably is functioning as a quencher of toxic singlet oxygen.

The provocative test for solar urticaria is the broad-spectrum fluorescent tube to which individual filters may be appended to transmit desired wavelengths.

Note that in cases of light-induced eruption, one must carefully inquire for and rule out a toxic basis to the disease. Prolonged sunburn reactions rather than wheals can be seen with drugs like the phenothiazines and demeclocycline and may mimic solar urticaria.

Vibratory Angioedema. Vibratory angioedema is an extremely rare disorder [32], described in a kinship, and occasionally seen in association with cholinergic urticaria. It occurs within minutes of a vibratory stimulus. Elevated serum histamine levels have been noted with experimental production of this disease. A positive provocative test, consisting of the application of a laboratory vortex to the patient's forearm for 4 min, is evidenced by pruritus and swelling. Therapy for vibratory angioedema is avoidance of incitatory stimuli and type I antihistamines.

Aquagenic Urticaria. Aquagenic urticaria is extremely rare. As its name implies, it is produced by water exposure [33]. It is not temperature-dependent. Lesions consist of small wheals, resembling cholinergic urticaria. A water compress applied to the forearm for several minutes is an adequate provocative test.

Heritable Disorders

Hereditary Angioedema. Hereditary angioedema is a rare cause of recurrent swelling, but a not uncommon diagnostic consideration. This type of angioedema is associated with considerable mor-

bidity and a relatively high mortality. Now that effective therapy is available, correct diagnosis is most important.

In hereditary angioedema, the swelling is *not* accompanied by urticaria. Lesions are characteristically nonpainful, nonerythematous, nonpruritic, and nonpitting. Swelling evolves over several hours and lasts 24 to 72 hr. It is not resolved by morning, like the usual acquired or allergic angioedema. There is usually no periodicity to the episodes, and lesions may occur singly or in any combination. The lesions occur most commonly on the extremities and face. Involvement of the gastrointestinal tract occurs in more than 50 percent of patients, with symptoms consisting of rather severe, crampy abdominal pain often accompanied by nausea and vomiting. The clinical picture may closely mimic small-bowel obstruction or appendicitis. Laryngeal swelling occurs at some time in 70 percent of patients and may lead to airway compromise. In several series airway obstruction was responsible for the demise of 20 to 25 percent of afflicted individuals. A nondescript, transient, serpiginous, erythematous rash precedes or accompanies the angioedema in about 25 percent of patients. The attacks usually begin in childhood, but the frequency of episodes increases during adolescence and into the third and fourth decades. For most episodes there are no apparent initiating factors, though minor trauma is a clear precipitant in many patients. Since hereditary angioedema is inherited in a dominant fashion, family history is usually positive.

Most patients have low levels of the C1 esterase inhibitor, a 90,000-dalton glycoprotein that, as one of its important functions, inhibits the first component of complement. It is normally present in concentrations of 15 to 20 mg/dL. Eighty-five percent of affected patients have levels lower than 6 mg/dL. Fifteen percent have normal or high levels of a nonfunctional protein with a prolonged half-life.

There are several puzzling features to the pathophysiology of hereditary angioedema. Because it is now reasonably clear that both patient groups (the low vs. the high C1 esterase inhibitor groups) possess one normal gene and one abnormal gene, there should be synthesis of 50 percent of both the normal and abnormal gene products. The unchecked cleavage of C4 and C2 by C1 is thought to underlie the local edema formation since there is evidence that a small C2-derived peptide has vasodilatory properties and may be responsible for the angioedema. In most patients this cleavage reaction is constantly ongoing, as evidenced by the chronically low C4, and, to a lesser degree, C2 levels. It is unclear why the angioedema is intermittent and localized and spontaneously subsides.

The description of the lesions by the patient, especially their nonassociation with hives, readily discriminates this entity from acquired angioedema. In patients with a compatible clinical picture for hereditary angioedema, the screening test of choice is a determination of C4. This widely available assay is below the limits of detectability by standard radioimmunodiffusion or rate nephelometry assays in over 80 percent of patients at all times, and is always low in association with an acute attack. In other words, with a normal or high C4, the disease is in all likelihood ruled out. If the C4 level is low, then a specific antigenic or functional C1 inhibitor assay needs to be performed to confirm the diagnosis. This confirmation is necessary since immune complex–mediated diseases can occasionally present with a combination of angioedema and low C4, thus mimicking hereditary angioedema.

The therapy of this disease will be only briefly summarized below [34,35,38]. The frequency and/or location of the swelling episodes in large part determine the morbidity in this disease, and the necessity for therapy. Many patients have relatively infrequent episodes and patient education is all that is necessary. Acute episodes not involving the airway will resolve without residua and no treatment is indicated. Swelling of the tongue, pharynx, or larynx demand that the patient go to a setting such as the emergency room where he/she can be carefully observed and an airway secured if necessary. Acute episodes associated with dental work present special problems. To prevent attacks following dental manipulation, these patients can be treated for 7 to 10 days prior to the dental work with an androgen (see below) in order to raise the levels of C1 inhibitor to protective levels or can be given several units of fresh frozen plasma (a source of the inhibitor) within a few hours of the procedure.

In patients (usually only adults) with frequent attacks or life-threatening ones, the episodes can be largely abrogated with antifibrinolytic agents [ε-aminocaproic acid (EACA) or tranexamic acid] or androgens. The mechanism whereby antifibrinolytic agents reduce the frequency of the attacks is unknown. The C1 inhibitor and C4 levels do not increase. The physician treating patients with EACA (tranexamic acid, the other antifibrinolytic agent used by some groups, is not commercially available) should review the appropriate papers detail-

ing the use of this drug [34,35]. The observation that various androgens not only prevent the clinical syndrome but also cause the C1 inhibitor levels to increase [36–38] represents a major breakthrough in the treatment of this disorder. As would be expected, the C4 levels increase in parallel to the increase in the C1 inhibitor. The mechanism underlying this biochemical correction is unknown. Except for unusual circumstances children should probably not be treated with these drugs. Impeded androgens such as danazol have proved to be acceptable to treat hereditary angioedema in females. Androgens have well-recognized side effects and these problems must be carefully looked for in patients receiving chronic therapy. The extensive experience of the NIH group with androgen therapy has recently been reported [38].

C3b Inactivator Deficiency. This defect of complement regulation has now been reported in detail in several patients [39,40]. These patients have a clinical picture of frequent infections and massive histamine release with urticaria on exposure to changes in temperature. Laboratory evaluation reveals erythrocytes coated with C3 without overt hemolysis. The patients' sera have low levels of serum C3 and properdin factor B, and C3b inactivator is absent. Absence of the C3b inactivator is associated with continuous activation of the alternative pathway, with resulting cleavage of C3. Some of the C3b cleavage fragments attach to erythrocytes, producing the Coombs-positive state, and C3a liberation may be responsible for the urticaria. Infusion of normal plasma, a source of C3b inactivator, temporarily corrects all the abnormalities.

Serum Carboxypeptidase B Deficiency. Serum carboxypeptidase B, a protein that rapidly inactivates C3a and C5a, was found to be reduced (20 percent of normal) in a 64-year-old male with a 10-year history of frequent angioedema [41]. He was discovered by screening the sera of 140 patients with chronic urticaria and angioedema. Studies indicate that the reduced serum level of this inhibitor is inherited.

Hereditary Forms of Physical Urticaria. Some types of physical urticaria, especially the cold and vibratory types, have been found among multiple family members and a genetic inherited causative factor has therefore been assumed but has not been elucidated.

Amyloidosis with Nerve Deafness and Limb Pain. This rare syndrome is probably inherited as an autosomal dominant trait and is associated with urticaria and angioedema. The urticaria may resemble the lesions of cholinergic urticaria.

Type VI Solar Urticaria (Erythropoietic Protoporphyria). This entity was previously discussed.

Systemic Diseases

Though the association of urticaria and angioedema with various systemic illnesses has been widely reported, the actual incidence of systemic disease as a causative factor to urticaria and angioedema, especially of the chronic type, is probably very low.

Serum sickness is a systemic illness often accompanied by urticaria and angioedema. It is classically seen with the use of heterologous antiserum or drugs such as penicillin, cephalosporins, sulfonamides, and streptomycin. Transient serum-sickness-like reactions probably occur frequently in association with many infectious diseases, especially viral illnesses, e.g., during the prodrome stage (antigen excess) of serum hepatitis. Patients characteristically present with fever, lymphadenopathy, arthralgias, arthritis, and skin lesions. The most frequent skin lesions of serum sickness are urticaria and angioedema, though occasionally morbilliform, purpuric, or erythema-multiforme-type rashes can be seen. The disease course is usually self-limited, with the discontinuance of the inciting agent in the case of drugs or at the onset of jaundice in the case of viral hepatitis.

Connective tissue disorders may be associated with urticaria and angioedema. At some time in their course, approximately 7 percent of patients with systemic lupus erythematosus will manifest urticarial lesions [42]. Patients with acute rheumatic fever and juvenile rheumatoid arthritis may exhibit nonpruritic urticaria-like lesions. There are now numerous reports of hypocomplementemic vasculitic syndromes in which chronic urticaria is a major clinical manifestation. This syndrome is seen predominantly in women and characterized by persistent urticaria, occasionally life-threatening angioedema, arthralgias and arthritis, abdominal pain, neurologic abnormalities such as seizures, mononeuritis, noninfectious meningitis, and rarely glomerulonephritis [43,44]. Skin biopsies in these patients reveal leukocytoclastic angiitis, with cellular infiltrates of dense polymorphonuclear leukocytes and mononuclear cells within and around vessel walls. There is nuclear dust or nuclear fragmentation and extravasation of red blood cells

from vessels. Immunofluorescence demonstrates immunoglobulin deposition. Laboratory tests disclose diminished C1q, C4, C2, and C3 and elevated erythrocyte sedimentation rate. Although these patients clinically resemble those with systemic lupus erythematosus, the antinuclear antibody test is negative. In practice, the systemic complaints and elevated sedimentation rate usually readily separate this group from patients with chronic idiopathic urticaria and angioedema.

There is also a subgroup of chronic urticaria patients with vasculitis, whose primary disease manifestation is longstanding urticaria, without the generalized signs and symptoms of vasculitis [45,46]. Hypocomplementemia may or may not be present. Diagnosis is established by the biopsy appearance of inflammatory cells such as neutrophils, lymphocytes, monocytes, or eosinophils, concentrated within vessel walls. Over a quarter of the patients demonstrate positive immunofluorescence for immunoglobulins.

There are case reports of urticaria and angioedema in association with carcinomas and lymphoreticular neoplasms. The more commonly reported ones are dysproteinemias, polycythemia vera, Hodgkin's disease, chronic lymphocytic leukemia, reticulum cell sarcoma, and cancer of the colon, rectum, and lung. Immune complex formation involving tumor antigens may be responsible for the urticaria and angioedema in some of these patients. An acquired C1 esterase inhibitor deficiency has been described in patients with lymphoma [47]. This group of patients clinically resembles those with hereditary angioedema and laboratory analysis reveals both low C1 esterase inhibitor and C4. The associated malignancy and low C1 titers (in hereditary angioedema the C1 titer is normal) help to separate this group from hereditary angioedema.

Urticaria pigmentosa and systemic mastocytosis are both mast cell diseases associated with urticaria. Skin biopsies of lesions of urticaria pigmentosa or systemic mastocytosis, when performed atraumatically to avoid mast cell degranulation and when appropriately stained, reveal mast cells in increased numbers. Urticaria pigmentosa is localized to the skin and presents as focal or diffuse pigmented lesions containing mast cells. These lesions, upon stroking, characteristically urticate (Darier's sign). Mast cells are concentrated in the skin, as well as bone marrow and gastrointestinal tracts, in systemic mastocytosis. Disease signs and symptoms include urticaria, flushing, hypotension, abdominal pain, nausea, vomiting, and diarrhea. Disease manifestations coincide with massive mast cell infiltration and mediator release. Mediators implicated in disease pathogenesis include histamine and arachidonic acid metabolites [48].

Uncommonly, certain endocrine disorders have been associated with urticaria and angioedema. These include reports of urticaria with thyrotoxicosis that resolves with therapy of hyperthyroidism [49] and of cycling of the severity of chronic urticaria with the menstrual cycle.

Idiopathic Disease

The majority of patients with chronic urticaria and angioedema must unfortunately be classified into the idiopathic group. In this patient population, despite a thorough initial evaluation and follow-up for several years, the physician can detect no etiologic factor responsible for the disease state. Although occasional series claim a greater than 50 percent success rate in unveiling a primary pathologic disorder, most investigators attain a 5 to 20 percent success in identifying a cause, such as infection, infestation, allergy, heredity, vasculitis, or malignancy. In many instances, even when other diseases are discovered in association with urticaria and angioedema, a causal relation is not demonstrated, as therapy or removal of the presumed "underlying etiology" does not result in resolution of urticaria and angioedema.

Chronic idiopathic urticaria and angioedema can occur at any age, but it more frequently presents in middle-aged females in the third and fourth decades of life. In this group there is no increased incidence of atopy. Typically, patients manifest no systemic symptoms such as fevers, arthralgias, or malaise. Though a vexing and frustrating problem to its sufferers, the natural history of the chronic idiopathic state is a benign one. To our knowledge there have been no reported deaths from laryngeal obstruction. Furthermore, the spontaneous remission rate is such that approximately 50 percent of patients are symptom-free by 6 months, 70 percent by 1 year, and 90 percent by 5 years.

The pathogenesis of idiopathic disease is poorly understood. With no underlying cause obvious, research emphasis has been devoted largely to mediators. There has been some suggestion that the skin histamine levels in such patients are elevated as compared with the normal population. Induced blisters over affected and nonaffected areas in patients with idiopathic urticaria contain high histamine levels. Fifty percent of patients demonstrate dermographia. Some patients demonstrate hyperresponsiveness to such mediators

as bradykinin and kallikrein on intradermal placement. However, no abnormality has been regularly detected in the majority of these patients that adequately accounts for the disease process.

It is likely that in the idiopathic subgroup we are dealing with a heterogeneous patient population with multiple and varied etiologies to account for their disease. Hopefully this group will become smaller as new environmental antigens, inflammatory mediators, genetic factors, and other etiologic agents are found to be responsible for this clinical syndrome.

Evaluation of the Patient with Urticaria and Angioedema

An unguided workup for the etiology of urticaria and angioedema would incur excessive costs, enormous time commitment, and undue frustration for the patient [50]. The physician should avoid unnecessary costs and invasive tests by individualizing each evaluation as directed by the history, physical examination, and suspected etiology (Table 6).

There is *no substitute* for the detailed, conscientious, compulsive, and time-consuming history. Review of systems should include inquiries of general physical and emotional health, activity status, travel, appetite, changes in weight, and symptoms suggestive of infection, infestation, or collagen-vascular conditions. A complete drug history should be obtained. Occupational exposures should be elicited. The temporal character of urticaria and angioedema should be determined, such as frequency of lesions, circadian variances, changes with the menstrual cycle, seasonal exacerbations, and relationship of lesions to food, activity, and work. Possible physical precipitants such as heat, cold, water, pressure, light, vibrations, and exercise should be queried.

A physical examination to rule out underlying or associated diseases is mandatory. During this examination, light stroking of the skin should be performed to assess for dermographia. The number, size, character, and position of all skin lesions should be noted and recorded. If symptoms are suggestive of a physical urticaria, provocative testing with the appropriate stimuli should be performed.

Screening laboratory tests for most patients include at least a blood count, urinalysis, chemistry profile, sedimentation rate, and chest x-ray. An elevated sedimentation rate is not found in most patients with chronic urticaria and should be an

Table 6   Evaluation of patient with urticaria and angioedema

History
    Description of present illness
    Past medical history
    Drugs
    Occupation
    Travel
    Family history
Physical examination

Provocative physical tests, if indicated
Screening laboratory
    Complete blood count with differential
    Chemistry profile
    Sedimentation rate
    Chest x-ray
    Urinalysis

Selective laboratory, if indicated

To rule out allergy:	Skin tests to aeroallergens and patch tests to contactants, IgE, RASTs for specific antigens, eosinophil count
To evaluate cold-induced disease:	Cryofibrinogens, cryoglobulins, cold agglutinins, VDRL, immune complexes
To rule out connective tissue disease:	Antinuclear antibody, rheumatoid factor, immune complexes, total hemolytic complement, C3, C4, cryoglobulins, skin biopsy
To rule out hepatitis:	Hepatitis antibody and antigen
To evaluate infections:	Stool for ova and parasites, appropriate radiographic studies
To rule out neoplasm:	Protein electrophoresis, appropriate radiographic and other studies
To evaluate food sensitivity:	Diary, RASTs to foods, elimination diet
For hereditary angioedema:	C4, C1 inhibitor

indication for the physician to carefully consider an underlying systemic illness.

Other laboratory procedures are reserved for appropriate indications as revealed through the history, physical examination, and likely etiologic factors. If viral hepatitis is suspected, hepatitis antigen and antibody should be checked. For the infrequent instance in which an atopic basis for the disease is entertained, skin tests for aeroallergens or patch tests to contactants should be done, or RASTs, IgE levels, and eosinophils should be measured. To assess for underlying collagen-vascular disease, antinuclear antibody, rheumatoid factor, serum immune complexes, total hemolytic complement, C3, C4, and cryoglobulins should be measured. Systemic complaints, elevated sedimentation rate, positive serology, or atypical lesions necessitate skin biopsy for microscopic and immunofluorescence analysis. For cold-induced lesions, cryofibrinogens, cryoglobulins, immune complexes, cold agglutinins, and syphilis serology should be drawn. For hereditary angioedema, C4 and C1 esterase inhibitor (if the C4 is low) are appropriate tests. For suspected underlying neoplasia, suitable radiographic and protein electrophoretic studies and biopsies should be undertaken. For infections, tests are performed as symptoms and signs dictate. Stools for ova and parasites are appropriately performed if the history and exam-

ination are suggestive of infestation. For suspected food-induced urticaria and angioedema, RASTs, food diary, and diagnostic elimination diet may be tried.

These aforementioned tests should not be ordered indiscriminately on all individuals with urticaria and angioedema. The history, physical examination, screening laboratory tests, and judicious use of additional tests and procedures allow for a sensible and accurate evaluation. A thorough reevaluation is indicated in patients with persistent disease, especially if any atypical features or new signs and symptoms develop.

Therapy

Therapy for the urticaria and angioedema patient must be as individualized as the diagnostic workup. For patients in whom an etiology for the urticaria and angioedema is found, avoidance of the causative agent or therapy of the underlying disease is obviously the treatment of choice. Then, if this is ineffective, or in cases of idiopathic disease where no etiology is recognized, the physician can usually provide adequate symptomatic relief. For purposes of determining the therapeutic approach we prefer to divide our patients into two groups—those with infrequent episodes and those with frequent episodes.

For those patients with "infrequent" episodes, that is, less often than approximately one attack per month, our philosophy is to observe and treat attacks as they occur. These are patients with infrequent occurrences of a non-life-threatening disease. Because of the minimal morbidity of the syndrome, high spontaneous remission rate, and difficulty in judging the effectiveness of therapy, prophylactic medication is usually not justified.

Patient education is a vital adjunct to the management of the person with infrequent urticaria and angioedema. Patients are frightened by the mysterious outbreaks of their "affliction" and are concerned with the possibility of underlying disease and the seriousness and future course of their illness. Better understanding often allays anxiety and lessens frustration. After the evaluation, most patients may be informed of the following: (1) Though the cause of their disease is unknown, no underlying disease has been detected. (2) Though attacks may be aggravating, they are not life-threatening. (3) The natural course of the disease is such that spontaneous remissions occur in most patients. (4) Until a remission ensues the lesions can usually be adequately controlled with medication.

In an effort to assess frequency and severity of episodes, patients are instructed to keep a diary. Patients are also advised to take hydroxyzine or cyproheptadine when episodes occur.

For patients with frequent episodes, that is, at least one per month to as many as one or more per week, our approach is as follows. Patient education and a several-week to several-month record of attack rate are prerequisites to initiating therapy. If lesions are not present at the time of the examination, the patient is requested to return during the next episode. A drug trial is then begun, with a goal of preventing and/or ameliorating episodes with prophylactic therapy rather than attempting to "chase" the attacks.

Antihistamines

There are many compounds to choose from, with two types (the H-1 and H-2 blockers) and six classes (the ethanolamines, the ethylenediamines, the alkylamines, the piperazines, the phenothiazines, and cimetidine). Antihistamines act by binding histamine receptor sites of effector cells. Clinically, they reduce itching of already present lesions and reduce the frequency and severity of

future lesions. Antihistamines do not hasten the resolution of the edema once the urticaria and angioedema are present. On intradermal injection of histamine, H-1 blockers alone reduce cutaneous reactivity to histamine, while H-2 blockers alone have no significant effect. In combination, however, H-1 and H-2 blockers behave synergistically to reduce the size of wheal and flare to intradermally injected histamine [51–53]. This recent observation has prompted clinical studies in patients with chronic urticaria. A percentage of patients who have not responded to type I antihistamines have demonstrated clinical improvement with combined H-1 and H-2 blockers [54,55]. About 50 percent of the patients do not improve with either type I or type I plus type II therapy.

Hydroxyzine or cyproheptadine is our usual first choice. These drugs seem to be less soporific, and they possess anticholinergic and antiserotonin properties in addition to their antihistaminic action. Cimetidine is reserved for use with H-1 blockers if type I antihistamines are ineffective singly.

Phosphodiesterase Inhibitors

These include any of the commercially available theophylline-containing preparations. These drugs act by inhibiting the enzyme required for conversion of $3',5'$-cAMP to $5'$-AMP. In experimental systems theophylline elevates intracellular cAMP and is a potent inhibitor of mast cell and basophil histamine release. Blood levels between 8 and 15 μg/mL are acceptable; higher concentrations such as would be used in some asthmatics are usually not indicated. The long-acting, slow-release theophylline capsules (such as Theodur) are convenient preparations. If antihistamines and phosphodiesterase inhibitors are both ineffective alone, a trial of both together is worthwhile.

Sympathomimetics

These include such agents as terbutaline and ephedrine. α-Receptor stimulation results in constriction of smooth muscles within vessels of the skin, viscera, and mucous membranes. β-Receptor stimulation results in dilatation of the vascular smooth muscle, bronchodilation, and possible inhibition of mediator release from mast cells and basophils. The untoward side effects of sympathomimetics are those of sympathetic stimulation. They should be used with caution in elderly patients and those with organic heart disease, hypertension, and hyperthyroidism. They are generally ineffective as single agents in treating urticaria and angioedema [56], but in combination with anti-histamines or phosphodiesterase inhibitors may act in concert to decrease disease activity.

Corticosteroids

Steroids are rarely if ever indicated for long-term therapy of chronic idiopathic disease but are often efficacious in patients who do not respond to the above agents. Some authors have reported success with every-other-day doses of prednisone.

In patients who for 6 weeks have had several episodes of urticaria and/or angioedema per week, have had appropriate evaluation of their disease, and have kept a diary account to document the frequency and severity of the lesions, the following sequential drug trial can be employed. Patients are instructed to proceed to the next step in their therapeutic trial if one or two episodes of urticaria and angioedema occur after 24 to 48 hr of therapy.

1. Cyproheptadine, 4 mg 3 to 4 times a day
2. Hydroxyzine, 20 to 50 mg 3 to 4 times a day
3. Hydroxyzine, 20 to 50 mg 4 times a day, and cimetidine, 300 mg 4 times a day
4. Hydroxyzine, 20 to 50 mg 4 times a day and a long-acting theophylline preparation, such as Theodur, 300 mg twice a day
5. Theophylline preparation plus terbutaline, 2.5 to 5 mg 3 times a day
6. Hydroxyzine, 20 to 50 mg 4 times a day, theophylline preparation, and terbutaline, 2.5 to 5 mg 3 times a day

It is the unusual patient who does not respond with either a decrease in frequency of the episodes or a complete remission to the single or combined therapy as described. However, some patients continue to have frequent attacks. For this group with severe disease and poorly tolerated morbidity, we administer prednisone beginning at a dose of ~1 mg/kg (40 to 80 mg in a single a.m. dose) for 1 week. It is rare that a patient does not note a resolution of his or her symptoms with this regimen. The steroids are rapidly tapered so that by 4 to 6 weeks they can be withdrawn. If the lesions recur, the level is reduced more slowly on an every-day or every-other-day schedule. The goal is to find the lowest dose that will control the lesions. Further, every 1 to 3 months attempts must be made to withdraw medication. Antihistamines and theophylline preparations are often used in conjunction with prednisone and continued following discontinuation of the steroids.

References

1. Champion RH et al: Urticaria and angioedema. *Br J Dermatol* **81**:588–597, 1969
2. Yecies LD, Kaplan AP: Urticaria, in *Clinical Immunology.* Edited by CW Parker. Saunders, Philadelphia, 1980, pp 1283–1315
3. Gigli I et al: Angioedema, in *Immunological Diseases.* Edited by M Samter. Little, Brown, Boston, 1978, pp 941–952
4. Kaplan AP: Urticaria and angioedema, in *Allergy: Principles and Practice.* Edited by E Middleton et al. Mosby, St Louis, 1978, pp 1080–1099
5. Mathews KP: Management of urticaria and angioedema. *J Allergy Clin Immunol* **66**:347–357, 1980
6. Warin RP, Champion RH: *Urticaria,* vol 1 of *Major Problems in Dermatology.* Saunders, Philadelphia, 1974, pp 1–164
7. Soter, NA, Wasserman SI: Urticaria/angioedema: a consideration of pathogenesis and clinical manifestations. *Int J Dermatol* **18**:517–532, 1979
8. Kaplan AP: Mediators of urticaria and angioedema. *J Allergy Clin Immunol* **60**:324–332, 1977
9. Mathews KP: A current view of urticaria. *Med Clin North Am* **58**:185–205, 1974
10. Kaplan AP: The pathogenic basis of urticaria and angioedema: recent advances. *Am J Med* **70**:755–758, 1981
11. Harnett JC et al: Aspirin idiosyncrasy. Asthma and urticaria, in *Allergy: Principles and Practice.* Edited by E Middleton et al. Mosby, St Louis, 1978, pp 1002–1022
12. Parker CW: Urticaria, in *Textbook of Immunopathology.* Edited by PA Miescher, HJ Muller-Eberhard. Grune & Stratton, New York, 1976, pp 369–376
13. Lewis T: *The Blood Vessels of the Human Skin and Their Responses.* Shaw & Sons, London, 1927, pp 1–293
14. Falkenhein SF et al: Effect of the 5-hydroperoxide of eicosatetraenoic acid and inhibitors of the lipoxygenase pathway on the formation of slow-reacting substance by rat basophilic leukemia cells. Direct evidence that slow-reacting substance is a product of the lipoxygenase pathway. *J Immunol* **125**:163–168, 1980
15. Parker CW et al: Hypersensitivity to penicillenic acid derivatives in human beings with penicillin allergy. *J Exp Med* **115**:821–838, 1962
16. Wide L, Juhlin L: Detection of penicillin allergy of the immediate type by radioimmunoassay of reagins (IgE) to penicilloyl conjugates. *Clin Allergy* **1**:171–177, 1971
17. Zeiss CR et al: Comparison of the radioallergosorbent test and a quantitative solid-phase radioimmunoassay for the detection of ragweed-specific immunoglobulin E antibody in patients undergoing immunotherapy. *J Allergy Clin Immunol* **67**:105–110, 1981
18. Wicher K, Reisman RE: Anaphylactic reaction to penicillin (or penicillin-like substance) in a soft drink. *J Allergy Clin Immunol* **66**:155–157, 1980
19. Warin RP, Smith RJ: Challenge test battery in chronic urticaria. *Br J Dermatol* **94**:401–406, 1976
20. Wraith DG et al: Recognition of food-allergic patients and their allergens by the RAST technique and clinical investigation. *Clin Allergy* **9**:25–36, 1979
21. American Academy of Allergy: Position statements—controversial techniques. *J Allergy Clin Immunol* **67**:333–338, 1981
22. Fisher AA: *Contact Dermatitis.* Lea & Febiger, Philadelphia, 1973

23. Braverman IM: Urticaria as a sign of internal disease. *Postgrad Med* **41**:450–454, 1967

24. James J, Warin RP: An assessment of the role of *Candida albicans* and yeasts in chronic urticaria. *Br J Dermatol* **84**:227–237, 1971

25. Soter NA, Wasserman SI: Physical urticaria/angioedema: an experimental model of mast cell activation in humans. *J Allergy Clin Immunol* **66**:358–365, 1980

26. Kaplan AP et al: In vivo studies of mediator release in cold urticaria and cholinergic urticaria. *J Allergy Clin Immunol* **55**:394–402, 1975

27. Wanderer AA et al: Primary acquired cold urticaria. Blind comparative study of treatment with cyproheptadine, chlorpheniramine, and placebo. *Arch Dermatol* **113**:1375–1377, 1977

28. Moore-Robinson M, Warin RP: Some clinical aspects of cholinergic urticaria. *Br J Dermatol* **80**:794–799, 1968

29. Herxheimer A: The nervous pathway mediating cholinogenic urticaria. *Clin Sci* **15**:195–205, 1956

30. Sams WM Jr et al: Solar urticaria. Investigation of pathogenetic mechanisms. *Arch Dermatol* **99**:390–397, 1969

31. Lim HW et al: Complement-derived chemotactic activity is generated in human serum containing uroporphyrin after irradiation with 405-nm light. *J Clin Invest* **67**:1072–1077, 1981

32. Patterson R et al: Vibratory angioedema: a hereditary type of physical hypersensitivity. *J Allergy Clin Immunol* **50**:174–182, 1972

33. Chalamidas SL, Charles CR: Aquagenic urticaria. *Arch Dermatol* **104**:541–546, 1971

34. Gelfand J et al: Hereditary angioedema. Clinical syndrome and its management. *Ann Intern Med* **84**:580–593, 1976

35. Atkinson JP: Diagnosis and management of hereditary angioedema (HAE). *Ann Allergy* **42**:348–352, 1979

36. Gadek JE et al: Response of variant hereditary angioedema phenotypes to danazol therapy: genetic implications. *J Clin Invest* **64**:280–286, 1979

37. Gelfand JA et al: Treatment of hereditary angioedema with danazol: reversal of clinical and biochemical abnormalities. *N Engl J Med* **295**:1444–1448, 1976

38. Hosea SW et al: Long-term therapy of hereditary angioedema with danazol. *Ann Intern Med* **93**:809–812, 1980

39. Ziegler JB et al: Restoration by purified C3b inactivator of complement-mediated function *in vivo* in a patient with C3b inactivator deficiency. *J Clin Invest* **55**:668–672, 1975

40. Thompson RA, Lachmann PJ: A second case of human C3b inhibitor (KAT) deficiency. *Clin Exp Immunol* **27**:23–29, 1977

41. Mathews KP et al: Familial carboxypeptidase N deficiency. *Ann Intern Med* **93**:443–445, 1980

42. Dubois EL: The clinical picture of systemic lupus erythematosus, in *Lupus Erythematosus*. Edited by E Dubois. Univ of Southern California Press, Los Angeles, 1974, pp 232–279

43. Zeiss RC et al: A hypocomplementemic vasculitic urticaria syndrome. Report of four new cases and definition of the disease. *Am J Med* **68**:867–875, 1980

44. Soter NA: Chronic urticaria as a manifestation of necrotizing venulitis. *N Engl J Med* **296**:1440–1442, 1977

45. Mathison DA et al: Hypocomplementemia in chronic idiopathic urticaria. *Ann Intern Med* **86**:534–538, 1977

46. Phanuphak P et al: Vasculitis in chronic urticaria. *J Allergy Clin Immunol* **65**:436–444, 1980

47. Gelfand J et al: Acquired C1 esterase inhibitor deficiency and angioedema: a review. *Medicine (Baltimore)* **58**:321–328, 1979

48. Roberts LJ et al: Increased production of prostaglandin D_2 in patients with systemic mastocytosis. *N Engl J Med* **303**:1400–1404, 1980

49. Isaacs NJ, Ertec NH: Urticaria and pruritus: uncommon manifestations of hyperthyroidism. *J Allergy Clin Immunol* **48**:73–81, 1971

50. Jacobson KW et al: Laboratory tests in chronic urticaria. *JAMA* **243**:1644–1646, 1980

51. Harvey RP, Schocket AL: The effect of H_1 and H_2 blockade on cutaneous histamine response in man. *J Allergy Clin Immunol* **65**:136–139, 1980

52. Plaut M: Histamine, H_1 and H_2 antihistamines, and immediate hypersensitivity reactions. *J Allergy Clin Immunol* **63**:371–375, 1979

53. Smith JA et al: The effect of cimetidine on the immediate cutaneous response to allergens. *Ann Allergy* **42**:353–354, 1979

54. Phanuphak P et al: Treatment of chronic idiopathic urticaria with combined H1 and H2 blockers. *Clin Allergy* **8**:429–433, 1978

55. Commens CA, Greaves MW: Cimetidine in chronic idiopathic urticaria: a randomized double-blind study. *Br J Dermatol* **99**:675–679, 1978

56. Spangler DL et al: Terbutaline in the treatment of chronic urticaria. *Ann Allergy* **45**:246–247, 1980

MUCOCUTANEOUS COMPLICATIONS OF CANCER CHEMOTHERAPY

Antoinette F. Hood

Harley A. Haynes

In today's war against cancer, chemotherapeutic agents are being used with increasing frequency. Originally established as effective treatment for hematologic malignancies, chemotherapy has recently assumed an important role in the treatment of many solid tumors—usually either in combination with surgery or radiation therapy or as "adjunctive" therapy in situations where tumor is no longer clinically detectable but where the probability of microscopic disease is high.

These cytotoxic drugs nonspecifically inhibit rapidly dividing cells and cannot differentiate between tumor cells and normal cells. It is not surprising therefore that the most common complications occur as a result of their action on rapidly dividing tissue such as bone marrow, gastrointestinal tract, and skin.

The adverse mucocutaneous reactions associated with the use of antineoplastic agents vary considerably in their clinical presentation (Table 1). While these cutaneous complications are rarely life-threatening or dose-limiting, the additional stress of overtly disfiguring changes such as alopecia and hyperpigmentation may be psychologically devastating to a patient already severely stressed by his or her underlying disease.

Unfortunately, only a few comprehensive articles on the subject of mucocutaneous side effects of antineoplastic drugs have been written [1–4]. The purpose of this chapter is to review the reported mucocutaneous complications of cancer chemotherapeutic agents in order to (1) increase

Table 1   Common cutaneous reactions associated with the administration of cancer chemotherapeutic agents

Stomatitis
  Actinomycin D
  Bleomycin
  Cyclophosphamide
  Cytarabine
  Daunorubicin
  Doxorubicin
  5-Fluorouracil
  6-Mercaptopurine
  Methotrexate
  Mithramycin
  Nitrosoureas
  Procarbazine
  Vinblastine

Alopecia
  Bleomycin
  Cyclophosphamide
  Decarbazine
  Doxorubicin
  5-Fluorouracil
  Hydroxyurea
  Nitrosoureas
  Methotrexate
  Procarbazine
  Vinblastine
  Vincristine

Hypersensitivity reactions
(urticaria, angioedema)
  L-Asparaginase
  Chlorambucil
  Cyclophosphamide
  Daunorubicin
  Doxorubicin
  Mechlorethamine
  Melphalan
  Methotrexate
  Procarbazine
  Triethylenethiophosphoramide

Chemical cellulitis
  Actinomycin D
  Daunorubicin
  Doxorubicin
  Mithramycin
  Nitrogen mustard
  Vinblastine
  Vincristine

Phlebitis
  Actinomycin D
  Daunorubicin
  Doxorubicin
  Vinblastine

Hyperpigmentation
  Skin
    Localized
      Bleomycin ("flagellate" and linear)
      Cyclophosphamide
      Doxorubicin
      5-Fluorouracil
      Mechlorethamine (topical)
      Nitrosoureas (topical)

Diffuse
  Busulfan
  Cyclophosphamide
  Hydroxyurea
  Methotrexate
Mucous membranes
  Cyclophosphamide
  Doxorubicin
  5-Fluorouracil
Nails
  Bleomycin
  Cyclophosphamide
  Daunorubicin
  Doxorubicin
  5-Fluorouracil
  Hydroxyurea

Inflammation of seborrheic or actinic keratoses
  Cytarabine
  5-Fluorouracil

Radiation enhancement and recall
  Actinomycin D
  Doxorubicin
  5-Fluorouracil
  Methotrexate

Photosensitivity
  Decarbazine
  5-Fluorouracil
  Methotrexate
  Vinblastine

Tenderness and/or erythema of palms and soles
  Bleomycin
  Cytosine arabinoside
  Methotrexate

Raynaud's phenomenon
  Bleomycin with vinblastine

Acral sclerosis
  Bleomycin

Ulceration over pressure areas
  Bleomycin
  Methotrexate

Folliculitis
  Actinomycin D
  Methotrexate

Onychodystrophy or onycholysis
  Bleomycin
  Cyclophosphamide
  Doxorubicin
  5-Fluorouracil
  Hydroxyurea

Erythema of face and neck
  5-Fluorouracil
  Mithramycin
  Procarbazine

Exfoliative dermatitis
  Chlorambucil/busulfan
  Methotrexate

Atrophy of skin and nails
  Hydroxyurea

awareness and recognition of these reactions and (2) assist the clinician faced with the problem of a rash developing in a patient on chemotherapy.

Before beginning a detailed discussion of reactions to individual cytotoxic agents one point should be stressed. It is often quite difficult to document the cause-and-effect relationship between one specific drug and the occurrence of a cutaneous complication. While the literature contains many references to cutaneous complications associated with antineoplastic drugs, concise descriptions of these changes are often lacking and rarely is there additional documentation with photography or histopathology. Furthermore, patients on chemotherapy are usually quite ill, often infected, and almost always on many other drugs such as antibiotics, analgesics, and antiemetics. In this complex environment it may be impossible to determine absolutely the causal relationship between a drug and a mucocutaneous reaction.

Alkylating Agents

The alkylating agents (Table 2) interfere with DNA replication and transcription by producing breaks in the DNA molecule and cross-linking of its twin strands. Although there are marked differences in clinical effects among these drugs, as a group alkylators are cell cycle phase–nonspecific and radiomimetic. The five chemical classes of alkylating agents include

Nitrogen mustard derivatives (cyclophosphamide, mechlorethamine, chlorambucil, melphalan)
Alkylsulfonates (busulfan)
Ethylenemine derivatives (thiotepa)
Triazine derivatives (decarbazine)
Nitrosureas (BCNU, CCNU, methyl-CCNU)

Nitrogen Mustard Derivatives

Cyclophosphamide (Cytoxan). Cyclophosphamide is the most widely used of the alkylating agents. As a cytotoxic it is used in the treatment of a variety of neoplastic diseases, including leukemia, lymphoma, and solid tumors. As a powerful immunosuppressive, it has been used successfully to prevent organ transplant rejection and in the treatment of nonneoplastic diseases such as rheumatoid arthritis, nephrotic syndrome, pemphigus vulgaris, lupus erythematosus, and Wegener's granulomatosis.

Table 2 Cutaneous complications secondary to alkylating agents

Cyclophosphamide
  Alopecia
  Stomatitis
  Hyperpigmentation
    Generalized
    Nails
    Palms and soles
    Teeth
  Urticaria

Mechlorethamine
  Systemic
    Angioedema
    Erythema multiforme (?)
  Topical
    Contact dermatitis
    Hyperpigmentation

Chlorambucil
  Urticaria with periorbital edema

Melphalan
  Urticaria
  Angioedema

Busulfan
  Diffuse hyperpigmentation with or without symptoms of adrenal cortical insufficiency
  Porphyria cutanea tarda
  Erythema multiforme (?)

Triethylenethiophosphoramide
  Urticaria
  Angioedema
  Hypopigmentation

Decarbazine
  Alopecia
  Facial flushing
  Photosensitivity

Nitrosoureas (BCNU)
  Alopecia
  Stomatitis
  Hyperpigmentation (topical application)

Alopecia is a common complication of cyclophosphamide therapy [5]. The alopecia, which is of the anagen effluvium type, is apparently dose related, occurring with increasing frequency in cumulated doses over 5.0 g [6]. Regrowth of hair occurs when cyclophosphamide is discontinued and occasionally even during maintenance therapy [6]. The new hair may be of a different texture or color. Mucosal ulcerations are less commonly seen with cyclophosphamide than with other chemotherapeutic agents.

Hyperpigmentation following cyclophosphamide administration has been reported by several authors. The hyperpigmentation may be widespread [7,8] or it may be localized to the palms and soles [7], nails [7,9–12], or teeth [12]. The nail hyperpigmentation appears at the base of the fingernails and toenails 2 to 4 weeks after the onset of cyclophosphamide therapy and disappears over a 6-month period. The bands move distally with nail growth. Transverse or horizontal bands are more commonly seen than longitudinal bands. The pigmented bands on the teeth do not disappear, even after medication is discontinued [12].

Although hypersensitivity reactions are rare, six cases of anaphylactic [13,14] and urticarial reactions to cyclophosphamide have been reported [15–18]. Lakin and Cahill [17] described generalized urticaria related to cyclophosphamide administration occurring on three separate occasions in a 6-year-old boy. Serum samples were found to contain homocytotropic antibody activity, which was of the IgE type.

One patient with a history of a hypersensitivity reaction to topical and intravenous mechlorethamine developed angioedema following intravenous administration of cyclophosphamide, which suggested a cross-sensitivity [15] among alkylators. However, this cross-sensitivity is variable since other patients with documented cyclophosphamide hypersensitivity who were subsequently treated with chlorambucil [14,18] and mechlorethamine and isophosphamide [16] did not have allergic reactions. Nevertheless, care must be exercised in administering a second alkylating agent to a patient with a known allergic reaction.

Mechlorethamine (Nitrogen Mustard). Mechlorethamine was one of the first anticancer drugs to be widely used clinically, but the indications for its use have become more restricted as new anticancer agents have been developed. It is used most often in the treatment of Hodgkin's disease and other lymphomas, as well as of solid tumors as part of the MOPP regimen [mechlorethamine, vincristine (Oncovin), procarbazine, and prednisone]. Used topically in dilute solution, it is effective in the treatment of mycosis fungoides.

Reactions to systemically administered mechlorethamine are uncommon. One patient with mycosis fungoides who had been previously sensitized to topical mechlorethamine developed angioedema and pruritus after intravenous administration of the medication [15]. He had a similar reaction when intravenous cyclophosphamide was given, indicating a cross-sensitivity between the two agents. Another patient developed a papular pruritic eruption on two occasions after receiving intravenous mechlorethamine [19]. The clinical course and histopathology were felt to be consistent with erythema multiforme.

Used topically, mechlorethamine may produce a primary irritant reaction [20], allergic contact dermatitis [20–22], hyperpigmentation [20,22–24], or anaphylaxis [25].

Chlorambucil (Leukeran). Chlorambucil is most frequently used in the treatment of chronic lymphocytic leukemia and is occasionally used to maintain a remission with lymphomas.

Cutaneous complications are rare; however, there are two reported cases of hypersensitivity characterized by a generalized, pruritic, urticarial eruption with pronounced periorbital edema [26,27]. The eruption recurred when the patient was rechallenged with the drug. A skin biopsy of an urticarial lesion revealed vascular dilatation and perivascular mononuclear cell infiltrate. Direct immunofluorescence was negative for immunoglobulin, complement, and fibrin deposition [27]. Patch, scratch, and intradermal tests to chlorambucil were uniformly negative.

Melphalan (Alkeran, L-PAM). Melphalan has long been used as a first-time drug in the treatment of multiple myeloma; it is also used in patients with ovarian carcinoma and breast carcinoma.

Skin reactions to melphalan are uncommon. One patient was reported who had repeated episodes of urticaria, angioedema, and anaphylaxis after receiving oral melphalan [28]. In a large series of multiple myeloma patients who were being treated with intravenous melphalan, there was a 3.9 percent incidence of allergic reactions attributed to the drug [29]. The allergic reactions included pruritus, urticaria, angioedema, flushing, a "tingling sensation," diaphoresis, chest pain, dyspnea, nausea, and anaphylaxis. Four of five patients who were rechallenged with oral melphalan developed symptoms of a type 1 hypersensitivity reaction. IgA kappa monoclonal gammopathy occurs with increased frequency among allergic individuals, suggesting that these patients are more susceptible to melphalan hypersensitivity [29].

Regional limb perfusion with intraarterial melphalan has been used in the treatment of malignant melanoma. Erythema of the perfused limb was commonly seen; blistering and desquamation occurred in one patient; and another patient developed extensive skin necrosis that required grafting [30].

Busulfan

Busulfan is a potent inhibitor of the growth of cells in the granulocytic series. For this reason it is widely used to treat patients with chronic myelocytic leukemia.

Widespread to diffuse hyperpigmentation may occur with prolonged administration of the drug [31–33]. Several patients have been reported who developed an Addisonian-like syndrome with fatigue, weight loss, diarrhea, and hyperpigmentation of the skin [34–36]. The diffuse brownish pigmentation was more pronounced on the trunk, face, and hands. There was no hyperpigmentation of the palmar creases and, except for one patient with linear pigmentation on the gingiva, the mucous membranes were spared [37]. Biopsies of involved skin showed increased melanin in the basal cell layers and melanin deposition in the upper dermis but no increase in the number of melanocytes [35]. Although the clinical picture resembles adrenal cortical insufficiency, endocrine abnormalities have never been documented. One patient with chronic myelogenous leukemia who received high daily doses of busulfan for 8 months developed generalized hyperpigmentation, generalized alopecia, anhydrosis, and glossitis [32].

Another patient with chronic myelocytic leukemia who was receiving busulfan developed well-documented porphyria cutanea tarda with diffuse hyperpigmentation and skin fragility but no bullae or milia [37].

Hypersensitivity reactions to busulfan are rare. There has, however, been one case report of a patient who developed multiple, clinically bullous lesions which were felt to represent erythema multiforme [38]. The biopsy in this case demonstrated the presence of a subepidermal bulla with necrosis and neutrophils, which also raised the possibility of acute neutrophilic dermatosis (Sweet's disease). The lesions improved when busulfan was discontinued and prednisone therapy was begun.

Triethylenethiophosphoramide (Thiotepa)

Thiotepa has a spectrum of toxicity and clinical use that is nearly identical to that of nitrogen mustard, but it is a more stable preparation. It is used topically (intracavitary, intravesicle, and intraocular) in patients with malignant pleural or pericardial effusions, bladder cancer, and following surgery for pterygium. Fever, urticaria, pruritus, and angioedema were observed in 5 of 164 patients who received intravesicle thiotepa for bladder carcinoma [39]. Hypopigmentation of the eyelashes and periorbital skin has been reported after topical intraocular application for pterygium [40,41].

Decarbazine (DTIC)

Decarbazine is an alkylating agent that has been used in the treatment of malignant melanoma, astrocytomas, Hodgkin's disease, as well as of some sarcomas and lymphomas.

Cutaneous complications include alopecia, facial flushing, and photosensitivity [42]. The photosensitivity reactions occurred in two patients who developed erythema and a burning sensation on sun-exposed skin shortly after receiving intravenous DTIC. The erythema recurred with repeated administration of the medication and could be reduced by appropriate covering of the areas. No attempt to prevent the reaction with sunscreening agents was described. DTIC requires biotransformation before it is capable of exerting cytotoxic effects. One form of biotransformation is through photodegradation [43]. Presumably one of the light activation products produced the reported phototoxic reactions.

Nitrosoureas [Carmustine (BCNU), Lomustine (CCNU), Semustine (methyl-CCNU)]

The nitrosoureas are a group of lipid-soluble alkylating agents with a wide therapeutic spectrum. BCNU has been used effectively in the treatment of melanoma, brain tumors, and multiple myeloma. CCNU is used in the treatment of lymphomas and lung cancer. Methyl-CCNU is available on an experimental basis only.

Cutaneous reactions attributable to nitrosoureas are uncommon but stomatitis [44], alopecia [44], and hyperpigmentation of skin in contact with BCNU [45] have been reported. BCNU causes severe local pain and occasionally phlebitis at the site of injection [44].

Antimetabolites

The antimetabolites (Table 3) inhibit the biosynthesis of the nucleic acids (1) by substituting for a metabolite normally incorporated into a key molecule, (2) by competing with a normal metabolite that acts as an enzyme regulatory site, or (3) by competing with a normal metabolite for occupation of the catalytic site of a key enzyme. The five antimetabolites that are widely used in oncology include

Methotrexate (MTX)
5-Fluorouracil (5-FU)

Table 3   Adverse cutaneous reactions produced by antimetabolites

Methotrexate
  Alopecia
  Stomatitis
  Erythema and desquamation over pressure points
  Macular and/or papular eruptions
  Radiation enhancement
  Photosensitivity
  Urticaria
  Hyperpigmentation
  Folliculitis
6-Mercaptopurine/6-Thioguanine
  Stomatitis
5-Fluorouracil
  Systemic
    Alopecia
    Stomatitis
    Erythema, bullae, desquamation
    Photosensitivity
    Hyperpigmentation
      Sun-exposed areas
      Over veins used for infusion
      Mucous membranes
      At radiation sites
      Nails
    Inflammation of actinic keratoses
  Topical
    Contact dermatitis
      Irritant and allergic
Cytarabine
Erythema, tenderness, exfoliation of palms and soles
  Stomatitis
  Inflammation of seborrheic keratoses

Cytarabine (Ara-C)
6-Mercaptopurine (6-MP)
6-Thioguanine (6-TG)

With the exception of 5-fluorouracil, these agents are all cell cycle phase–specific.

Methotrexate (MTX)

The folate antagonist methotrexate is an important drug in the treatment of acute leukemia, choriocarcinoma, squamous cell carcinoma of the head and neck, and in the adjuvant setting following surgical resection of osteogenic sarcoma or breast carcinoma. The administration of leucovorin (citrovorum factor) following high-dose MTX significantly reduces many of the cytotoxic effects on normal tissue. In low doses MTX is effectively used in the treatment of nonneoplastic diseases such as psoriasis, psoriatic arthritis, and polymyositis.

Many mucocutaneous complications have been reported with MTX. The buccal mucosa in partic-

ular is vulnerable to cytotoxic effects of MTX and stomatitis is common [46–50] (Fig. 1). The changes may range from mild erythema to severe and extensive ulcerations. Since stomatitis may be prognostic of a more severe reaction if the drug is continued, ulcerative stomatitis is considered an indication for discontinuing therapy. The severity of stomatitis may be reduced by altering the dose or the frequency of administration. With regard to its effect on mucosal ulcerations, various authors have found leukovorin rescue diminishes lesions [46,51], is unpredictable [52], or is of no significant benefit [53].

Transient alopecia is frequently observed with MTX therapy [47–50]. As with other chemotherapeutic agents, regrowth occurs when the medication is discontinued and sometimes even during repeated courses [49].

Erythema, with or without edema, followed by superficial desquamation or sloughing of the entire epidermis has been described by many authors [42,51,54–56]. These reactions occur more frequently in pressure areas such as the hands, feet, and elbows and in intertriginous areas (Fig. 2). They have been reported in patients who have received oral MTX and intravenous MTX. One case was labeled vasculitis [54] but this diagnosis was not substantiated by a biopsy.

Erythematous macular or macular and papular eruptions are reported [51,55]. These lesions appear 2 to 3 days after MTX is given and resolve in 2 to 11 days. Most of the eruptions occurred only during the first treatment course; recurrence with subsequent administration was uncommon [55]. Biopsies of the lesions showed parakeratosis, focal epidermal spongiosis, and a perivascular lymphohistiocytic and eosinophilic infiltrate [55].

Fig. 1.   Severe stomatitis secondary to methotrexate. (From Adrian et al [3], with permission.)

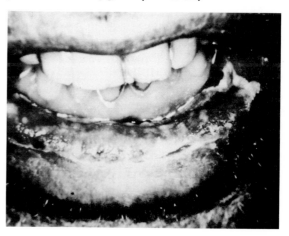

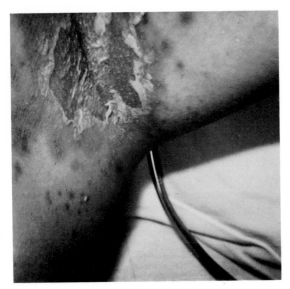

Fig. 2. Erythema and desquamation in the axilla due to methotrexate toxicity.

A synergistic effect between ionizing radiation and high-dose MTX may occur [51,57]. If MTX is administered within 3 weeks after the completion of radiation therapy, marked erythema, sometimes progressing to epidermal necrosis, is seen in the irradiated area. The reaction may be elicited with subsequent doses of MTX [57]. One illustrative example of how devastating this process can be was described in a patient with acute undifferentiated leukemia. He had received intravenous, intrathecal, and oral MTX as well as cranial irradiation. Three days after the completion of the irradiation he developed alopecia and blisters over his entire scalp which progressed to necrosis and widespread ulcerations [58].

The interaction between MTX and ultraviolet radiation may produce either a phototoxic reaction or a reactivation of preexisting sunburn [59]. With the phototoxic reaction, a patient who is on MTX develops a sunburn after exposure to what is a normally suberythrogenic dose of sunlight [50]. In the second reaction, a so-called false photosensitization, a patient is exposed to ultraviolet radiation with or without ensuing sunburn, receives MTX 2 to 5 days later, and develops severe erythema occasionally with blisters localized to the exposed areas [50,60,61]. The duration of time between the initial exposure and the administration of MTX is critical [62] and there is no recurrence with subsequent doses of drug [60,61].

Isolated cases of urticaria have been reported in patients receiving both oral and parenteral MTX [63,64], and severe anaphylaxis with high-dose MTX has been reported by several authors [65,66].

Other uncommon cutaneous complications associated with MTX administration include hyperpigmentation [49], folliculitis [51], and exacerbation of acne [51].

5-Fluorouracil (5-FU)

5-Fluorouracil is a structural analogue of the DNA precursor thymine which works by inhibiting the enzyme thymidylate synthetase. It is useful in the treatment of carcinoma of the breast and gastrointestinal tract and is used topically in the treatment of some premalignant skin diseases.

Mucocutaneous complications are seen quite frequently when 5-FU is given systemically. Stomatitis and alopecia (Fig. 3) are both common [67–70]. Diffuse erythema, scaling, desquamation, or bullae formation was described in 13 percent of patients receiving 5-FU in one series [67]. Erythema and ulcerations developing in an area of radiation damage [67], severe seborrheic dermatitis [70,71], and dryness of the palms and soles with fissuring [72] have also been reported.

A variety of different reactions to sunlight have been described in patients receiving 5-FU. Exposure to suberythemogenic doses of sunlight resulted in marked erythema limited to sun-exposed areas in 57 percent of patients receiving 5-FU in one series [71]. The erythema developed within half an hour of ultraviolet exposure and persisted for several days. Extensive erythema in exposed areas of the skin, often followed by hair loss, hyperpigmentation, and cutaneous atrophy, was described in three other patients [70]. One patient was reported who developed plaque-type poly-

Fig. 3. Diffuse alopecia associated with 5-FU chemotherapy.

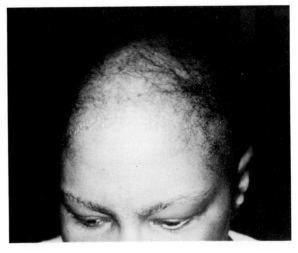

morphous light eruption localized to her face with each course of systemic 5-FU [71]. Marked hyperpigmentation in sun-exposed areas without preceding clinically apparent erythema has also been noted [71]. This hyperpigmentation may persist for months after exposure to sunlight.

Other interesting hyperpigmentation problems include hyperpigmentation limited to irradiation portal sites [71] and serpiginous hyperpigmentation overlying the veins used for multiple 5-FU infusions [73] (Fig. 4). Similar changes were not present on the opposite, noninfused arm. Patients on 5-FU may develop hyperpigmentation of the nails, either diffusely or in transverse bands [71].

Other nail changes reported with 5-FU include proximal onycholysis, increased brittleness with cracking, and ridge formation (Beau's lines) [67].

Systemic 5-FU may produce inflammation and clearing of actinic keratosis [74]. It may also ''light up'' areas of recurrence or metastasis. There is a single case report of a patient with carcinoma of the breast who received 5-FU on three occasions and each time developed a macular and papular pruritic erythematous eruption on the chest. After the rash had subsided biopsies were taken from clinically normal skin which revealed tumor cells in the dermis [75].

An irritant dermatitis characterized by intense erythema and scaling frequently occurs in areas of topically applied 5-FU. Actinically damaged skin responds most dramatically. Actual allergic contact dermatitis reactions have been reported [76,77]. These reactions are eczematous and pruritic and may be widespread or localized to the area of applied medication [77].

Persistent telangiectasia at the site of application [78], reactivation of herpes labialis [78], hypertrophic scarring [79], and the development of bullous pemphigoid [80] are other uncommon complications reported in association with topical 5-FU.

Hypersensitivity reactions to 5-FU are rare; however, in patients previously treated with topical 5-FU, systemic administration may be associated with a generalized papular eruption or with a pruritic erythematous eruption localized to sun-exposed areas [81].

Cytarabine (Cytosine Arabinoside, Ara-C)

This nucleoside analogue is antineoplastic, antiviral, and immunosuppressive. It is used clinically combined with other drugs in the treatment of acute myelogenous leukemia.

Mucocutaneous complications are rare. Stomatitis has been reported [83] as well as inflammation of preexisting seborrheic keratoses [84]. High-dose cytarabine can cause painful erythema and subsequent desquamation of the skin of the palms and soles.

6-Mercaptopurine and 6-Thioguanine

The purine analogues 6-mercaptopurine (6-MP) and 6-thioguanine (6-TG) are used almost exclusively in the treatment of acute leukemia. Except for oral ulceration [82], cutaneous complications are uncommon.

Antibiotics

The antibiotics (Table 4) used in cancer chemotherapy are natural products of various strains of the *Streptomyces*. They act by binding to DNA and inhibiting DNA and RNA synthesis. The antibiotics act on different phases of the cell cycle and therefore behave as cell cycle phase–nonspecific agents.

The clinically useful antibiotics include

Bleomycin
Actinomycin D (Dactinomycin)
Doxorubicin (Adriamycin)
Daunorubicin
Mithramycin (Mithracin)
Mitomycin C (Mutamycin)

Bleomycin

Bleomycin inhibits synthesis of DNA, RNA, and proteins and induces single-strand breaks in DNA [85]. It reaches high concentrations in the skin, lungs, kidney, peritoneum, and lymphatics. Bleomycin shows significant antitumor activity against

Fig. 4. Hyperpigmentation over a vein used to inject 5-FU. *(From Adrian et al [3], with permission.)*

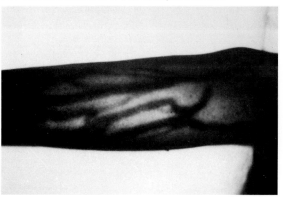

Table 4   Mucocutaneous complications associated with antineoplastic antibiotics

Bleomycin
  Alopecia
  Stomatitis
  Palmar erythema, edema, vesiculation, and hyperkeratosis
  Erythema, plaques, and nodules over pressure areas
  Raynaud's phenomenon
  Acral sclerosis
  Penile calcification
  Linear "flagellate" hyperpigmentation
  Onychodystrophy

Actinomycin D
  Alopecia
  Stomatitis
  Chemical cellulitis plus ulceration
  Radiation enhancement and recall
  Acneform eruption
  Erythema multiforme

Daunorubicin
  Stomatitis
  Nail hyperpigmentation
  Chemical cellulitis
  Localized urticaria

Doxorubicin
  Alopecia
  Stomatitis
  Hyperpigmentation
    Nails
    Palms and soles
    Buccal mucosa
  Chemical cellulitis plus ulceration
  Radiation enhancement and recall
  Urticaria
    Localized
    Generalized
  Contact dermatitis

Mithramycin
  Stomatitis
  Macular erythema of face and neck
  Chemical cellulitis
  Toxic epidermal necrolysis

squamous cell carcinomas of the head and neck, testicular neoplasms, and lymphomas.

Because the drug reaches high concentrations in the skin, cutaneous reactions are commonly encountered. Stomatitis, which may be severe enough to be dose-limiting, occurs in 20 to 40 percent of patients [85–88]. Alopecia beginning 3 weeks after initiation of bleomycin treatment develops in 10 to 40 percent of patients [85–87]. Regrowth is seen in 2 to 3 months and occasionally new hair may be darker in color than previously [86].

Hyperesthesia, edema, and erythema of the palms often followed by vesiculation and hyperkeratosis have been reported in two series of patients [88,89].

Erythema over pressure sites such as elbows,

scapulae, scrotum, and vulva progressing to ulceration was described by Yagoda et al. [86]. They also noted a morbilliform eruption in 11 percent and pruritus in 9 percent of their patients. Some, but not all, patients in their series who had received previous x-ray therapy developed erythema or "radiation recall" in irradiated areas.

Werner and Tornberg [89] followed eight patients with squamous cell carcinoma who received systemic bleomycin and who developed occasionally painful red plaques on the elbows (Fig. 5), knees, and face. Despite the fact that there was no ulceration observed clinically, biopsies of these lesions showed dyskeratosis, epidermal necrosis, dermal edema, and a perivascular mononuclear cell infiltrate.

Infiltrated nodules and plaques were also seen in the series of Cohen et al. [90]; however, these lesions were most commonly found on the hands. Histologically these lesions showed dermal sclerosis and appendageal entrapment similar to scleroderma. Blood vessel thickening was also noted. Although usually reversible when the medication was discontinued, one patient's sclerosis progressed to gangrene of the fingertips.

Raynaud's phenomenon occurs in patients who receive combination therapy with bleomycin and vincristine [91–94]. Whether this reaction is ac-

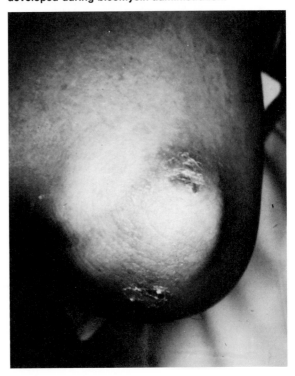

Fig. 5.   Crusted papules and nodules on the elbow that developed during bleomycin administration.

tually due to the bleomycin, the vincristine, or a synergism between the two drugs is uncertain at this time.

Reversible penile calcifications were described in one patient with lymphoma and hypercalcemia who was treated with bleomycin [95]. The possibility that the metastatic calcification observed was due to the tumor and the hypercalcemia rather than the bleomycin was also raised [96].

Hyperpigmentation may occur with bleomycin therapy. Generalized hyperpigmentation [87], hyperpigmentation over pressure areas such as joints [87,90], and pigmented banding of the nails [97] are well-documented complications. Linear streaks or "flagellate" hyperpigmentation is an unusual pigmentary reaction that has not been described with other chemotherapeutic agents (see Fig. 1, color plate). Some authors noted the progression of erythematous or urticarial pruritic swelling and subsequent hyperpigmentation of the excoriations due to scratching [86,87]. Attempts to reproduce these marks by scratching the skin while the patient was receiving bleomycin have been unsuccessful [90].

Onychodystrophy has also been reported with bleomycin therapy [86,90].

Actinomycin D (Dactinomycin)

Actinomycin D acts by binding to the guanine residues of DNA and thus inhibiting DNA-primed RNA synthesis. It is widely used in the treatment of Wilms' tumor, rhabdomyosarcomas, choriocarcinoma, lymphomas, testicular tumors, and Ewing's sarcoma.

Erythema and soreness of the buccal mucosa and tongue with or without ulcerations is a common complication of actinomycin therapy [98–101]. The severity of stomatitis increases with frequent administration of the drug [102]. Alopecia is usually noted 7 to 10 days after an intravenous course of actinomycin [101] and is inevitably transient in nature [98–100]. One patient who had dark, straight hair prior to her actinomycin-induced alopecia, regrew hair that was lighter in color and wavy [98].

Actinomycin D is an irritating chemical substance which may produce phlebitis along veins used for injection (see Fig. 2, color plate). Inadvertent extravasation of actinomycin D into normal tissue will produce severe local reaction (chemical cellulitis) with tissue necrosis [98,100].

Actinomycin D is frequently used in conjunction with radiation therapy and the occurrence of "ra-diation recall" and radiation hypersensitivity has been noted by several authors [98,100,101]. If the x-ray therapy is given simultaneously with the actinomycin, the degree of erythema at the portal site is much greater than would be expected from x-ray alone [101]. In fact, prospective studies demonstrated that in the presence of actinomycin D it takes only 25 percent of a normal dose of radiation to produce significant erythema [100]. Actinomycin D can also reactivate latent radiation effects in tissues that have been irradiated previously but have returned to normal appearance [103]. This radiation recall may occur a long time after the radiation has been administered, up to 17 months in one patient [101].

An unusual eruption, seemingly unique to actinomycin D, is an acneform eruption that was first described in 1969 by Epstein and Lutzner [104] (Fig. 6). The authors described nine patients receiving actinomycin D for testicular carcinoma or Ewing's sarcoma who developed erythema of the face on the fifth day of administration. Subsequently, over a 2- to 3-day period, papules and

Fig. 6.   Acneform eruption with pustules and papules secondary to actinomycin D therapy. *(From Adrian et al [3], with permission.)*

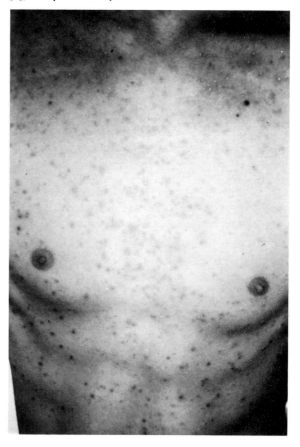

pustules appeared and the eruption spread to involve the chest, back, and occasionally the buttocks. The eruption resolved after 10 days, leaving only mild hyperpigmentation or discolored plugged follicles. Histologically, fully developed lesions showed invasion and replacement of the pilosebaceous units by neutrophils.

A syndrome characterized by fever, lethargy, and rash was reported to occur in 13 of 15 patients who were treated for Wilms' tumor with surgery, actinomycin D, and supervoltage irradiation [105]. The eruption, which was described as maculopapular, began on the abdomen or face, became generalized, and persisted for 5 to 10 days. In two patients the fever and eruption recurred with subsequent courses of actinomycin D.

Hypersensitivity characterized by urticaria has not been reported with actinomycin D; however, erythema multiforme has been described in two patients receiving the drug [98].

Doxorubicin (Adriamycin)

Doxorubicin is an anthracycline antitumor antibiotic that intercalates into the DNA helix and thus inhibits both DNA and RNA synthesis. It also is capable of preventing DNA repair and can damage preformed DNA. An agent with a broad antitumor spectrum, it is effective against acute leukemia, lymphomas, soft tissue sarcomas, breast carcinoma, and bladder carcinoma.

Severe alopecia occurs in almost all patients who receive doxorubicin [106,107]. Axillary and pubic hair may be lost in addition to scalp hair. Because doxorubicin is widely used and because chemotherapy-induced alopecia may be psychologically and emotionally debilitating, investigators have attempted to minimize this complication by a variety of techniques aimed toward reducing blood flow to the scalp during drug administration. Using a special pneumatic scalp tourniquet prior to, during, and for 15 min after injection of doxorubicin, Lovejoy [108], in a very small series of patients, was able to demonstrate significantly less hair loss than in a control group. In a larger series reported by Soukop and coworkers [109], the use of a scalp tourniquet merely delayed the development of doxorubicin-induced alopecia by 6 weeks.

Vasoconstriction produced by local scalp hypothermia has been reported to be effective in preventing severe hair loss with doxorubicin [110,111]. The use of crushed ice in plastic bags [110] seemed to be easier and less expensive than the use of cryogel packs [111]. These techniques may be useful when administering doxorubicin against solid tumors. However, the use of either the scalp tourniquet or hypothermia is not recommended for patients with hematologic malignancies because of the possible presence of malignant cells in the scalp.

The incidence of doxorubicin-induced stomatitis ranges from 12 to 80 percent [46,106]. This complication appears to be a function of the dose schedule, occuring less frequently as the interval increases between doses [106].

Hyperpigmentation may occur with doxorubicin therapy. This abnormality most commonly affects the nails [112–114] and appears as a longitudinal band of hypermelanosis 6 to 8 weeks after the initiation of chemotherapy [113] (see Fig. 3, color plate). Vertical banding has also been noted [115]. Hyperpigmentation may also occur in the palmar creases [122], palms and soles [114,116,117], dorsa of the knuckles [98], buccal mucosa [114], and tongue [118]. Doxorubicin-induced pigmentary changes occur more frequently in black patients [112] and are not associated with measurable alterations in serum α-MSH levels [117].

Doxorubicin is a potent vesicant and may produce a severe chemical cellulitis if inadvertently injected into the paravenous tissue [107,119,120]. Tissue reaction progresses from erythema and induration to ulceration (Fig. 7). If the extravasation occurs near joints, contractures may result. The ulcers that form are indolent and heal slowly, or not at all. Histologically these ulcers demonstrate epidermal necrosis, granulation tissue, fibrosis, and adjacent epidermal atrophy [121]. Progression to ulceration is not always prevented by early infiltration with steroids [122], and the

Fig. 7. Severe tissue necrosis after extravasation of doxorubicin. (Courtesy of Dr. Harris Blackman.)

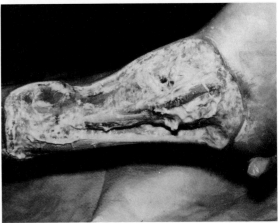

ulcers may require surgical excision and grafting [119,120].

An interesting tissue-injury recall phenomenon was reported by Cohen and coworkers [123]. They described a patient who developed chemical cellulitis and ulceration at the site of doxorubicin extravasation. Two months after the original extravasation, doxorubicin was readministered in a different extremity. Within 2 days the patient experienced pain, erythema, and increased tissue necrosis at the site of the original injury.

Another patient, who developed painful phlebitis at the site of doxorubicin injections in her right arm, was subsequently given daunorubicin in another extremity and developed a reexacerbation of the original phlebitis. This extends the spectrum of recall phenomenon to include any inflammatory reaction produced by doxorubicin and also suggests that daunorubicin and doxorubicin may cross-react with regard to this reaction [124].

Like actinomycin D, doxorubicin may enhance or recall radiation reactions [125,126]. If doxorubicin is administered before radiation, an eruption may occur at the portal site. This eruption appears 8 to 18 days after beginning radiation therapy and varies from mild desquamation and hyperpigmentation to a more severe eruption progressing from erythema and vesiculation to desquamation and hyperpigmentation [126]. When doxorubicin is given after radiation, erythema, edema, and pain may occur in the radiation portal [125] (Fig. 8). This phenomenon is more likely to occur if there was a preceding radiation dermatitis. Activation of this recall phenomenon may occur as late as 15 years after initial radiation [127].

Fig. 8. "Radiation recall." Severe erythema and blistering in a site of radiation, following administration of doxorubicin. *(From Adrian et al [3], with permission.)*

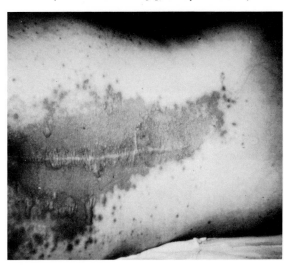

Solberg et al. [128] described a patient with leukemia cutis who received whole-body electron-beam irradiation followed by doxorubicin. She subsequently developed a generalized toxic epidermal necrolysis (TEN) and toxic megacolon and died. The TEN was thought to be a direct result of the electron beam–doxorubicin interaction; however, the patient had received multiple other medications, including antibiotics, which have been implicated in the causation of TEN. A direct cause-and-effect relationship can be only speculative.

Hypersensitivity reactions to doxorubicin have been documented, including generalized urticaria [129–131] and angioedema [132]. More commonly seen, however, is a localized urticaria in the area of drug injection [129,130,133]. The reaction is characterized by localized erythema and edema, with or without accompanying pruritus, occurring over the injected vein. The frequency of this so-called flare was 3 percent of administered doses in one series [133]. The reaction may or may not recur with the subsequent administration of doxorubicin; recurrences were not totally prevented by premedication with antihistamine. The mechanism by which this local urticaria is produced is not known. Because the reaction may occur with the initial exposure to the drug [129], it is difficult to postulate an allergic mechanism; however, a nonfatal episode of anaphylaxis has also been reported following a local flare [129], making it difficult to ignore the possibility of an IgE-mediated allergic reaction. Currently, the appearance of a localized urticarial reaction following doxorubicin administration is not considered an indication for discontinuing or changing the medication.

A case of contact dermatitis was reported in a laboratory technician who handled doxorubicin and daunomycin [134]. Both these agents fluoresce with exposure to ultraviolet radiation with a wavelength of 254 nm, and the characteristic red-orange fluorescence was observed in the patient's involved skin.

An uncommon reaction to doxorubicin described in one patient was characterized by onycholysis with blistering and desquamation of the palms and soles [135].

Daunorubicin (Daunomycin)

Daunorubicin is structurally similar to doxorubicin, lacking only a hydroxyl group at the C14. It is used almost exclusively in the treatment of acute leukemia.

Severe stomatitis is common with daunorubicin

[46]. Other mucocutaneous complications are infrequent. Pigmented transverse bands of hyperpigmentation involving the nails have been observed, similar to those seen with use of doxorubicin and other chemotherapeutic agents [136]. Extensive necrosis of skin and subcutaneous tissue of the fingers occurred in one patient to whom daunomycin was infused intravenously distal to an arteriovenous fistula [137]. The authors hypothesize that there was retrograde venous flow from the fistula into digital vessels, resulting in a high tissue concentration of the medication. Hypersensitivity reactions include generalized urticaria and angioedema localized to the arm of injection [138].

Mithramycin

Mithramycin is an antibiotic that inhibits the synthesis of RNA and is used in the treatment of testicular tumors, especially embryonal cell carcinoma.

Kennedy [139] followed 56 patients through 126 courses of mithramycin therapy and noted a unique dermatologic reaction in over 35 percent. This reaction began as macular erythema on the face and neck and progressed to deeper erythema with coarsening of the facial features. Scattered papules were also noted. The eruption gradually faded with desquamation and residual hyperpigmentation. Another transient rash, described as discrete erythematous papules on the face, neck, and upper trunk, was reported by Koons and colleagues [140] in 3 of 14 patients receiving mithramycin for embryonal carcinoma.

Stomatitis is seen in approximately 15 percent of patients on this drug [139]. Chemical cellulitis and ulceration may occur at the site of mithramycin extravasation [141,142]. Reactivation of tissue injury was precipitated by sun exposure in one patient 3 months after the initial extravasation [143].

A more serious complication of mithramycin therapy is the development of TEN. Reported in two patients, it proved fatal in one case [144,145].

Vinca Alkaloids

The *Vinca* alkaloids (Table 5), vincristine (Oncovin) and vinblastine (Velban), are derived from the periwinkle, a perennial plant widely cultivated in gardens throughout the world. These large and complex molecules interrupt cell division in metaphase by interfering with microtubule function. The *Vinca* alkaloids are thought to be cell

Table 5 Cutaneous reactions secondary to the *Vinca* alkaloids

Vincristine
  Alopecia
  Chemical cellulitis
Vinblastine
  Alopecia
  Stomatitis
  Chemical cellulitis
  Phlebitis
  Photosensitivity

cycle phase–specific. Structurally quite similar, the two drugs share many clinical uses and toxicities.

Vincristine (Oncovin)

Vincristine is used principally in combination with prednisone and other chemotherapeutic agents to treat Hodgkin's disease, non-Hodgkin's lymphomas, and acute lymphoblastic leukemia.

Reversible alopecia is a common complication of vincristine therapy [146], and regrown hair may be more pigmented and curly than previously [147]. Stomatitis is uncommon [146,147].

Chemical cellulitis at the site of extravasation may result in vesiculation and ulceration of the epidermis [147]. If vincristine is administered to a patient with a fresh surgical wound, a significant amount of the drug may ooze into the wound. This results in inflammation, induration, necrosis, and impaired wound healing [148].

Vinblastine (Velban)

Vinblastine is used in the treatment of Hodgkin's disease, some testicular tumors, other lymphomas, histiocytic malignancies, and breast cancer.

Variable, mild alopecia and stomatitis may occur, as with vincristine. As with vincristine, extravasation of vinblastine may produce painful erythema, edema, and induration which may take weeks to resolve [149,150]. Phlebitis limited to the vein used to inject vinblastine has also been reported [151].

A photosensitivity reaction occurred in a patient with Hodgkin's disease who was receiving vinblastine. Spectrophotometric studies demonstrated that the absorption for vinblastine was in the UVB range [152]. The important implication is that patients receiving this drug should be warned about possible sun intolerance and advised to use an appropriately protective sunscreen.

As mentioned in the section on bleomycin, Raynaud's phenomenon has been reported in patients receiving the combination of vinblastine and bleomycin [91].

Verified hypersensitivity to the *Vinca* alkaloids has not yet been reported [153].

Miscellaneous Agents (Table 6)

Procarbazine

Procarbazine is a derivative of methylhydrazine, which was originally synthesized as a monoamine oxidase inhibitor. Although the exact mechanism of action of procarbazine as a chemotherapeutic agent has not yet been clearly defined, it is thought that metabolites of procarbazine inhibit DNA synthesis. This drug is cell cycle phase–nonspecific. Procarbazine is used primarily in combination drug therapy for patients with advanced Hodgkin's disease.

Cutaneous complications associated with procarbazine administration are uncommon but include alopecia [154], stomatitis, urticaria [153,155,156], and a maculopapular rash [154,157]. One patient receiving procarbazine developed urticaria, angioedema, and arthralgias which were associated with a marked fall in serum complement activity [158].

L-Asparaginase

L-Asparaginase, a polypeptide enzyme with antitumor activity, is derived from *Escherichia coli*. By destroying extracellular supplies of L-aspara-

gine, L-asparaginase indirectly contributes to the demise of cancer cells that are unable to produce this amino acid. Although it may block some cells in G or S phase, this drug is considered to be cell cycle phase–nonspecific. L-Asparaginase is primarily useful in treating acute lymphocytic leukemia.

Of all anticancer drugs, L-asparaginase has the highest prevalence of hypersensitivity reactions [153]. Urticaria is a common manifestation of hypersensitivity but other reactions include respiratory symptoms, hypotension, dyspnea, serum sickness–like reactions, and anaphylaxis [159–161]. L-Asparaginase hypersensitivity is mediated by IgE [162] but IgG and IgM antibodies have also been detected in the serum of patients receiving this agent [160]. Interestingly, hypersensitivity reactions occur more commonly in patients receiving L-asparaginase as a single agent [159,161]. It is hypothesized that the additional chemotherapeutic agents in combination regimens are capable of producing sufficient immunosuppression to prevent the development of hypersensitivity [152,163].

Generalized and localized "rashes" as well as itching and swelling of the feet have been reported [163].

Hydroxyurea

Hydroxyurea is an antineoplastic agent that inhibits ribonucleotide reductase, an enzyme essential to DNA synthesis. It is cytotoxic to cells that are synthesizing DNA and is therefore an S phase–specific agent. Hydroxyurea is used primarily by oncologists in the treatment of busulfan-resistant chronic myelogenous leukemia and occasionally by dermatologists in the treatment of psoriasis.

Most cutaneous complications from hydroxyurea have been described in patients on long-term maintenance therapy who were receiving daily rather than intermittent doses of the drug. Kennedy and coworkers [164] described cutaneous changes in 7 of 20 patients receiving daily hydroxyurea for chronic myelogenous leukemia; these changes consisted of alopecia, hyperpigmentation, scaling, violaceous papular, and/or atrophic lesions resembling lichen planus, and onychodystrophy. Biopsies of the violaceous lesions revealed hyperkeratosis, hypergranulosis, epidermal atrophy, basilar vacuolization, and scattered dyskeratotic cells.

Moschella and Greenwald [165] treated 60 psoriatic patients with hydroxyurea and reported the occurrence of a palpable purpuric eruption on the lower extremities of two patients. These patients

Table 6   Reactions associated with miscellaneous chemotherapeutic agents

Procarbazine
  Alopecia
  Stomatitis
  Urticaria
  Angioedema
  Maculopapular rash

L-Asparaginase
  Urticaria
  Generalized or localized rashes
  Pruritus and swelling of the feet

Hydroxyurea
  Lichen planus–like eruption
  Hyperpigmentation
  Palpable purpura
  Onychodystrophy
  Alopecia

also experienced a flulike syndrome consisting of fever, chills, malaise, and myalgia. Biopsies of these lesions revealed a necrotizing venulitis. Similar lesions were also reported in the absence of systemic symptoms [166].

Fixed drug eruption has been reported in one patient [165].

Conclusion

In conclusion, the cutaneous complications associated with chemotherapeutic agents are numerous and varied in their presentations. Because of the multiplicity of medications patients are often receiving, it may be difficult to ascribe a particular reaction to one particular drug. Verification of reactions will occur with the gradual accumulation of data and careful documentation of cutaneous changes with photography and histology. Hopefully by studying such reactions we will learn more about the pharmacokinetics of these powerful medications as well as the capacity of the skin to react to injury and stimulus.

References

1. Levantine A, Almeyda J: Cutaneous reactions to cytostatic agents. *Br J Dermatol* **90**:239–242, 1974
2. Levine N, Greenwald ES: Mucocutaneous side effects of cancer chemotherapy. *Cancer Treat Rep* **5**:67–84, 1978
3. Adrian RM et al: Mucocutaneous reactions to antineoplastic agents. *CA* **30**:143–157, 1980
4. Nixon DW et al: Dermatologic changes after systemic cancer therapy. *Cutis* **27**:181–194, 1981
5. Spear PW, Patno ME: A comparative study of the effectiveness of HN₂ and cyclophosphamide in bronchogenic carcinoma, Hodgkin's disease and lymphosarcoma. *Cancer Chemother Rep* **16**:413–415, 1962
6. Wall RL, Conrad FG: Cyclophosphamide therapy. *Arch Intern Med* **108**:456–482, 1961
7. Romankiewicz JA: Cyclophosphamide and pigmentation. *Am J Hosp Pharm* **31**:1074–1075, 1974
8. Thurman WG et al: Cyclophosphamide therapy in childhood neuroblastoma. *N Engl J Med* **270**:1336–1340, 1964
9. Inalsingh CH: Melanonchia after treatment of malignant disease with radiation and cyclophosphamide. *Arch Dermatol* **106**:765–766, 1972
10. Shah PC et al: Cyclophosphamide-induced nail pigmentation. *Lancet* **2**:548–549, 1975
11. Markerson AL et al: Hyperpigmentation after cancer chemotherapy. *Lancet* **2**:128, 1975
12. Harrison BM, Wood CBS: Cyclophosphamide and pigmentation. *Br Med J* **1**:352, 1972
13. Murti L, Horsman LR: Acute hypersensitivity reaction to cyclophosphamide. *J Pediatr* **94**:844–845, 1979
14. Karchmer RK, Hansen VL: Possible anaphylactic reaction to intravenous cyclophosphamide: report of a case. *JAMA* **237**:475, 1977
15. Ross WE, Chabner BA: Allergic reaction to cyclophosphamide in a mechlorethamine-sensitive patient. *Cancer Treat Rep* **61**:495–496, 1977
16. Legha SS, Hall S: Acute cyclophosphamide hypersensitivity reaction: possible lack of cross-sensitivity to mechlorethamine and isophosphamide. *Cancer Treat Rep* **62**:180–181, 1978
17. Lakin JD, Cahill RA: Generalized urticaria to cyclophosphamide: type I hypersensitivity to an immunosuppressive agent. *J Allergy Clin Immunol* **58**:160–171, 1976
18. Krutchik AN et al: Cyclophosphamide-induced urticaria: occurrence in a patient with no cross-sensitivity to chlorambucil. *Arch Intern Med* **138**:1725–1726, 1978
19. Brauer MJ et al: Hypersensitivity to nitrogen mustards in the form of erythema multiforme: a unique adverse reaction. *Arch Intern Med* **120**:499–503, 1967
20. Van Scott EJ, Winters PL: Responses of mycosis fungoides to intensive external treatment with nitrogen mustard. *Arch Dermatol* **102**:507–514, 1970
21. Waldorf DS et al: Cutaneous hypersensitivity and desensitization to mechlorethamine in patients with mycosis fungoides lymphoma. *Ann Intern Med* **67**:282–290, 1967
22. Epstein EH Jr, Ugel AR: Effects of topical mechlorethamine on skin lesions of psoriasis. *Arch Dermatol* **102**:504–506, 1970
23. Mandy S et al: Topically applied mechlorethamine in the treatment of psoriasis. *Arch Dermatol* **103**:272–276, 1971
24. Flaxman BA et al: Changes in melanosome distribution in Caucasoid skin following topical application of nitrogen mustard. *J Invest Dermatol* **60**:321–326, 1973
25. Daughters D et al: Urticaria and anaphylactoid reactions after topical application of mechlorethamine. *Arch Dermatol* **107**:429–430, 1973
26. Knisley RE et al: Unusual reaction to chlorambucil in a patient with CLL. *Arch Dermatol* **104**:77–79, 1971
27. Millard LG, Rajah SM: Cutaneous reaction to chlorambucil. *Arch Dermatol* **113**:1298, 1977
28. Lawrence BV et al: Anaphylaxis due to oral melphalan. *Cancer Treat Rep* **64**:731–732, 1980
29. Cornwell GG et al: Hypersensitivity reactions to iv melphalan during treatment of multiple myeloma: cancer and leukemia group B experience. *Cancer Treat Rep* **63**:399–403, 1979
30. Irvine WT, Luck RJ: Review of regional limb perfusion with melphalan for malignant melanoma. *Br Med J* **1**:770–774, 1966
31. Galton DA: Myleran in chronic myeloid leukemia: results of treatment. *Lancet* **1**:208–213, 1953
32. Haut A et al: Busulfan in the treatment of chronic myelocytic leukemia. The effect of long term intermittent therapy. *Blood* **17**:1–19, 1961
33. Feingold ML, Koss LG: Effects of long-term administration of busulfan. *Arch Intern Med* **124**:66–71, 1969
34. Dahlgren S et al: Clinical and morphological side-effects of busulfan (Myleran) treatment. *Acta Med Scand* **192**:129–135, 1972
35. Kyle RA et al: A syndrome resembling adrenal cortical insufficiency associated with long term busulfan (Myleran) therapy. *Blood* **18**:497–510, 1961
36. Harrold BP: Syndrome resembling Addison's disease following prolonged treatment with busulfan. *Br Med J* **1**:463–464, 1966
37. Kyle RA, Dameshek W: Porphyria cutanea tarda associated with chronic granulocytic leukemia treated with busulfan. *Blood* **23**:776–785, 1964
38. Dosik H et al: Bullous eruption and elevated leukocyte

alkaline phosphatase in the course of busulfan-treated chronic granulocytic leukemia. *Blood* **35:**543–548, 1970

39. Veenema RJ et al: Thiotepa bladder instillations: therapy and prophylaxis for superficial bladder tumors. *J Urol* **101:**711–715, 1969

40. Asregadoo ER: Surgery, thio-TEPA, and corticosteroid in the treatment of pterygium. *Am J Ophthalmol* **74:**960–963, 1972

41. Howitt D, Karp EJ: Side-effect of topical thio-TEPA. *Am J Ophthalmol* **68:**473–474, 1969

42. Beck TM et al: Photosensitivity reaction following DTIC administration: report of two cases. *Cancer Treat Rep* **64:**725–726, 1980

43. Bono VH Jr: Studies on the mechanism of action of DTIC (NSC-45388). *Cancer Treat Rep* **60:**141–148, 1976

44. Wasserman TH: The nitrosoureas: an outline of clinical schedules and toxic effects. *Cancer Treat Rep* **60:**709–711, 1976

45. Frost P, DeVita VT: Pigmentation due to a new antitumor agent: effects of topical application of BCNU. *Arch Dermatol* **94:**265–268, 1966

46. Dreizens S et al: Chemotherapy-induced oral mucositis in adult leukemia. *Postgrad Med* **69:**103–112, 1981

47. Weinstein GD: Drugs five years later: methotrexate. *Ann Intern Med* **86:**199–204, 1977

48. Ratnam SS et al: Methotrexate for prophylaxis of choriocarcinoma. *Am J Obstet Gynecol* **111:**1021–1027, 1971

49. Delmonte L, Jukes TH: Folic acid antagonists in cancer chemotherapy. *Pharmacol Rev* **14:**91–135, 1962

50. Vogler WR et al: Toxicity and antitumor effect of divided doses of methotrexate. *Arch Intern Med* **115:**285–293, 1965

51. Jaffe N et al: Favorable response of metastatic osteogenic sarcoma to pulse high-dose methotrexate with citrovorum rescue and radiation therapy. *Cancer* **31:**1367–1373, 1973

52. Djerassi I, Rominger J: Phase I study of high doses of methotrexate with citrovorum factor in patients with lung cancer. *Cancer* **30:**22–30, 1972

53. Berkowitz RS et al: Methotrexate with citrovorum factor rescue: reduced chemotherapy toxicity in the management of gestational trophoblastic neoplasms. *Cancer* **45:**423–426, 1980

54. Lanzkowsky P et al: Vasculitis as a complication of high-dose methotrexate in the treatment of acute leukemia. *Am J Dis Child* **130:**675, 1976

55. Bell R et al: Toxic rash associated with high dose methotrexate therapy. *Clin Exp Pharmacol Physiol* **5:**57–61, 1979

56. Lyell A: Psoriasis and folic acid antagonists. *Br J Dermatol* **79:**367, 1967

57. Rosen G et al: Combination chemotherapy and radiation therapy in the treatment of metastatic osteogenic sarcoma. *Cancer* **35:**622–630, 1975

58. Kim YH et al: Radiation necrosis of the scalp: a complication of cranial irradiation and methotrexate. *Radiology* **124:**813–814, 1977

59. Vogler WR, Jacobs J: Toxic and therapeutic effects of methotrexate-folinic acid (leukovorin) in advanced cancer and leukemia. *Cancer* **28:**894–900, 1971

60. Corder MP, Stone WH: Failure of leukovorin rescue to prevent reactivation of a solar burn after high dose methotrexate. *Cancer* **37:**1660–1662, 1976

61. Korossy KS, Hood AF: Methotrexate reactivation of sunburn reaction. *Arch Dermatol* **117:**310–311, 1981

62. Möller H: Reactivation of acute inflammation by methotrexate. *J Invest Dermatol* **52:**437–441, 1969

63. Weinstein GD, Frost P: Methotrexate for psoriasis: a new therapeutic schedule. *Arch Dermatol* **103:**33–38, 1971

64. Van Scott EJ et al: Parenteral methotrexate in psoriasis. *Arch Dermatol* **89:**550–556, 1964

65. Goldberg NH et al: Anaphylactoid type reactions in two patients receiving high-dose methotrexate. *Cancer* **41:**52–55, 1978

66. Gluck-Kuyt I, Irwin LE: Anaphylactic reaction to high-dose methotrexate. *Cancer Treat Rep* **63:**797–798, 1979

67. Kennedy BJ, Theologides A: The role of 5-fluorouracil in malignant disease. *Ann Intern Med* **55:**719–730, 1961

68. Ansfield FJ et al: Five years clinical experience with 5-fluorouracil. *JAMA* **181:**295–299, 1962

69. Ivy HK: Treatment of breast cancer with 5-fluorouracil. *Ann Intern Med* **57:**598–605, 1962

70. Vaitkevicius VK et al: Clinical evaluation of cancer chemotherapy with 5-fluorouracil. *Cancer* **14:**131–152, 1961

71. Falkson G, Schulz EJ: Skin changes in patients treated with 5-fluorouracil. *Br J Dermatol* **74:**229–236, 1962

72. Greenwald ES: Fluorouracil. *JAMA* **232:**1126–1127, 1975

73. Hrushesky WJ: Serpentine supravenous 5-fluorouracil hyperpigmentation. *Cancer Treat Rep* **60:**639, 1976

74. Omura EF, Torre D: Inflammation of actinic keratoses due to systemic fluorouracil therapy. *JAMA* **208:**150–151, 1969

75. Schlang HA, Curtin R: Inflammation of malignant skin involvement with fluorouracil. *JAMA* **238:**1722, 1977

76. Sams WM: Untoward response with topical fluorouracil. *Arch Dermatol* **97:**14–19, 1968

77. Goette DK et al: Allergic contact dermatitis from topical fluorouracil. *Arch Dermatol* **113:**196–198, 1977

78. Burnett JW: Two unusual complications of topical fluorouracil therapy. *Arch Dermatol* **111:**398, 1975

79. Kaplan LA et al: Hypertrophic scarring as a complication of fluorouracil therapy. *Arch Dermatol* **115:**1452, 1979

80. Bart BJ, Bean SF: Bullous pemphigoid following topical use of fluorouracil. *Arch Dermatol* **102:**457–460, 1970

81. Bernstein T: Skin reactions to 5-fluorouracil. *N Engl J Med* **297:**337–338, 1977

82. Ellison RR et al: Comparative study of 6-chloropurine and 6-mercaptopurine in acute leukemia in adults. *Ann Intern Med* **51:**322–338, 1959

83. Nitschke R et al: Toxicity study of cytosine arabinoside and methotrexate in the maintenance therapy of childhood leukemia. *J Clin Pharmacol* **18:**131–135, 1978

84. Kechijian P et al: Cytarabine-induced inflammation in the seborrheic keratoses of Leser-Trelat. *Ann Intern Med* **91:**868–869, 1979

85. Blum RH et al: A clinical review of bleomycin—a new antineoplastic agent. *Cancer* **31:**903–914, 1973

86. Yagoda A et al: Bleomycin, an antitumor antibiotic. *Ann Intern Med* **77:**861–870, 1972

87. Ohnuma T et al: Clinical study with bleomycin: tolerance to twice weekly dosage. *Cancer* **30:**914–922, 1972

88. Shastri S et al: Clinical study with bleomycin. *Cancer* **28:**1142–1146, 1971

89. Werner Y, Tornberg B: Cutaneous side effects of bleomycin therapy. *Acta Derm Venereol (Stockh)* **56:**155–158, 1976

90. Cohen IS et al: Cutaneous toxicity of bleomycin therapy. *Arch Dermatol* **107:**553–555, 1973

91. Teutch C et al: Raynaud's phenomenon as a side effect of chemotherapy with vinblastine and bleomycin for testicular carcinoma. *Cancer Treat Rep* **61:**925–926, 1977

92. Soble AR: Chronic bleomycin-associated Raynaud's phenomenon. *Cancer Treat Rep* **62**:570, 1978

93. Chernicoff DP et al: Raynaud's phenomenon after bleomycin treatment. *Cancer Treat Rep* **62**:570–571, 1978

94. Rothberg H: Raynaud's phenomenon after vinblastine-bleomycin chemotherapy. *Cancer Treat Rep* **62**:569–570, 1978

95. Ihde DC et al: Reversible penile calcifications associated with bleomycin-induced pulmonary toxicity. *Cancer Chemother Rep* **59**:1039–1041, 1975

96. Gorshein D: Soft tissue metastatic calcification and bleomycin therapy. *Cancer Treat Rep* **60**:963, 1976

97. Shetty MR: Case of pigmented banding of the nail caused by bleomycin. *Cancer Treat Rep* **61**:501–502, 1977

98. Keidan SE: Actinomycin D in the treatment of carcinoma in children. *Br J Surg* **53**:614–618, 1966

99. Berkowitz RS et al: Methotrexate with citrovorum factor rescue: reduced chemotherapy toxicity in the management of gestational trophoblastic neoplasms. *Cancer* **45**:423–426, 1980

100. Frei E III: The clinical use of actinomycin. *Cancer Chemother Rep* **58**:49–54, 1974

101. Tan CTC et al: The effect of actinomycin D on cancer in childhood. *Pediatrics* **24**:544–561, 1959

102. Petrilli ES, Morrow CP: Actinomycin D toxicity in the treatment of trophoblastic disease: a comparison of the five-day course to single-dose administration. *Gynecol Oncol* **9**:18–22, 1980

103. D'Angio GJ et al: Potentiation of x-ray effects by actinomycin D. *Radiology* **73**:175–177, 1959

104. Epstein EH, Lutzner MH: Folliculitis induced by actinomycin D. *N Engl J Med* **281**:1094–1096, 1969

105. Cassady JR et al: Fever, lethergy and rash complicating treatment for Wilms' tumor—a new syndrome. *Radiology* **115**:171–174, 1975

106. Blum RH, Carter SK: Adriamycin. A new anticancer drug with significant clinical activity. *Ann Intern Med* **80**:249–259, 1974

107. Wang JJ et al: Therapeutic effect and toxicity of adriamycin in patients with neoplastic disease. *Cancer* **28**:837–843, 1971

108. Lovejoy NC: Preventing hair loss during adriamycin therapy. *Cancer Nurs* **2**:117–121, 1979

109. Soukop M et al: Adriamycin, alopecia and the scalp tourniquet. *Cancer Treat Rep* **62**:489–490, 1978

110. Dean JC et al: Prevention of doxorubicin-induced hair loss with scalp hypothermia. *N Engl J Med* **301**:1427–1429, 1979

111. Edelstyn GA, MacRae KD: Doxorubicin-induced hair loss and possible modification by scalp cooling. *Lancet* **2**:253–254, 1977

112. Pratt CB, Shanks EC: Hyperpigmentation of nails from doxorubicin. *JAMA* **228**:460, 1974

113. Morris D et al: Horizontal pigmented banding of the nails in association with adriamycin chemotherapy. *Cancer Treat Rep* **61**:499–501, 1977

114. Rothberg H et al: Adriamycin toxicity: unusual melanotic reaction. *Cancer Chemother Rep* **58**:749–751, 1974

115. Priestman TJ, James KW: Adriamycin and longitudinal pigmented banding of fingernails. *Lancet* **1**:1337–1338, 1975

116. Law IP: Doxorubicin and unusual skin manifestations. *Arch Dermatol* **113**:379–380, 1977

117. Kew MC et al: Melanocyte-stimulating-hormone levels in doxorubicin-induced hyperpigmentation. *Lancet* **1**:811, 1977

118. Rao SP et al: Pigmentation of the tongue after treatment with adriamycin. *Cancer Treat Rep* **60**:1402–1404, 1976

119. Reilly JJ et al: Clinical course and management of accidental adriamycin extravasation. *Cancer* **40**:2053–2056, 1977

120. Rudolph R et al: Skin ulcers due to adriamycin. *Cancer* **38**:1087–1094, 1976

121. Rudolph R et al: Experimental skin necrosis produced by adriamycin. *Cancer Treat Rep* **63**:529–537, 1979

122. Cohen MH: Amelioration of adriamycin skin necrosis: an experimental study. *Cancer Treat Rep* **64**:1003–1004, 1979

123. Cohen SC et al: Recall injury from adriamycin. *Ann Intern Med* **83**:232, 1975

124. Baer D, Wilkinson LS: Daunomycin, adriamycin and recall effect. *Ann Intern Med* **85**:259–260, 1976

125. Donaldson SS et al: Adriamycin activating and recall phenomenon after radiation therapy. *Ann Intern Med* **81**:407–408, 1974

126. Greco FA et al: Adriamycin and enhanced radiation reaction in normal esophagus and skin. *Ann Intern Med* **85**:294–298, 1976

127. Burdon J et al: Adriamycin-induced recall phenomenon 15 years after radiotherapy. *JAMA* **10**:931, 1978

128. Solberg LA Jr et al: Doxorubicin-enhanced skin reaction after whole-body electron-beam irradiation for leukemia cutis. *Mayo Clin Proc* **55**:711–715, 1980

129. Etcubanas E, Wilbur JR: Uncommon side effects of adriamycin. *Cancer Chemother Rep* **58**:757–758, 1974

130. Souhami L, Feld R: Urticaria following intravenous doxorubicin administration. *JAMA* **240**:1624–1626, 1978

131. Fallah-Sohy E, Figueredo AT: Allergic reaction to doxorubicin. *JAMA* **241**:1108–1109, 1979

132. Maldonado JE: Angioneurotic edema from doxorubicin. *N Engl J Med* **301**:386, 1979

133. Vogelzang NJ: "Adriamycin flare": a skin reaction resembling extravasation. *Cancer Treat Rep* **63**:11–12, 1979

134. Reich SD, Bachur NR: Contact dermatitis associated with adriamycin (NSC-123127) and daunorubicin (NSC-82151). *Cancer Chemother Rep* **59**:677–678, 1975

135. Manalo FB et al: Doxorubicin toxicity. Onycholysis, plantar callus formation and epidermolysis. *JAMA* **233**:56–57, 1975

136. deMarinis M et al: Nail pigmentation with daunorubicin therapy. *Ann Intern Med* **89**:516–517, 1978

137. Dragon LH, Braine HG: Necrosis of the hand after daunorubicin infusion distal to an arteriovenous fistula. *Ann Intern Med* **91**:58–59, 1979

138. Freeman AI: Clinical note: allergic reaction to daunomycin. *Cancer Chemother Rep* **54**:475–476, 1970

139. Kennedy BJ: Metabolic and toxic effects of mithramycin during tumor therapy. *Am J Med* **49**:494–503, 1970

140. Koons CR et al: Clinical studies of mithramycin in patients with embryonal cancer. *Bull Johns Hopkins Hosp* **118**:462–475, 1966

141. Duvall E, Baumann B: An unusual accident during the administration of chemotherapy. *Cancer Nurs* **3**:305–306, 1980

142. Ignoffo RJ, Friedman MA: Therapy of local toxic extravasation of cancer chemotherapeutic drugs. *Cancer Treat Rev* **7**:17–27, 1980

143. Fuller B et al: Mitomycin C extravasation exacerbated by sunlight. *Ann Intern Med* **94**:542, 1981

144. Purpora D et al: Toxic epidermal necrolysis after mithramycin. *N Engl J Med* **299**:1412, 1978

145. Eyster FE et al: Mithramycin as a possible cause of toxic epidermal necrolysis. *Calif Med* **114**:42–43, 1971

146. Heyn RM et al: Vincristine in the treatment of acute leukemia in children. *Pediatrics* **38**:82–91, 1966

147. Holland JF et al: Vincristine treatment of advanced cancer: a cooperative study of 392 cases. *Cancer Res* **33**:1258–1264, 1973

148. Forte FA: Vincristine neuropathy. *JAMA* **227**:325, 1974

149. Sohier WF Jr et al: Vinblastine in the treatment of advanced Hodgkin's disease. *Cancer* **22**:467–472, 1968

150. Lacher MJ: Vinblastine sulfate in Hodgkin's disease. *NY State J Med* **69**:808–814, 1969

151. Martin VH, Schubert JCF: Behandlung der Lymphogranulomatose mit Vincaleukoblastin. *Blut* **16**:157–160, 1967

152. Breza TS et al: Photosensitivity reaction to vinblastine. *Arch Dermatol* **111**:1168–1170, 1975

153. Weiss RB, Bruno S: Hypersensitivity reactions to cancer chemotherapeutic agents. *Ann Intern Med* **94**:66–72, 1981

154. Stolinsky DC et al: Procarbazine HCl in Hodgkin's disease, reticulum cell sarcoma, and lymphosarcoma. *Proc Am Assoc Cancer Res* **10**:88, 1969

155. Brunner KW, Young CW: A methylhydrazine derivative in Hodgkin's disease and other malignant neoplasms: therapeutic and toxic effects studied in 51 patients. *Ann Intern Med* **63**:69–86, 1965

156. Jones SE et al: Hypersensitivity to procarbazine (Matulane) manifested by fever and pleuropulmonary reaction. *Cancer* **29**:498–500, 1972

157. Lokich JJ, Moloney WC: Allergic reaction to procarbazine. *Clin Pharmacol Ther* **13**:573–574, 1972

158. Glovsky MM et al: Hypersensitivity to procarbazine associated with angioedema, urticaria and low serum complement activity. *J Allergy Clin Immunol* **57**:134–140, 1976

159. Oettgen HF et al: Toxicity of *E. coli* L-asparaginase in man. *Cancer* **25**:253–278, 1970

160. Killander D et al: Hypersensitive reactions and antibody formation during L-asparaginase treatment of children and adults with acute leukemia. *Cancer* **37**:220–228, 1976

161. Haskell CM et al: L-Asparaginase. Therapeutic and toxic effects in patients with neoplastic disease. *N Engl J Med* **281**:1028–1034, 1969

162. Khan A, Hill JM: Atopic hypersensitivity to L-asparaginase. *Int Arch Allergy* **40**:463–469, 1971

163. Ertel IJ et al: Effective dose of L-asparaginase for induction of remission in previously treated children with acute lymphocytic leukemia: a report from Childrens Cancer Study Group. *Cancer Res* **39**:3893–3896, 1979

164. Kennedy BJ et al: Skin changes secondary to hydroxyurea therapy. *Arch Dermatol* **111**:183–187, 1975

165. Moschella SL, Greenwald MA: Psoriasis with hydroxyurea: an 18-month study of 60 patients. *Arch Dermatol* **107**:363–368, 1973

166. Roe LD, Wilson JW: Hydroxyurea therapy. *Arch Dermatol* **108**:426–427, 1973

PRIMARY MELANOMA OF THE SKIN
Recognition of Precursor Lesions and Estimation of Prognosis in Stage I

Arthur J. Sober

Arthur R. Rhodes

Calvin L. Day, Jr.

Thomas B. Fitzpatrick

Martin C. Mihm, Jr.

For reasons that are not yet clear, primary melanoma of the skin of white people has increased in incidence by more than 500 percent in the past 4 decades (Connecticut Tumor Registry). No type of therapy (chemotherapy, immunotherapy, or radiation therapy) of stage II* and stage III melanoma has improved the survival rates. Yet the overall survival rate has increased from a 67 percent 5-year survival rate in 1967 to an 82 percent 5-year survival rate in 1980. This is most probably related to increased recognition of early stage I disease with excision of the primary. Excision of early primary melanoma of the skin and possibly prophylactic elective regional node dissections are the only therapies at present that affect the prognosis of this neoplasm, one that is still increasing at an alarming rate.

The recognition of early melanoma has been championed for the past decade and now the concentration is on one step earlier—the precursor lesions of primary melanoma: (1) lentigo maligna, (2) congenital melanocytic nevi, and a newly discovered lesion, (3) the dysplastic nevus. Dysplastic nevi are especially important as they occur in families as well as sporadically; it is the obligation of every physician to learn to identify these unique pigment cell neoplasms that are distinctive in their clinical features and in their histology from the common melanocytic nevus cell nevi.

---

* For explanation of the clinical and histologic stages of melanoma, see Table 1.

The prognosis of stage II and stage III melanoma is quite clear at present: (1) All patients with stage III disease (distant metastases) will die of their disease despite any existing therapy, and (2) nearly all patients with regional nodes large enough to detect by palpation (stage II) will die by 10 years. What is not yet clear is the prognosis of stage I disease (primary melanoma without palpable lymph nodes). Using sophisticated statistical analyses (Cox proportional hazards multivariate analyses) of large numbers of patients, there are now new diagnostic criteria of the primary melanoma in addition to the thickness of the lesion; these include: (1) body location of the primary, (2) presence or absence of ulceration, (3) the mitotic rate, (4) the lymphocytic response, and (5) the number of positive regional lymph nodes. These criteria are essential in the selection of those patients who require radical lymph node dissection or immunotherapy and chemotherapy.

Precursor Lesions for Melanoma

Among the numerous pigmented lesions confronting the physician there are several distinct types known or suspected to be capable of developing into malignant melanoma, as noted above. These precursor lesions are described and the relative risk and weight of evidence for each assessed.

Lentigo Maligna

Historically, the lentigo maligna (LM) was the first precursor lesion to be delineated [1–3], although the first case of melanoma reported in the English literature, that of Norris [4] in 1920, probably arose within a congenital nevus in the context of familial melanoma (see below). The LM is a flat (macular) pigmented lesion which occurs nearly exclusively on sun-exposed surfaces in elderly patients with sun-damaged atrophic skin [5]. It begins as a tan, freckle-like lesion of irregular shape. The vast majority of LM occur on the head and neck or on the upper extremities. They appear late in life, usually in the fifth or sixth decades. The lesion is tan-brown to black with a highly irregular pigment pattern and border. Regression is also a prominent feature. The lesion grows by apparent radial spread, increasing in size and assuming a variety of irregular shapes (Fig. 1). In its preinvasive phase, the LM is flat. Grossly, the lesion may look like a "stain" in the skin. Different pigmentation patterns include the appearance of dark brown, reticulate shapes or the appearance of irregular dark brown or black freckling. Amelanoic lesions have been reported (rare event) [6]. The lesion may grow slowly and develop into lentigo maligna melanoma (LMM) with a latency period of from 5 to 50 years. The median age at diagnosis for patients with LMM in the Melanoma Clinical Cooperative Group (MCCG) series was 70 years (range: 47 to 94 years) [7]. It has been estimated that perhaps only 30 percent of LM ever develop into invasive melanoma [8,9]. In the MCCG series, LMM represented only 5 percent of all cases of melanoma [7].

The histopathology is characterized by an atrophic epidermis with thinning and loss of rete ridges, containing increased numbers of highly atypical basilar melanocytes. One to another, these melanocytes are very different in appearance, vary in size and shape, and have nuclei of different sizes that are irregularly hyperchromatic. The cytoplasm of these cells, which is usually shrunken around the nucleus, leaving a space between the cell borders and adjacent melanocytes, is pink to purple to red-brown and is irregularly granular. These cells may extend down hair follicles and

Fig. 1. Lentigo maligna displaying irregular borders and irregular pigment pattern.

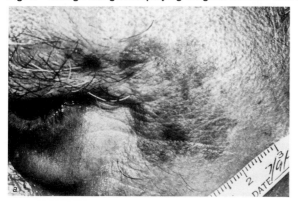
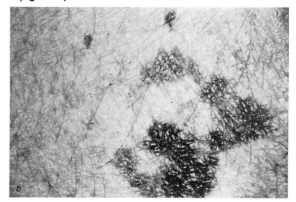

skin appendages, making the lesion difficult to erradicate by superficial therapies. A mononuclear cell infiltrate is characteristically present in the superficial lesions below the proliferated melanocytes. The dermis shows elastotic changes of the connective tissue from chronic sun damage.

Diagnosis can usually be established by biopsy of the darkest portion or any palpable portion. Occasionally the histopathology will not be diagnostic, and rebiopsy will be necessary or repeat biopsy over time with close observation [10].

Management ranges from no therapy (may be acceptable in very elderly patients in poor health) to superficial removal (grenz, 5-fluorouracil, dermabrasion, cryotherapy), which often results in recurrence, to surgical excision [10] or irradiation with standard orthovoltage techniques [11].

Congenital Melanocytic Nevi

The second lesion with an established premalignant potential is the "giant" congenital melanocytic nevus. Numerous series have been reported in which the frequency of malignant degeneration ranged from 2 to 30 percent [12–18]. While it is acknowledged that the melanoma cases arising in giant congenital nevi might tend to be overreported, nonetheless the malignant potential of the precursor is clearly established.

Congenital melanocytic nevi are found in 1 percent of newborns [19–22]. Giant hairy nevi may range in size to cover areas such as the dorsum of the hand, the shoulder, the buttocks, the entire arm, or the entire trunk. Such lesions are descriptively called *coat sleeve, capelike, nestlike,* or *bathing trunk nevi.* They often lie in the distribution of a dermatome [18]. The color of these lesions varies from brown to black. The intensity of the hue increases during childhood, until adolescence, and then may tend to fade. The lesions may be quite markedly raised and they frequently demonstrate small papillomatous projections studding the entire surface. As the patient matures, the lesions become even more raised and irregular in surface contour. The hairs, which characterize many giant nevi, become coarser, darker, and more numerous in late childhood [23]. Two principal histopathologic patterns are noted in giant congenital nevi: In one pattern, the melanocytes have the characteristics of those seen in typical compound nevi and dermal nevi. In the other, the histology is that of dermal nevi possessing numerous neural-like structures. In both patterns, areas may be found that are similar to blue nevi or areas characteristic of compound melanocytoma (Spitz's juvenile melanoma) [18,24]. Congenital nevi have been characterized as having nevus cells

that penetrate to the lower two-thirds of the reticular dermis or that surround blood vessel walls, nerve sheaths, or epidermal appendages [25]. Histologic findings in the small congenital nevus are similar to those found in the giant nevus. Fewer than 10 percent of congenital nevi are larger than 3 to 4 cm, a size cutoff below which nevi are usually designated as *small* [21]. *Giant* is a term [26] generally reserved for lesions not easily excised and where the defect cannot be closed primarily without flaps or skin grafts, but definitions vary [27]. Lesions 10 cm or more in their greatest dimension are found in fewer than 1 in 20,000 newborns [21]. The term *gigantic,* or *garment,* is used to describe congenital nevi covering a major anatomic area of the body [27].

There is little debate about the risk of melanoma associated with giant congenital nevi, estimated to be at least 6.3 percent over a lifetime [27]. In melanomas arising within the giant nevi, malignant degeneration may occur early in life. For 21 cases in which metastatic melanoma in prepuberal children had been associated with giant nevi, 60 percent were diagnosed within the first 3 years of life [12]. Melanomas arising in giant congenital nevi are difficult to detect early for several reasons: (1) The origin of the melanoma in two-thirds of cases has been reported to be dermal or subcutaneous [27]. (2) The giant congenital nevus may have a very irregular surface and an irregular pigment pattern which obscures recognition of small early malignant changes [18]. We advocate early full-thickness removal for prophylactic purposes. Consideration should be given to prophylactic excision of giant nevi as soon as the problem is recognized, balancing the known risks of surgery (including general anesthesia) against the theoretical risks of the development of malignant melanoma. Dermabrasion may reduce the surface pigmentation of congenital nevi but it is not recommended as the nevus cells may penetrate to the fat, muscle fascia, and even muscle or bone in some cases, occasionally giving rise to melanoma from these sites [27]. We have reported one patient in whom the melanoma arose in the subcutaneous location below an area that had been surgically excised with split-thickness removal [27].

Head and neck involvement by giant nevi may be associated with leptomeningeal melanocytosis, sometimes causing hydrocephalus, seizures, and even leptomeningeal melanoma [18,28–30]. Diagnosis of leptomeningeal melanocytosis may be confirmed by computerized tomographic (CT) scan [31,32].

There are divergent opinions regarding the mel-

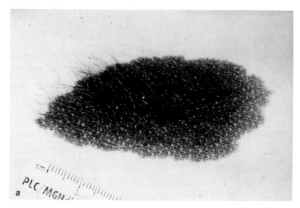
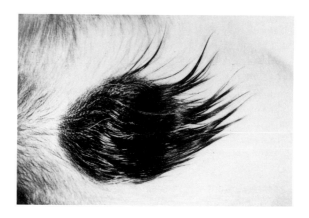

Fig. 2.   Congenital melanocytic nevi.

anoma risk associated with small congenital nevi [26,33–35], lesions that are easily excised and where the defect is usually closed with adjacent tissues in a single operation (Fig. 2). Recent data from the Harvard Melanoma Registry suggest a significant association and increased melanoma risk with small congenital nevi [33].

The chance finding of a melanoma and a small congenital nevus in contiguity (Fig. 3) in any series of consecutive cases may be estimated to be less than 1 in 100,000 [33]. Also, the chance of finding congenital nevi in adults is expected to be no greater than for newborns, i.e., 1 percent [19,22]. The melanoma arising in contiguity with small congenital nevi has been observed to be 15 percent (20/136) in melanoma patients questioned about preexisting pigmented lesions at the tumor site [34,36] and 8 percent (19/234) of melanoma specimens examined for tumor-associated nevi with histologic changes as noted in congenital melanocytic nevi [34]. These observed rates of asso-

ciation are more than 1000 times greater than the expected association based on chance alone [34].

First approximations of relative risk, using the historic and histologic data as compared with observations in newborns, may be converted to cumulative melanoma risks of 1 in 20 by history and 1 in 25 to 1 in 38 by histology for persons born with congenital nevi who live to the age of 60 years [36]. These estimates are highly dependent on the specificity of methods used for ascertainment of congenital nevi. Nonetheless, the data suggest that at least some cases of melanoma arise in small congenital melanocytic nevi.

Small congenital nevi may be a greater hazard than giant congenital nevi in the epidemiology of melanoma, since giant nevi represent a rare association in most series of consecutive cases of melanoma (approximately 1 per 1000) compared to the 7 to 15 percent rate of association described for small congenital nevi [37].

Congenital melanocytic nevi of any size should

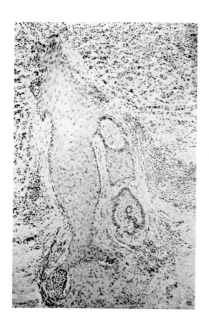

Fig. 3.   Melanoma arising in association with a congenital nevus. (a) Low-power photomicrograph demonstrating nevus cell nest in hair follicle and melanoma above. X 100. (b) High-power photomicrograph of 3a showing cellular detail of nevus cell nest in hair follicle. X 200.

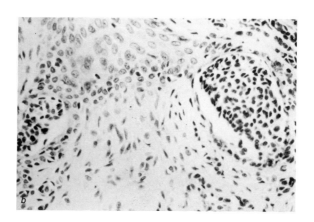

be considered for prophylactic excision, but management decisions should be balanced by the theoretical risks. Because prepuberal melanoma is rare, small congenital nevi may be observed if follow-up is adequate until they can be excised, using local anesthesia, at the end of the first decade of life. Alternatively, small lesions may be excised under local anesthesia during the newborn period, especially if marked hyperpigmentation or uneven surface prevents evaluation of malignant change.

Dysplastic Nevi

Another precursor for cutaneous melanoma which has been recognized only recently is the dysplastic nevus, a unique form of nevocellular nevus with irregular and/or indistinct borders, variegation of color (varying shades of brown, red, and flesh tones), and a slightly raised or almost flat surface [38] (Figs. 4 and 5). Although 75 to 80 percent of normal Caucasian postpuberal adults have one or more nevocellular nevi, only 1 to 2 percent have one or more dysplastic nevi [37–42]. By history, most dysplastic nevi appear at the end of the first and during the second decades of life [38,40].

Dysplastic nevi may also continue to appear during adulthood.

Compared to the low prevalence rate of dysplastic nevi in normal adults, 30 percent of patients with sporadic melanoma have been observed to have one or more dysplastic nevi [37,41,43]. In patients with familial melanoma (two or more blood relatives diagnosed as having melanoma), up to 90 percent of the melanoma patients and 40 percent of the nonmelanoma relatives have been described as having one or more dysplastic nevi [38,40]. The first case of cutaneous melanoma reported in the English language was probably a familial case [4]. Familial melanoma constitutes about 10 percent of all melanoma cases [38,44,45]. Familial melanoma associated with dysplastic nevi is thought to be transmitted in an autosomal dominant fashion [38,40]. Striking family pedigrees have been reported in which up to 15 cases of melanoma in a single family have been reported [40,46]. The most convincing evidence for the malignant potential of dysplastic nevi are the several published cases in which invasive melanoma has been documented

Fig. 5. Dysplastic nevi. Note irregularity of borders and pigment pattern.

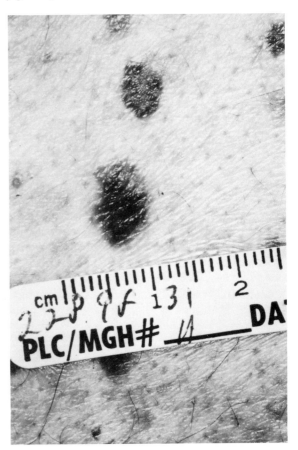

Fig. 4. Multiple dysplastic nevi. Note variation in sizes and irregularity of borders. This patient has had two melanomas.

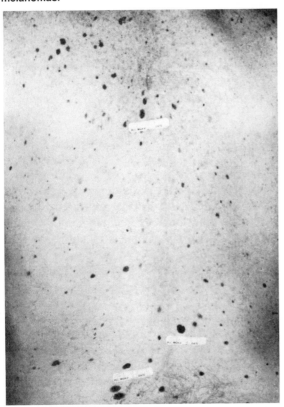

to arise in previously photographed dysplastic nevi [38,40,41]. There were 34 reports of familial melanoma covering 165 different kindreds and 490 cases, an average of 3.0 cases per family at the time of Greene and Fraumeni's recent summary [40]. In 47 percent of families, tumors developed in a parent and one or more children. In an additional 30 percent, the tumors occurred in siblings only. The remaining 20 percent occurred in more distant relatives. When familial cases are compared to sporadic melanoma, the familial cases are (1) younger (mean age: 42 years vs. 50 years) [40], (2) have lesions more frequently located on the trunk (38 vs. 30 percent), (3) have lesions disproportionately of the superficial spreading type (86 vs. 68 percent), and (4) have lesions more superficially invasive (100 percent level II or III vs. 53 percent) [40]. The latter observation may represent a less aggressive biologic behavior than sporadic melanoma or may represent earlier diagnosis in subsequent familial cases once the initial family member has been diagnosed.

The histopathology of dysplastic nevi formerly had been interpreted as "active junctional nevi" (Fig. 6). Dysplastic nevi that are removed for diagnosis should be reviewed by a pathologist familiar with the syndrome; otherwise, the interpretation may be "within the spectrum of normal" or an erroneous diagnosis of melanoma may be made. The most striking histopathologic changes in dysplastic nevi are proliferation and variable atypism of epidermal melanocytes [38,41]. The microscopic features of dysplastic nevi appear to fall into two classes [41]. The first (epithelioid cell melanocytic dysplasia) is characterized by intraepidermal nevus cells in the form of nests with horizontally oriented epithelioid melanocytes. In the second (lentiginous melanocytic dysplasia) there is irregular basal proliferation of pleomorphic hyperchromatic melanocytes that show prominent cytoplasmic retraction artifact. The hyperplastic melanocytes are commonly disposed at the margin of elongated rete ridges [41]. An additional feature is the presence of a dermal inflammatory host response consisting of a focal or diffuse lymphocytic infiltrate with delicate fibroplasia and new vessel formation [41]. These latter features resemble those of immunologic regression in melanoma or halo nevi. Lamellar fibroplasia, a condensation of collagen about elongated rete ridges containing hyperplastic melanocytes, was also commonly present [47]. Cytologic appearances that were common to all dysplastic nevi were nuclear pleomorphism and hyperchromatism, seen in a few or many cells of each lesion [41]. A dermal nevus

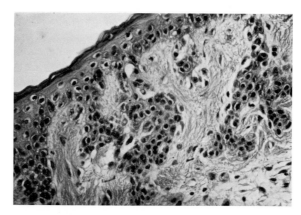

Fig. 6. Dysplastic nevus. High-power photomicrograph showing lentiginous downward projection of the epidermal rete ridges with fibrosis of the papillary body and increased frequency of slightly atypical melanocytes. X 400.

cell component is often present in the dysplastic lesion. The dermal nevus cells are of the epithelioid or small cell type. The pathologist who examines the histology of a dysplastic nevus may be the first to call attention to the problem. Dysplastic nevi are frequently removed because they are considered ugly (darkly pigmented, large, irregular border).

The 1 to 2 percent prevalence of dysplastic nevi in white adults may be an important factor in the epidemiology of melanoma. A total skin examination should be considered a routine part of the physical examination. Any pigmented lesion that is extremely dark in color or markedly irregular in pigmentation should be considered for diagnostic excision. Size is the least helpful criterion for diagnosing dysplastic nevi. In general, dysplastic nevi measure 5 mm or larger. Individual nevi out of step (appearance or rate of growth) with the majority of pigmented lesions in a given patient should also be considered for removal. The routine examination of sites of infrequent melanoma occurrence (scalp, buttock) are warranted in patients with dysplastic nevi since melanomas arising from dysplastic nevi have been observed in these locations [47]. Multiple dysplastic nevi (hundreds) are common in patients with multiple primary melanomas and also in their family members [38–40], a situation requiring close photographic observation with follow-up every 3 months and excision of the most atypical lesions. Dermabrasion, electrodesiccation, or cryotherapy are contraindicated for dysplastic nevi, since gross and microscopic identification are obliterated by these modalities. 5-Fluorouracil has been used with variable success [48] but at present cannot be recommended. Early recognition, surgical excision, histologic identification, and examination of family members are the main goals of current management for patients with dysplastic nevi with or without a family history of melanoma; the significance of isolated dysplastic nevi in individuals without a personal or family history of melanoma needs further clarification.

Conclusions

Precursors for cutaneous melanoma* include lentigo maligna, giant congenital nevi, small congenital nevi, and dysplastic nevi. Presumably, early recognition and prophylactic removal of precursor lesions may eventually reduce the morbidity and mortality associated with metastatic melanoma. However, the impact of routine screening and excision of all congenital and dysplastic nevi is unknown. Clinical judgment is required to balance the presumed risk of melanoma associated with these lesions and the known risks of surgical excision for a given patient.

Prognostic Factors in Cutaneous Melanoma†

The determination of prognosis in malignant melanoma is important for three reasons. First, most patients naturally want some idea of what the future holds for them. An accurate assessment of prognosis allows them either peace of mind or, conversely, the option of changing their life-style to accomplish more limited goals when the prognosis is guarded. Second, the physician must outline a treatment plan that is appropriate to the severity of disease. No physician would subject melanoma patients to unnecessary anesthesia for elective removal of regional lymph nodes or administer an experimental drug with unknown long-term side effects to a patient with a very high likelihood of survival following local excision alone. Conversely, a patient with little chance of cure deserves the benefit of considering the most promising available chemo- and/or immunotherapies.

---

* Also required for consideration as potential precursors of melanoma are the very dark pigmented lesions on the soles. Lewis noted a high correlation of these lesions and the incidence of melanoma in Ugandan blacks. The histopathology of these lesions has been observed to be a lentiginous melanocytic proliferation. (Lewis MG: Malignant melanoma in Uganda: the relationship between pigmentation and malignant melanoma on the soles of the feet. *Br J Cancer* **21**:483–495, 1967)

† This section is reprinted by permission from *Ca-A Cancer Journal for Clinicians* (Ca 32:113–122) © American Cancer Society 1982.

Table 1   Clinical and histologic stages of melanoma

	Clinical	Histologic
Stage I	Localized disease (no clinically palpable nodes)	Absence of histologic evidence of tumor in regional lymph nodes
Stage II	Palpable regional lymph nodes	Histologic evidence of melanoma in regional lymph nodes
Stage III	Presence of distant metastases	Histopathologic documentation of distant metastases

The third and perhaps most important reason for continuing to seek new methods to estimate prognosis is the corollary that the better we are at predicting melanoma clinical behavior, the closer we are to understanding the clinicopathologic events associated with neoplasia. Since there are several available staging systems for melanoma, Table 1 defines the system used in the following discussions.

Survival Rates for Stage III Patients

It is not difficult to assess the outcome for cutaneous melanoma patients with distant metastases (clinical stage III) or for patients with regional node metastases that are large enough to detect by palpation (clinical stage II, pathologic stage II). Nearly all patients in both of these groups eventually die of disease [49–51]. Patients with distant metastases that can be surgically resected and who are judged to be clinically free of disease have a median survival of 16 months, as compared to 5 months for patients with unresectable distant metastases [49].

Survival Rates for Clinical Stage II, Pathologic Stage II Patients

No more than 30 percent of clinical stage II, pathologic stage II patients live 5 years, and 10-year survivors are uncommon [50,51]. Mundth et al. [50] showed a 3 percent 10-year survival, and Balch and associates [51] had no 10-year survivors among patients in this group. Balch et al. [51], in their multivariate analysis of prognostic factors for melanoma patients with regional lymph node metastases, showed the highest survival rate for patients with only one positive lymph node and a nonulcerated primary melanoma. It should be noted that in this series all of the 10-year melanoma survivors with regional lymph node metastases had "micrometastases" (clinical stage I, pathologic stage II) rather than metastases that were large enough to detect by palpation of the involved lymph node group (clinical stage II, pathologic stage II). Thus, the number and percentage of involved lymph nodes, histologic ulceration of the primary melanoma, and primary tumor thickness [52] are important prognostic factors for clinical stage I, pathologic stage II patients. However, these variables have little bearing on the final outcome of clinical stage II, pathologic stage II patients because nearly all such patients eventually die of disease.

Survival Rates for Clinical Stage I Patients

The outcome is far less clear-cut for individuals who have clinically localized disease (clinical stage I). No single test or prognostic factor currently exists that will accurately predict the outcome for all these patients. For this reason, optimal combinations of single variables (prognostic models) have been generated using multivariate analyses [52–63] (see Table 2). These analyses of clinical stage I patients showed that thickness of the primary melanoma was the best determinant for outcome even if regional lymph nodes contained "micrometastases" (clinical stage I, pathologic stage II). Furthermore, there was general agreement among different centers on survival rates as determined by primary tumor thickness [53,54] (Tables 3 and 4). Previous inconsistencies can be traced to the mixing of clinical stage I and stage II patients and the use of different outcomes (i.e., metastases, recurrence, melanoma death, death from all causes, etc.).

There was also general agreement in the reported prognostic models that the location of the primary melanoma had a significant effect on survival even after correcting for thickness. All but 2 of the 10 multivariate analyses in Table 2 contained location as an important additive prognostic factor to thickness: (1) The multivariate analysis of clinical stage I patients wih clinically occult regional lymph node metastases (clinical stage I, pathologic stage II) conducted by the Massachusetts General Hospital–New York University Melanoma Clinical Cooperative Group (MGH–NYU MCCG) [52] did not include location. However, that same study showed that nearly all patients with volar, subungual, head, or neck melanomas died of disease when regional lymph nodes contained tumor. When grouped in this fashion, specific location ("subsite") was an important prognostic factor. (2) The other study that did not include location as an important interacting covariate was the WHO multivariate

analysis [55]; their Cox model selected only thickness and sex. Six subsequent analyses by the MGH–NYU MCCG showed that most of the previously observed effects of sex, age, ulceration, and type of biopsy were secondary to specific location or subsite. For example, nearly all patients with melanoma of the hands and feet died of disease if their primary tumor was greater than 2.75 mm in thickness [63]. Such patients, as a group, were older, more often had ulcerated melanomas with a poor lymphocyte response, and more often had incisional rather than excisional biopsies when compared to melanomas of similar thickness located elsewhere. We found no significant sex differences in survival after correcting for subsite and thickness [61–63]. Moreover, these MGH–NYU MCCG studies indicated that the customary grouping of patients into the broad location categories of extremities, trunk, head, and neck did not accurately reflect the biologic behavior of the disease. Rather, each subsite had its own natural history with respect to thickness (Table 5 and Figs. 7 to 9).

There was less agreement for other variables selected by the various multivariate analyses from different centers for at least four reasons: First, the variable subset tested in the above analyses were not identical. Balch et al. [54], for example, did not test mitoses or microscopic satellites [58] in their multivariate analysis. Second, the concordance among pathologists for the various histologic parameters other than thickness is only about 70 percent [64]. Thus, some of the differences in the prognostic models probably represent differences in pathologic interpretation. Third, the prognostic usefulness of a particular histologic parameter depends on the specific criteria used to test that variable. For example, the prospective MGH–NYU MCCG study was unable to reproduce the findings of the Balch et al. studies for histologic ulceration until ulceration width was measured [58]. Those patients with only focal ulceration less than 3 mm in width had the same prognosis as those patients with no ulceration [58]. Mitoses per mm^2 were the most useful when the microscope slides were first scanned on low power to find the area of highest concentration of mitoses; the mitotic counts were then performed in that area. Lymphocyte response was both more reproducible and more useful prognostically when the response was estimated only at the most deeply invasive portion of the tumor [52,63].

A fourth reason for different models is the nature of the Cox multivariate proportional hazards model itself. We have demonstrated, for example, that

Table 2 Important prognostic factors for clinical stage I melanoma patients selected by multivariate analyses from four different centers

Centers	Göteborg, Sweden [53]	Univ. of Alabama [54]	WHO [55]	MGH-NYU [52]	MGH-NYU [57]	MGH-NYU [56]	MGH-NYU [59]	MGH-NYU [61]	MGH-NYU [62]	MGH-NYU [63]
Qualifying factors	All sites	All sites	All sites	Regional lymph nodes contained microscopic deposits of tumor	Upper extremity	Lower extremity	Trunk	0.76–1.69 mm thick	1.51–3.99 mm thick	>3.60 mm thick
Important prognostic variables	Thickness Location Ulceration Size Level of invasion	Thickness Ulceration Surgical treatment Location	Thickness Sex	Thickness ≥4 positive nodes or ≥20% of nodes removed were positive Lymphocyte response	Thickness "Subsite" Ulceration	Thickness "Subsite" Mitotic rate	Thickness "Subsite" Mitotic rate Lymphocyte response	"Subsite" Level of invasion	Mitoses/mm² "Subsite" Ulceration Microscopic satellites	"Subsite" Lymphocyte response Histologic type Pathologic stage

Table 3 Five-year survival rate comparisons by primary tumor thickness for clinical stage I melanoma patients

Thickness, mm	University of Gö-teborg, Sweden [53]*	MGH–NYU MCCG†
≤0.75	98%	99%
0.76–1.50	90%	94%
1.51–2.25	83%	84%
2.26–3.00	72%	77%
>3.00	46%	46%

* None of these patients had an elective regional node dissection.
† Nearly all of the 598 patients in the prospective study who were candidates for elective regional node dissection had the procedure.
Note: % = Percent surviving 5 years.

Table 4 Five-year survival rate comparisons by primary tumor thickness for clinical stage I melanoma patients, all of whom had an elective regional node dissection

Thickness, mm	University of Alabama	MGH–NYU MCCG
≤0.75	100%	100%
0.76–1.50	94%	94%
1.51–3.99	83%	76%
≥4.0	40%	41%

Note: % = Percent surviving 5 years.

alternate models of comparable power can be produced from the same data set [63]. This suggests that a comparison of results from different centers be done, using those variables for which there is highest concordance (i.e., thickness and subsite).

The survival rates in Table 5 by subsite and thickness are intended for use by physicians and patients (Figs. 7–9). The thickness categories used (i.e., less than 0.85 mm, 0.85 to 1.69 mm, 1.70 to 3.64 mm, and greater than or equal to 3.65 mm) were chosen over previously published ranges because we demonstrated that the thickness-survival relationship was not perfectly linear [65], as assumed by investigators who published survival rates using regular thickness intervals [66–68]. Statistical techniques to find optimal thickness "cut points" demonstrated that "quantum jumps" occurred with increasing thickness, analogous to a rising staircase consisting of four-stair steps or categories with natural biologic boundaries of 0.85

mm, 1.70 mm, and 3.65 mm [69]. The second point to be gleaned from Table 5 is that deaths rarely occur in clinical stage I patients with melanomas 0.85 mm to 1.69 mm thick located on the face, anterior neck, lower trunk, and extremities excluding the posterolateral upper arm. Melanomas in these locations so rarely metastasize that they have about the same prognosis as melanomas less than about 0.85 mm in thickness. Third, "thick" melanomas of the hands and feet metastasize and cause death much more frequently than other-extremity melanomas [63]. Only one of 17 clinical stage I patients with a hand or foot melanoma greater than 2.75 mm thick remains alive. This again emphasizes the subsite concept: Namely, broad location categories of axial vs. extremity do not accurately reflect the clinical behavior of this disease. Fourth, those clinical stage I patients with micrometastases in either more than 4 or so lymph nodes or more than 20 percent or so of electively excised lymph nodes nearly all die of disease, as do patients with lymph node micrometastases who have primary melanomas of the head and neck

Table 5 Survival by primary tumor thickness and specific location in 598 patients with clinical stage I melanoma from the MGH–NYU MCCG

Primary melanoma thickness, mm	Specific location	Risk of death from melanoma within 7½ years after diagnosis	No. of MGH–NYU patients in this category
<0.85	Any site	1%	202
0.85–1.69	Non-BANS*	2%	111
	BANS	20%	55
1.70–3.64	Non-BANS extremities, excluding hands and feet	14%	49
	Non-BANS trunk	23%	27
	Non-BANS head and neck	36%	13
	Hands or feet	40%	16
	BANS	42%	46
>3.65	Non-Bans extremities, excluding hands and feet	17%	17
	Non-BANS head and neck	35%	10
	BANS	67%	21
	Non-BANS trunk	78%	22
	Hands or feet	100%	9

* BANS = upper back, posterolateral upper arm, posterior and lateral neck, or posterior scalp.

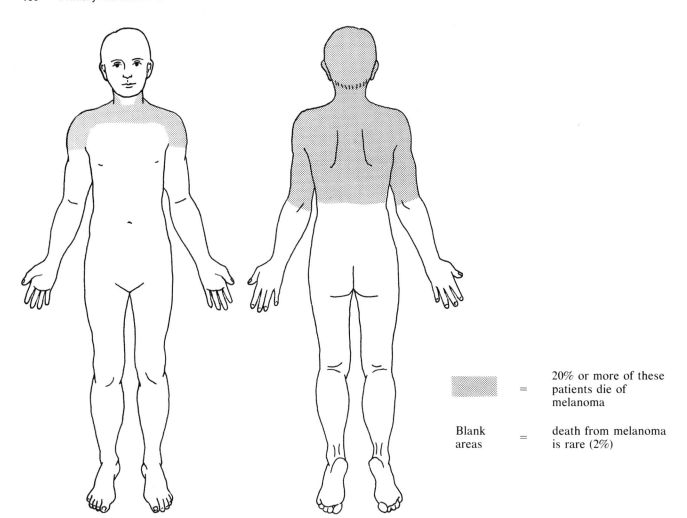

20% or more of these patients die of melanoma

Blank areas = death from melanoma is rare (2%)

Fig. 7. Risk of death from melanoma within the first 7½ years after diagnosis for patients with clinical stage I melanoma 0.85 through 1.69 mm thick. (Death from clinical stage I melanoma within the first 7½ years after diagnosis is uncommon at any location (<2%) in lesions that are <0.85 mm in thickness, even if regression is present.)

and volar or subungual areas [52]. Other than these situations, clinical stage I patients with microscopic metastases in regional lymph nodes have approximately the same survival rate as clinical stage I patients with pathologically negative nodes when matched for thickness and subsite.

The survival rates in Table 5 also apply to patients who are treated initially with only wide local excision (WLE) of the primary melanoma as well as those treated with WLE plus elective regional node dissection (ERND). Balch et al., in a retrospective analysis, showed a 0 percent 8-year survival for 24 patients with primary melanomas 1.51 to 3.99 mm thick treated with WLE only [54]. However, one retrospective study and two prospective studies showed 8-year survival rates of 70 percent (J. Eldh, University of Göteborg, personal communication), 68 percent [69], and 67 percent (N. Cascinelli, World Health Organization, personal communication) for these same

patients (Table 6). The two prospective studies showed that for patients with melanomas 1.51 to 3.99 mm thick, survival rates were 5 to 10 percent higher for those treated with ERND as compared with those treated only with WLE ([70], N. Cas-

Table 6   Survival rates for clinical stage I patients with melanomas 1.51 through 3.99 mm thick treated only with wide local excision of the primary tumor

Study	No. of patients in the study	Seven-year survival rate
Göteborg*	106	70%
WHO†	88	67%
MGH–NYU [69]	47	68%
University of Alabama [54]	24	0%‡

* Eldh J: University of Göteborg, Sweden, personal communication.
† Cascinelli N: World Health Organization results, personal communication.
‡ Eight-year results.

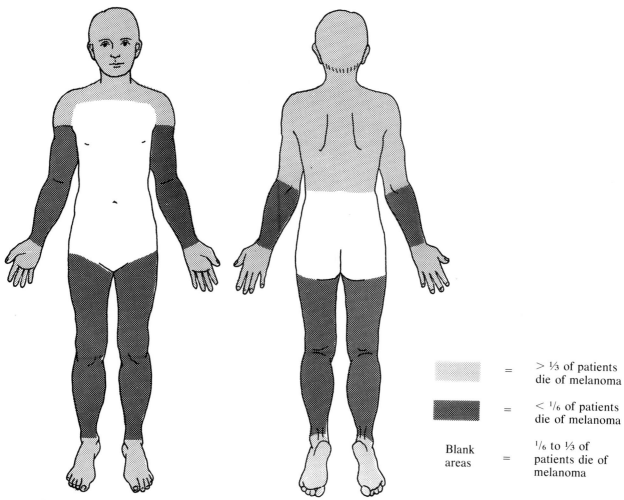

$=$ > ⅓ of patients die of melanoma

$=$ < ⅙ of patients die of melanoma

Blank areas $=$ ⅙ to ⅓ of patients die of melanoma

Fig. 8. Risk of death from melanoma within the first 7½ years after diagnosis for patients with clinical stage I melanoma 1.70 through 3.64 mm thick.

cinelli, personal communication). Thus, the benefit from ERND is probably real but much smaller than that noted in the study by Balch et al. [54].

Conclusions

1. Thickness in millimeters of the primary melanoma is the dominant variable for clinical stage I patients (without clinical lymphadenopathy) [52–63], even when regional lymph nodes contain metastases [52].
2. Statistical techniques to determine optimal "cut points" showed that the thickness-survival relationship was best characterized when melanomas were categorized into the following four thickness groups [65]: *a*. less than 0.85 mm *b*. 0.85 through 1.69 mm *c*. 1.70 through 3.64 mm *d*. greater than 3.65 mm.
3. Broad location categories (e.g., leg, trunk, etc.) do not accurately reflect melanoma clinical behavior. Specific location (subsite) plus primary tumor thickness is superior to any other two variable combinations for predicting recurrence and death [56,57,59,61–63] in clinical stage I patients.

   a.Clinical stage I melanomas 0.85 mm through 1.69 mm in thickness on the face, anterior neck, extremities (excluding the posterolateral upper arm), and lower trunk rarely metastasize and have the same excellent survival as melanomas less than 0.85 mm located anywhere (i.e., 95 percent survival) [62].

   b.Clinical stage I patients with melanomas greater than or equal to 3.65 mm on the trunk or with melanomas greater than 2.75 mm on the hands or feet nearly all die of melanoma [63].
4. The clinical stage I patients most likely to benefit from elective regional node dissection are (1) those with melanomas 0.85 through 1.69 mm on the upper back, posterolateral upper

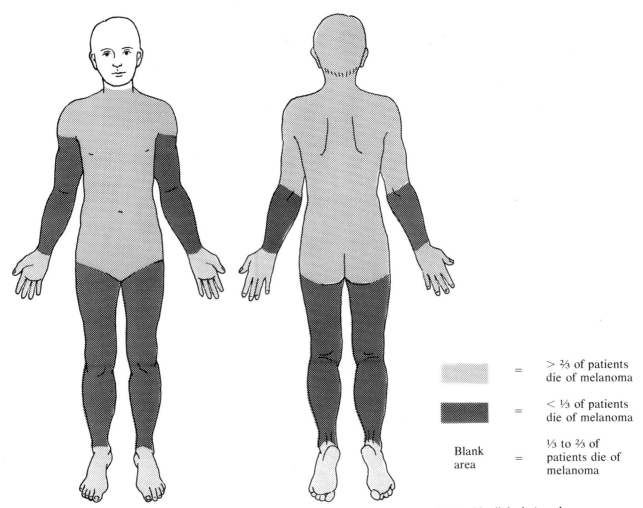

Fig. 9. Risk of death from melanoma within the first 7½ years after diagnosis for patients with clinical stage I melanoma >3.60 mm thick.

arm, posterior and lateral neck, and scalp [62] and (2) most patients with melanomas 1.70 mm through 3.64 mm [61]. Benefit for these groups of patients has not been established. Prospective randomized trials are necessary to establish the therapeutic value.

5. Patients with distant metastases surgically resected and judged to be clinically free of disease have a median survival of 16 months, as compared with 5 months for patients with unresectable distant metastases [49].

6. Only about 30 percent of clinical stage II, pathologic stage II patients survive 5 years, and 10-year survivors in this subgroup are uncommon (less than 10 percent) [50,51].

References

1. Hutchinson J: On cancer. *Arch Surg* **4**:61–65, 1892
2. Hutchinson J: Lentigo melanosis. A further report. *Arch Surg* **5**:253–256, 1894
3. Dubreuilh MW: Lentigo malin des vieillards. Société de Dermatologie, 4 Août, 1894
4. Norris W: A case of fungoid disease. *Edinb Med Surg J* **16**:562–565, 1920
5. Clark WH Jr, Mihm MC Jr: Lentigo maligna and lentigo maligna melanoma. *Am J Pathol* **55**:39–67, 1969
6. Su WPD, Bradley RR: Amelanotic lentigo maligna. *Arch Dermatol* **116**:82–83, 1980
7. Sober AJ et al: Primary malignant melanoma of the skin—1130 cases from the Melanoma Clinical Cooperative Group, in *Proceedings of the XVth International Congress of Dermatology, Mexico City, 16–22 October, 1977.* Excerpta Medica, Amsterdam, 1979
8. Davis J et al: Melanotic freckle of Hutchinson. *Am J Surg* **113**:457–463, 1967
9. Wayte DM, Helwig EB: Melanotic freckle of Hutchinson. *Cancer* **21**:893–911, 1968
10. Michalik EE et al: Rapid progression of lentigo maligna to deeply invasive lentigo maligna melanoma: report of two cases. *Arch Dermatol*, in press
11. Dancuart F et al: The radiotherapy of lentigo maligna and lentigo maligna melanoma of the head and neck. *Cancer* **45**:2279–2283, 1980
12. Trozak DJ et al: Metastatic malignant melanoma in prepubertal children. *Clin Pediatr (Phila)* **55**:191–204, 1974

13. Kaplan EN: The risk of malignancy in large congenital nevi. *Plast Reconstr Surg* **53:**421–428, 1974

14. Russell JL, Reyes RG: Giant pigmented nevi. *JAMA* **171:**2083–2086, 1959

15. Pers AM: Nevus pigmentosa giganticus. *Ugeskr Laeger* **125:**613–619, 1963

16. Lanier VC et al: Congenital giant nevi: clinical and pathological considerations. *Plast Reconstr Surg* **58:**48–54, 1976

17. Greeley PW et al: Incidence of malignancy in giant pigmented nevi. *Plast Reconstr Surg* **36:**26–37, 1965

18. Reed WB et al: Giant pigmented nevi, melanoma and leptomeningeal melanocytosis. *Arch Dermatol* **91:**100–119, 1965

19. Walton RG et al: Pigmented lesions in newborn infants. *Br J Dermatol* **95:**389–396, 1976

20. Alper J et al: Birthmarks with serious medical significance: nevocellular nevi, sebaceous nevi, and multiple café-au-lait spots. *J Pediatr* **95:**696–700, 1979

21. Castilla EE et al: Epidemiology of congenital pigmented nevi; incidence rates and relative frequencies. *Br J Dermatol* **104:**307–315, 1981

22. Pratt AG: Birthmarks in infants. *Arch Dermatol* **67:**302–306, 1953

23. Rook A: Nevi and other developmental defects, in *Textbook of Dermatology*. Edited by A Rook et al. Blackwell, Oxford, 1969, pp 73–111

24. Spitz S: Melanomas of childhood. *Am J Pathol* **24:**591–609, 1948

25. Mark GJ et al: Congenital melanocytic nevi of the small and garment type: clinical, histologic and ultrastructural studies. *Hum Pathol* **4:**395–418, 1973

26. Kopf AW et al: Congenital nevocytic nevi and malignant melanoma. *J Am Acad Dermatol* **1:**123–130, 1979

27. Rhodes AR et al: Non-epidermal origin of malignant melanoma associated with giant congenital nevocellular nevus. *Plast Reconstr Surg* **67:**782–790, 1981

28. Lamas E et al: Neurocutaneous melanocytosis. Report of a case and review of the literature. *Acta Neurochir (Wien)* **36:**93–105, 1977

29. Slam R: Primary malignant melanoma of the cerebellum. *J Pathol Bacteriol* **94:**196–200, 1967

30. Savitz MH, Anderson PJ: Primary melanoma of the leptomeninges: a review. *Mt Sinai J Med (NY)* **41:**774–791, 1974

31. Flodmark O et al: Neuroradiological findings in a child with primary leptomeningeal melanoma. *Neuroradiology* **18:**153–156, 1979

32. Kudel TA et al: Computed tomographic findings of primary malignant leptomeningeal melanoma in neurocutaneous melanosis. *AJR* **133:**950–951, 1979

33. Rhodes AR et al: Primary cutaneous malignant melanoma and congenital nevocellular nevi: histologic association and estimation of relative risk (abstr). *J Invest Dermatol* **76:**319, 1981

34. Rhodes AR et al: The malignant potential of small congenital nevocellular nevi: an estimate of association based on a histologic study of 234 primary cutaneous melanomas. *J Am Acad Dermatol*, **6:**230–241, 1982

35. Solomon LM: The management of congenital melanocytic nevi. *Arch Dermatol* **116:**1017, 1980

36. Rhodes AR, Melski JW: Small congenital nevi risk of cutaneous melanoma. *J Pediatr*, **100:**219–224, 1982

37. Rhodes AR et al: Possible risk factors for primary cutaneous malignant melanoma. *Clin Res* **28:**252A, 1980

38. Reimer RR et al: Precursor lesions in familial melanoma: a new genetic pre-neoplastic syndrome. *JAMA* **239:**744–746, 1978

39. Lynch HT et al: Familial atypical mole-melanoma syndrome. *J Med Genet* **15:**352–356, 1978

40. Greene MH, Fraumeni JF: Hereditary variant of malignant melanoma, in *Human Malignant Melanoma*. Edited by WH Clark Jr et al. Grune & Stratton, New York, 1979, pp 139–166

41. Elder DE et al: Dysplastic nevus syndrome: a phenotypic association of sporadic cutaneous melanoma. *Cancer* **46:**1787–1794, 1980

42. Greene MH et al: Precursor nevi in cutaneous malignant melanoma: a proposed nomenclature. *Lancet* **2:**1024, 1980

43. Rahbari H, Mehregan AH: Sporatic atypical mole syndrome. *Arch Dermatol* **117:**329–331, 1981

44. Wallace DC et al: Familial malignant melanoma. *Ann Surg* **177:**15–20, 1973

45. Sutherland CM et al: Familial melanoma, in *Pigment Cell*, vol 2. Edited by V Riley. Karger, Basel, 1976, pp 421–426

46. Anderson DE et al: Hereditary aspects of malignant melanoma. *JAMA* **200:**741–746, 1967

47. Greene MA et al: New observations in hereditary melanoma. American Society of Clinical Oncology abstracts p 323, March 1980

48. Bondi EE et al: Topical chemotherapy of dysplastic melanocytic nevi with 5% fluorouracil. *Arch Dermatol* **117:**89–92, 1981

49. Feun LG et al: The natural history of stage IVA melanoma (abstr). *Proc Am Soc Clin Oncol* **22:**C-372, 1981

50. Mundth ED et al: Malignant melanoma: a clinical study of 427 cases. *Ann Surg* **162:**15–28, 1965

51. Balch CM et al: A multifactorial analysis of melanoma. III. Prognostic factors in melanoma patients with lymph node metastases. *Ann Surg* **193:**377–388, 1981

52. Day CL et al: Melanoma patients with positive nodes and relatively good prognoses: microstaging retains prognostic significance in clinical stage I patients with regional node metastases. *Cancer* **47:**955–962, 1981

53. Eldh J et al: Prognostic factors in cutaneous malignant melanoma in stage I. *Scand J Plast Reconstr Surg* **12:**243–255, 1978

54. Balch CM et al: A multifactorial analysis of melanoma. II. Prognostic features of clinical stage I disease. *Surgery* **86:**343–351, 1979

55. Cascinelli N et al: Prognosis of stage I melanoma of the skin. *Int J Cancer* **26:**733–739, 1980

56. Day CL et al: A prognostic model for clinical stage I melanoma of the lower extremity: location on the foot is an independent risk factor for recurrent disease. *Surgery* **89:**599–603, 1981

57. Day CL et al: A prognostic model for clinical stage I melanoma of the upper extremity: the prognostic importance of anatomic subsites in predicting recurrent disease. *Ann Surg* **193:**436–440, 1981

58. Day CL et al: Malignant melanoma: the prognostic significance of microscopic satellites in the reticular dermis and subcutaneous fat. *Ann Surg* **194:**108–111, 1981

59. Day CL et al: A prognostic model for clinical stage I melanoma of the trunk: location near the midline is not an independent risk factor for recurrent disease. *Am J Surg* **142:**247–251, 1981

60. Day CL et al: A new approach for predicting recurrent disease in melanomas: the prognostic value of melanoma photographs. *J Invest Dermatol* **76:**316, 1981

61. Day CL et al: Prognostic factors for patients with clinical stage I melanoma of intermediate thickness (1.51–3.99 mm): a conceptual model for tumor growth and metastases. *Ann Surg* **195:**35–43, 1982

62. Day CL et al: Prognostic factors for melanoma patients with lesions 0.76 to 1.65 mm in thickness: an appraisal of thin level IV lesions. *Ann Surg* **195**:30–34, 1982

63. Day CL et al: A multivariate analysis of prognostic factors for melanoma patients with lesions >3.6 mm in thickness: the importance of revealing alternate Cox models. *Ann Surg* **195**:44–49, 1982

64. Larsen TE et al: International pathologists congruence survey on quantitation of malignant melanoma. *Pathology* **12**:245–253, 1980

65. Day CL et al: The natural breakpoints for primary tumor thickness in clinical stage I melanoma. *N Engl J Med* **305**:1155, 1981

66. Wanebo HJ et al: Malignant melanoma of the extremities: a clinico-pathologic study using levels of invasion (microstage). *Cancer* **35**:666–676, 1975

67. Breslow A: Tumor thickness, level of invasion, and node dissection in stage I cutaneous melanoma. *Ann Surg* **182**:572–575, 1975

68. Veronesi U et al: Stage I melanoma of the limbs. Immediate versus delayed node dissection. *Tumori* **66**:373–396, 1980

69. Day CL et al: Prognosis in malignant melanoma. *J Am Acad Dermatol* **3**:525–526, 1980

70. Balch CM et al: Tumor thickness as a guide to surgical management of clinical stage I melanoma patients. *Cancer* **43**:883–888, 1979

HERITABLE DISEASES WITH INCREASED SENSITIVITY TO CELLULAR INJURY

Kenneth H. Kraemer

A group of heritable diseases with differing clinical features share the common characteristics of in vitro or in vivo cellular hypersensitivity to damage by several physical or chemical agents [1–15]. Diseases with autosomal recessive, X-linked, and autosomal dominant inheritance fall into this group [16–18]. Clinical abnormalities in these disorders involve cutaneous, ocular, nervous, immune, hemopoietic, skeletal, or gastrointestinal systems. Some are associated with increased incidence of neoplasia. Several have a primary feature of progressive degeneration of previously normal bodily function [19]. This cellular hypersensitivity is often of diagnostic utility. Further, it may suggest pathogenic mechanisms and measures for therapeutic or prophylactic intervention. Very little is presently known of the molecular basis of the cellular hypersensitivity in most of these disorders. This chapter is divided into two portions: one outlining the major tests used to assess cellular hypersensitivity and the other portion describing the clinical features and cellular abnormalities found in each disorder.

Use of Cultured Cells for Assessment of Hypersensitivity

Cells for study are usually maintained in liquid culture medium [20]. This consists of a mixture of inorganic salts (calcium chloride, sodium chloride, magnesium sulfate, and others), vitamins, amino acids, and an energy source (most often glucose).

113

Buffers such as bicarbonate may be used to stabilize the pH at 7.1 to 7.4. A dilute solution of phenol red is often included to act as a visual pH indicator (phenol red turns from yellow to red in the pH range 6.6 to 8.0). Most cultured cells require the addition of serum to the medium. The serum provides as yet unidentified growth factors to the cells. Fetal bovine serum, calf serum, horse serum, or human serum is utilized, depending on the requirements of the particular cell type. Cultured cells are maintained at 37°C in temperature-regulated incubators. Some cells require 5% to 10% CO_2 for optimal growth.

Cells obtained directly from patients and grown in culture medium are termed *primary cultures*. Primary cultures are used in studies utilizing peripheral blood lymphocytes, epidermal cells, or differentiated tumor cells. These cells generally go through a very limited number of divisions in culture. Lymphocytes may be stimulated to divide by means of mitogens such as phytohemagglutinin, a plant lectin. Primary cultures of differentiated, adherent cells (such as epidermal keratinocytes) generally cannot be successfully subcultured (removed from their original tissue culture dish, separated, diluted in fresh medium, and placed in new dishes where growth is resumed).

Dermal fibroblasts, in contrast, generally grow well in culture and can be subcultured. These skin fibroblast cultures may be frozen (in medium containing glycerol) at liquid nitrogen temperatures and stored indefinitely in a state of suspended animation. When thawed, most of the cells recover and resume growth in fresh culture medium. These features have made skin fibroblasts very popular for studies of human genetic diseases. However, skin fibroblasts generally have a limited life span (approximately 40 subcultures). Their growth rate then slows dramatically and they cannot be successfully subcultured.

In order to avoid this cellular senescence, techniques have been developed to immortalize cultured cells. Transformation of lymphocytes with Epstein-Barr (E-B) virus (or fibroblasts with SV_{40} virus) results in cultures of cells that grow indefinitely without senescence [21]. The virus generally grows within these transformed cells without killing the cell and without being released into the culture medium. Such transformed lymphocytes have an appearance resembling immature lymphoid cells and have been termed *lymphoblastoid cell lines*. These cells readily grow to high cell density in suspension culture. They also may be stored indefinitely in liquid nitrogen. Lymphoblastoid cell lines have also become popular for studies of human genetic diseases.

Primary cultures of skin dermal fibroblasts can generally be established with a few cubic millimeters of sterile tissue, as from a 3- to 4-mm punch biopsy. The inner surface of the upper arm has proved to be a suitable site because this area heals easily, the resulting scar is not readily visible, the site is shielded from ultraviolet (UV) radiation, and a large proportion of the attempts to establish cultures have been successful. Lymphoblastoid cell lines generally can be established by E-B virus treatment of 5 to 10 mL of sterile, heparinized whole blood.

A nomenclature for cultured cells from patients with xeroderma pigmentosum has gained worldwide acceptance. The strain is identified by a name of the form: *XP*, followed by a number, which is followed by two letters indicating the location of the laboratory establishing the culture. Thus XP12BE indicates xeroderma pigmentosum strain number 12 established in Bethesda. Strains from heterozygotes are designated *XPH*. By analogy, ataxia-telangiectasia strains begin with *AT*, Cockayne's syndrome strains with *CS*, and Fanconi anemia strains with *FA*. In the United States, cultures of human cells are received by and are available for research from the Human Genetic Mutant Cell Repository, Camden, New Jersey; The American Type Culture Collection, Rockville, Maryland; and the Naval Biosciences Laboratory, Naval Supply Center, Oakland, California.

Assessment of Cellular Hypersensitivity

Tests to assess cellular hypersensitivity to physical or chemical agents may be divided into tests of intact cellular function or of chromosome integrity (Table 1) and tests which measure the mechanism of impairment of cell function such as DNA repair (Table 2).

Tests of Intact Cell Function

Tests of cellular function measure the capacity of the intact cell to recover from the damage induced.

Table 1   Tests of cellular sensitivity to physical or chemical agents

Intact cell function
  Growth rate
  Colony-forming ability
  Viral host cell reactivation
  Mutagenesis

Chromosome integrity
  Chromosome breakage
  Sister chromatid exchanges

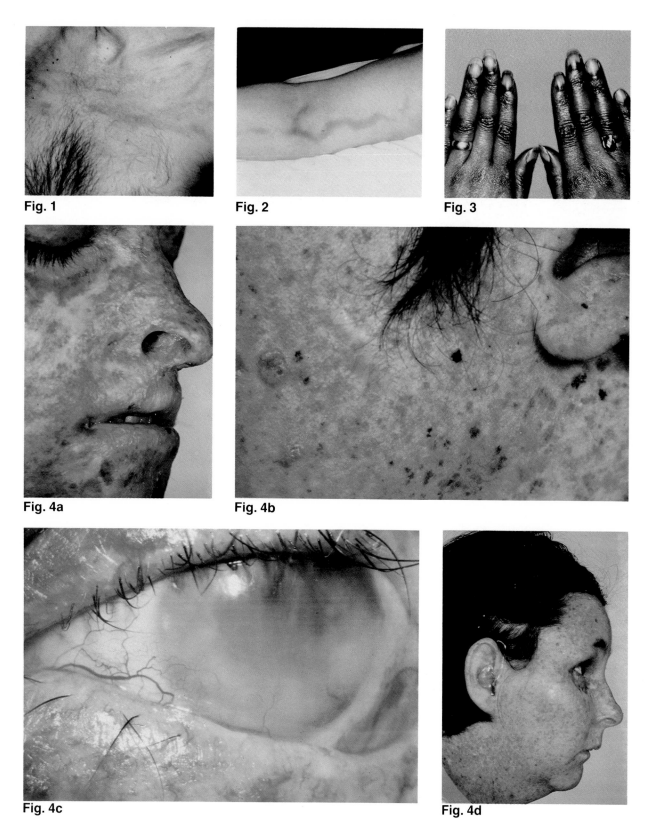

Fig. 1 Linear, "flagellate" hyperpigmentation following bleomycin therapy. *(From Adrian RM et al: Mucocutaneous reactions to antineoplastic agents. CA 30:143–157, 1980 with permission.)* **Fig. 2** Phlebitis secondary to actinomycin-D injections. **Fig. 3** Horzontal hyperpigmentation of the nails associated with doxorubicin. *(Courtesy of Dr. Harris Blackman.)* **Fig. 4** Xeroderma pigmentosum. **(a)** Pigmentary and atrophic changes in the skin of a 16-year-old patient. **(b)** Cheek of a 14-year-old patient with pigmentary abnormalities, actinic keratoses, and basal cell carcinoma. **(c)** Corneal clouding, prominent conjunctival blood vasculature, and loss of lashes. **(d)** A 26-year-old patient with deafness and mental retardation.

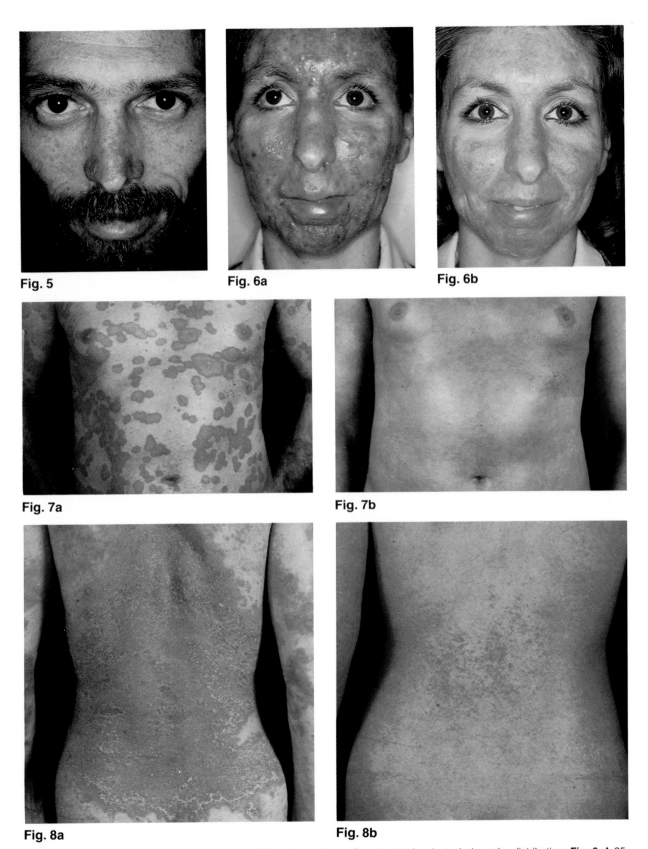

Fig. 5 Bloom's syndrome. Prominent telangiectasia in malar distribution. **Fig. 6** A 35-year-old female with severe cystic acne before **(a)** and after **(b)** 4 months of treatment with isotretinoid 60 mg/day. **Fig. 7** A 37-year-old male with extensive psoriasis vulgaris before **(a)** and after **(b)** 6 weeks of treatment with etretinate. *(Courtesy of Dr. C. Orfanos, Berlin.)* **Fig. 8** A 31-year-old female with generalized pustular psoriasis before **(a)** and after **(b)** 2 1/2 months of treatment with etretinate. *(Courtesy of Dr. C. Orfanos, Berlin.)*

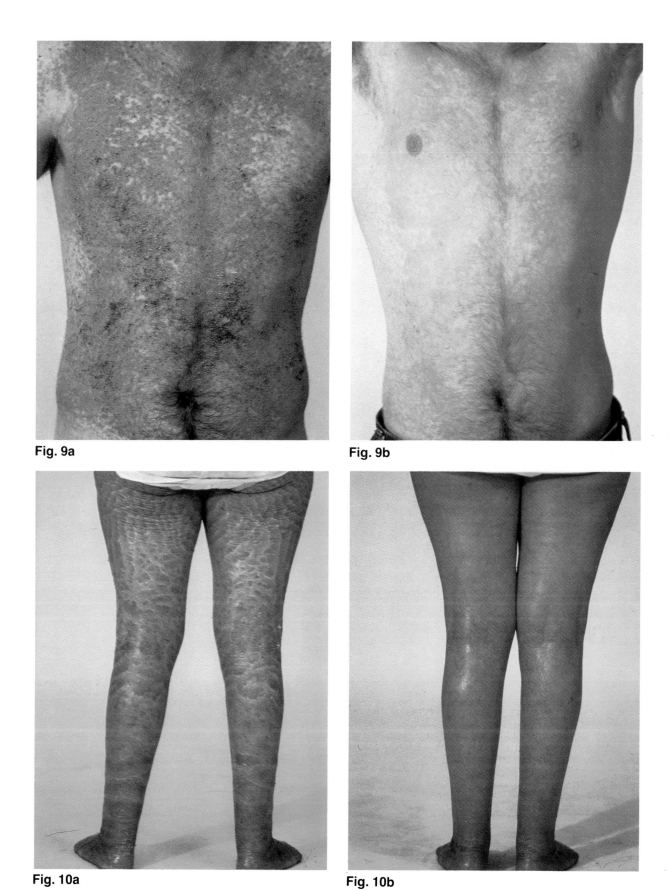

Fig. 9 A 26-year-old male with Darier's disease before **(a)** and after **(b)** 1 month of treatment with isotretinoin 60 mg/day. **Fig. 10** A 23-year-old female with lamellar ichthyosis before **(a)** and after **(b)** 1 month of treatment with isotretinoin 120 mg/day.

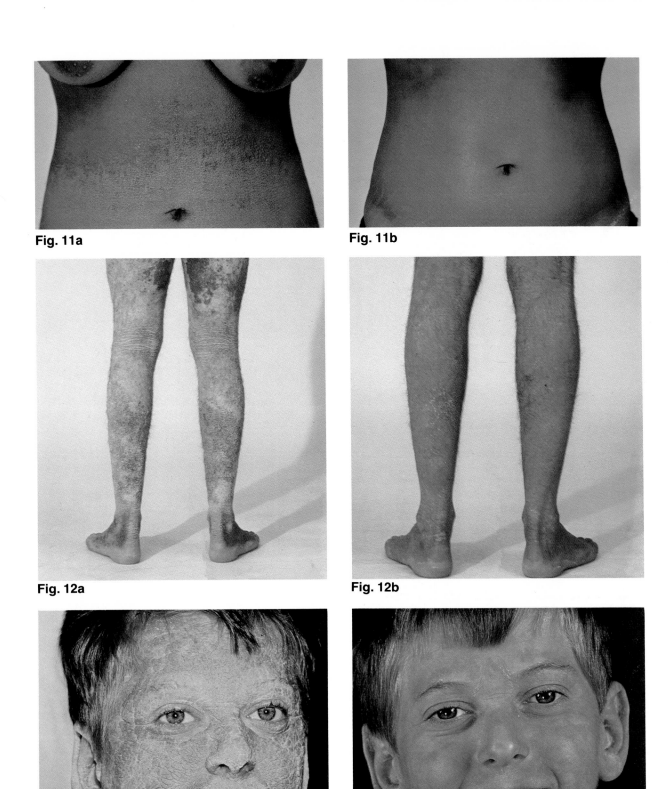

Fig. 11a

Fig. 11b

Fig. 12a

Fig. 12b

Fig. 13a

Fig. 13b

Fig. 11 A 33-year-old female with pityriasis rubra pilaris before **(a)** and after **(b)** 4 months of treatment with isotretinoin 160 mg/day. **Fig. 12** An 18-year-old male with epidermolytic hyperkeratosis before **(a)** and after **(b)** 2 months of treatment with isotretinoin 60 mg/day. **Fig. 13** A 13-year-old boy with erythrokeratodermia figurata variabilis before **(a)** and after **(b)** treatment with etretinate. *(Reprinted from Der Hatuarzt **30**:161–163, 1979.)*

Table 2   Tests of DNA repair function

Repair system	Step measured	Assay
Nucleotide excision repair	Endonuclease	Alkaline sucrose gradient Alkaline elution
	Endonuclease plus exonuclease	Direct dimer measurement Loss of endonuclease-sensitive sites Loss of antibody-reactive sites
	Endonuclease plus exonuclease plus polymerase	Repair replication (isopyknic CsC1 gradient) Unscheduled DNA synthesis (UDS) (autoradiography) Hydroxyurea-resistant thymidine incorporation Bromodeoxyuridine photolysis repair BND cellulose column chromatography
Postreplication repair	Gap formation plus gap filling	Rate of increase of molecular weight of newly replicated DNA after damage (alkaline sucrose gradient)
Base excision repair	Glycosylase action AP endonuclease	Release of altered base AP endonuclease activity
Photoreactivation repair	In situ repair	Photoreactivating enzyme activity

These tests do not provide information as to the specific damage resulting in cellular injury or the mechanism of cellular recovery but do form the basis for identifying cells as hypersensitive.

Growth Rate. One of the simplest tests of cellular function is the assessment of the growth rate of cells in mass culture. This method has been applied to cultured fibroblasts and to lymphoblastoid cell lines. Suspended cells are counted in a hemocytometer under a microscope (or by means of a Coulter counter) and the cell concentration determined. Daily changes in the cell concentration reflect cell growth. A variation of this assay involves treating the suspended cells with the vital dye, trypan blue [23]. The population is then scored for the concentration of unstained cells (termed *viable cells*) and stained cells (nonviable cells). Figure 1a shows growth of lymphoblastoid cell lines derived from a normal individual and from a patient with xeroderma pigmentosum. The initial concentration was 100,000 viable cells per mL. The untreated cells showed an exponential increase in concentration of viable cells as assessed by daily hemocytometer counts. Ultraviolet-irradiated normal lymphoblastoid cells had a 1-day growth lag followed by an exponential increase in viable cell concentration. In marked contrast, the viable cell concentration in the UV-treated xeroderma pigmentosum lymphoblastoid cell line fell exponentially with no recovery. This indicates that the xeroderma pigmentosum lymphoblastoid cell line was hypersensitive to the growth-inhibiting effects of UV radiation [1,2,9]. Figure 1b illustrates an analogous experiment using ataxia-telangiec-

tasia and normal lymphoblastoid cells treated with x-radiation. The untreated ataxia-telangiectasia and normal lymphoblastoid cells grow at a similar rate. It is apparent that the ataxia-telangiectasia cells were more sensitive to x-ray-induced growth inhibition than the normal cells.

Fig. 1.   Growth rate assay of cell sensitivity. (a) Ultraviolet sensitivity of xeroderma pigmentosum and normal lymphoblastoid cell lines. (b) X-ray sensitivity of ataxia-telangiectasia and normal lymphoblastoid cell lines.

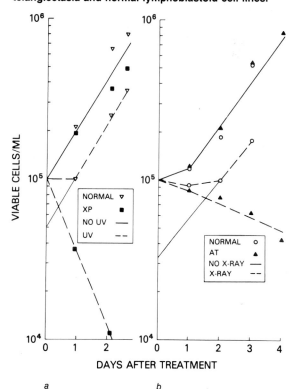

The shape of the growth curve may be utilized as a quantitative measure of cell survival under certain circumstances. If the treated population resumes growth at the same exponential rate as the untreated population, then the ratio of their intercepts at day zero may be interpreted as the surviving fraction. Thus, in Fig. 1a the treated normal cells resumed exponential growth at a similar rate as the untreated cells. Back extrapolation shows that this may be considered to represent the growth of 50,000 cells per mL at day zero. Thus, since the original population contained 100,000 cells per mL, the UV treatment resulted in 50,000/100,000 = 50 percent survival. The UV-treated xeroderma pigmentosum cells did not resume exponential growth. Though it is apparent that they were more sensitive than the normal cells, the extent of cell killing cannot be quantitated by this method.

Colony-Forming Ability. Colony-forming ability assesses the capacity of a single cell to proliferate enough to form a visible colony. This differs from the growth rate analysis, which measures the proliferative ability of a population of cells. Quantitation of survival by growth curves is subject to the criticism that the lag in growth following treatment (c.f. treated normals in Figs. 1a and b) may represent growth delay in the entire population rather than cell killing with a fraction of the cells surviving. Single-cell colony-forming ability measurements avoid this objection.

Colony-forming ability assessment has been utilized with fibroblasts and with lymphoblastoid cell lines [21,23,24]. With adherent fibroblasts, cells are treated and then placed in tissue culture dishes at appropriate dilutions so that the final number of colonies per dish is in a countable range (generally less than 100 colonies per 100-mm tissue culture plates). The treated cultures are incubated for 2 to 3 weeks at 37°C to permit the isolated cells to divide sufficiently to form visible colonies. The dishes are then stained and the number of colonies (aggregates of at least 15 to 30 cells of similar morphology) per plate counted with a dissecting microscope. The results of typical experiments are shown in Fig. 2. Normal and xeroderma pigmentosum fibroblasts were exposed to 254-nm UV radiation and colony-forming ability determined. The mean colony-forming ability for the unirradiated cells ranged from 3.1 to 27 percent. The colony-forming ability of the treated cells is plotted relative to that of the untreated cells. We see that both xeroderma pigmentosum fibroblast strains were more sensitive than the normal strain

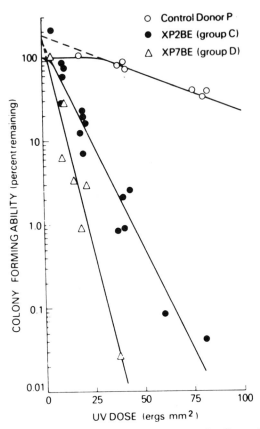

Fig. 2. Colony-forming ability assay of cell sensitivity. Ultraviolet sensitivity of two xeroderma pigmentosum and one normal fibroblast strain. *(Reproduced from Kraemer et al [24].)*

to UV-induced inhibition of colony-forming ability. Colony-forming ability of lymphoblastoid cells may be similarly measured by growth in agar or in microtiter wells [23].

Viral Host Cell Reactivation. This assay relies on the fact that many DNA viruses do not have the ability to repair damage to their DNA but depend on cellular repair systems [22,25]. Thus, damaged viruses would be expected to grow better on cells with normal repair capacity than on cells with reduced repair capacity. In practice, a virus suspension is treated with the damaging agent and then appropriate dilutions of virus are inoculated onto a "lawn" of confluent fibroblasts in a tissue culture plate. Next, the cells are overlaid with nutrient-containing agar (to immobilize extracellular virus particles) and incubated at 37°C for 1 to 2 weeks. After staining, visible "plaques" are apparent in areas where the virus underwent several cycles of replication and spread to adjacent cells. Figure 3 shows an experiment measuring the ability of normal and xeroderma pigmentosum fibroblasts to repair damage to adenovirus 2 treated

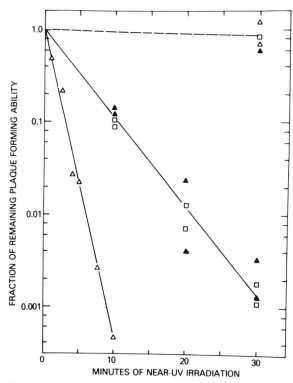

Fig. 3. Viral host cell reactivation assay of cell sensitivity. Relative ability of xeroderma pigmentosum and normal fibroblast strains to repair TMP plus near-UV-damaged adenovirus 2. Solid lines indicate data obtained in the presence of 4,5′,8-trimethylpsoralen, dashed line indicates data obtained with near-UV in the absence of TMP (△ XPILO, complementation group A; □ XP4BE, variant; ▲ normal). *(Reproduced from Day [25].)*

with 4,5′,8-trimethylpsoralen (TMP) followed by long-wavelength ultraviolet (UVA) irradiation. This treatment is known to produce binding of the TMP to the viral DNA. Thirty minutes of irradiation in the absence of trimethylpsoralen did not affect viral plaque-forming ability on any of the fibroblast strains. After pretreatment with TMP, plaque-forming ability at a given UVA exposure was reduced to a greater extent using the xeroderma pigmentosum complementation group A fibroblasts as hosts than with the normal or xeroderma pigmentosum variant strains as host. This decreased host cell reactivation in the xeroderma pigmentosum strain is strong evidence that these cells lack the ability to repair DNA damage induced by TMP plus UVA [25].

Mutagenesis. Assays of induced mutations measure the frequency of induction of mutated cells following treatment with damaging agents [22]. At present there are a limited number of mutated characteristics that have been examined in culture: thioguanine resistance [resulting from loss of activity

of the enzyme hypoxanthine-guanine phosphoribosyl transferase (HGPRT)], ouabain resistance (due to alteration in membrane ATPase), and diphtheria toxin resistance. In practice, a cell population is treated with a sublethal dose of damaging agent, grown for an interval (hours to days) in normal medium to permit "expression" of the mutation within the population, then grown under selective conditions which kill nonmutated cells and permit only mutated cells to grow. The growing cells presumably have mutations induced in their DNA. Such somatic mutations are thought to be related to induction of cancer in vivo. For example, at a given dose of UV radiation the frequency of mutation to HGPRT$^-$ per surviving cell is higher in xeroderma pigmentosum than in normal fibroblasts [2,9].

Tests of Chromosome Integrity

Chromosome Breakage. Chromosome breakage is usually assessed in primary cultures of mitogen-stimulated peripheral blood leukocytes or in long-term cultures of fibroblasts or lymphoblastoid cell lines [22,26]. Cell cycle progression is stopped at metaphase by treatment of the cells with a mitotic inhibitor such as colchicine. The cells are swollen in hypotonic salt solution and then fixed and lysed on glass slides. With this procedure, the metaphase chromosomes from a single cell are separated and spread over a discrete area of the slide. The preparation is stained, usually with Giemsa, and examined under oil immersion. For karyotypic analysis, photomicrographs are obtained and the individual chromosomes cut out and arranged in sequence. Some staining procedures permit discrimination of characteristic light and dark bands on each chromosome, facilitating identification of specific regions within each of the 23 pairs of human chromosomes.

Chromosome preparations may be analyzed for the number of chromosomes per metaphase, the morphology of the individual chromosomes, and the attachments or rearrangements of chromosomes with each other. Chromosome aberrations include breaks, gaps, translocations, dicentrics, and quadriradials. Figure 4 shows examples of spontaneous chromosomal aberrations in peripheral blood lymphocytes from patients with Bloom's syndrome. Spontaneous chromosome breakage is seen in Bloom's syndrome, ataxia-telangiectasia, and Fanconi anemia. These disorders are also associated with a high rate of neoplasia.

Chromosome breakage may also be assessed after treatment of cells with damaging agents.

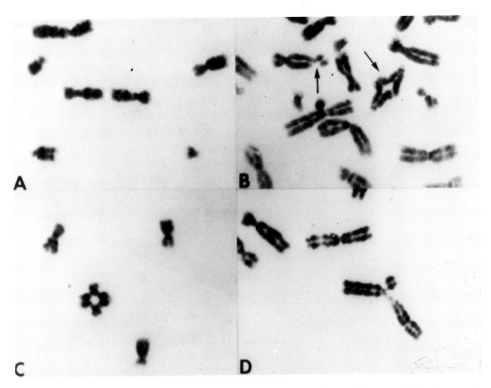

Fig. 4.   Chromosome breakage assay of cell sensitivity (Bloom's syndrome peripheral blood lymphocytes). (A) Terminal association of telomeres of homologous chromosomes. (B) and (C) Quadriradial configuration of homologous chromosomes. (D) A triradial configuration, seen less often than A-C. G-banding. (*Photographs courtesy of James L. German and Steven Schonberg.*)

Xeroderma pigmentosum cells are hypersensitive to chromosome breakage following UV irradiation [2,9].

Sister Chromatid Exchange. During cell growth, chromatids occasionally exchange positions along the arms of a chromosome. This "sister chromatid exchange" (SCE) may be detected by permitting the cells to grow through two cycles of replication in medium containing the nucleic acid analogue bromodeoxyuridine (BrUdR) (Fig. 5) [22,26–28]. After the first cycle of replication, the DNA of the newly synthesized chromatid strand is labeled with BrUdR while the older strand is unlabeled. Such chromosomes appear uniformly dark with Giemsa's stain. After a second cycle of replication in BrUdR-containing medium, one arm of a chromosome will contain two labeled chromatids while the other will contain one labeled and one unlabeled chromatid. Under appropriate staining the doubly substituted arm will stain lightly while the singly substituted arm will stain darkly. If a SCE occurred during replication, a portion of each chromosome arm would be doubly substituted and the remainder singly substituted with BrUdR. The resulting Giemsa-stained appearance is of light and dark areas and has been termed a *harlequin chromosome,* after the famous clown costume. Sister chromatid exchanges are thought to be related to DNA damage and repair although their precise significance is not understood. Figure 6 shows the appearance of mitogen-stimulated peripheral blood lymphocytes from a patient with Bloom's syndrome which have been treated to reveal spontaneous SCEs. Lymphocytes from normal individuals generally have 8 to 10 SCEs per metaphase. The Bloom's syndrome metaphase shown has 152 SCEs. This dramatically increased spontaneous rate of SCEs per metaphase is characteristic of Bloom's syndrome [29,30]. Xeroderma pigmentosum cells have an abnormally great increase in the SCE rate after treatment with UV radiation [2,9,31].

DNA Repair. Many environmental physical and chemical agents kill cells by damaging the cellular DNA. Some of the agents commonly used in laboratory studies on human cells and the type of damage induced are shown in Table 3 [8,22]. Normal cells contain enzyme systems which repair DNA damage. In bacteria, mutants with defective DNA repair have been shown to be hypersensitive to killing by physical agents (UV, x-ray) or chem-

**STAGE OF
CELL CYCLE**

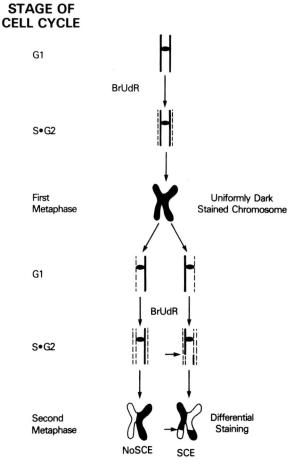

Fig. 5.   Schematic diagram of SCE assay of cell sensitivity. Cultured cells are permitted to go through two cycles of replication in medium containing bromodeoxyuridine. Staining with Giemsa's or Hoechst dye number 33258 differentiates singly substituted from doubly substituted chromosomes, thus permitting recognition of SCEs.

icals. Some of these hypersensitivity characteristics have been found in cells from patients. This has fueled the notion that the patients might also have defective DNA repair.

Figure 7 is a schematic diagram of DNA repair pathways in prokaryotes or eukaryotes [2,8,32]. Several pathways remove or reverse lesions in DNA; one pathway results in cell functioning with DNA lesions persisting. This schematic diagram will probably need to be modified as further information is obtained in this area of active research.

The "nucleotide excision repair" pathway is known to act on DNA damaged with UV radiation (forming thymine dimers and other photoproducts) or damaged with certain carcinogens [such as acetoxyacetoaminofluorene (AAAF)] (Table 3). In this pathway the damaged nucleotide is removed along with a number of adjacent nucleotides,

leaving a gap in one strand of the DNA. The gap is filled using the opposite strand as a template. This pathway results in repaired DNA with damage removed.

Another pathway, the "base excision repair" pathway, may also function on UV-induced lesions and other lesions such as alkylations, induced by carcinogens (e.g., dimethylsulfate). The initial step in the base excision repair pathway results in removal of the damaged base leaving the sugar-phosphate backbone of the DNA strand intact. Other enzymes then split the DNA at this base-free [apurinic (AP)] site. In vitro, certain basic tripeptides have been shown to possess this AP-endonuclease activity. This pathway then feeds into the end of the nucleotide excision repair pathway. Alternatively an "insertase" may directly replace the excised base without cutting the DNA backbone. DNA with methylated bases [produced by carcinogens such as methylnitronitro-soguanidine (MNNG)] may be repaired by removal of the methyl group (via a methyltransferase) without removal of the base.

A third pathway involves direct reversal of UV-induced thymine dimers. This "photoreactivation repair" is mediated via a photoreactivating enzyme (or a basic tripeptide in vitro) which is activated by visible light. The nucleotide excision repair, base excision repair, and photoreactivation repair pathways result in repaired DNA with the damage removed.

The "postreplication repair" pathway enables the cell to bypass the damaged bases during DNA replication. The ensuing gap is filled, resulting in replicated DNA with damage present.

Each step of the DNA repair pathways may be analyzed separately (Table 2). More extensive descriptions of these assays may be found [22]. One of the tests, unscheduled DNA synthesis (UDS), will be described. This test has been used to measure DNA repair in intact human skin, in cultured epidermal or dermal cells, and in blood cells and for prenatal diagnosis on amniotic fluid cells.

Unscheduled DNA synthesis measures the combined action of endonuclease, exonuclease, and polymerase in the nucleotide excision repair system. Cells are treated with UV radiation or other DNA-damaging agent and then incubated in medium containing radioactive thymidine. During the process of nucleotide excision repair the damage is removed and the radioactive thymidine is incorporated into the repaired region. The cells are treated with fixative, coated with autoradiographic (photographic) emulsion, and kept in the dark for

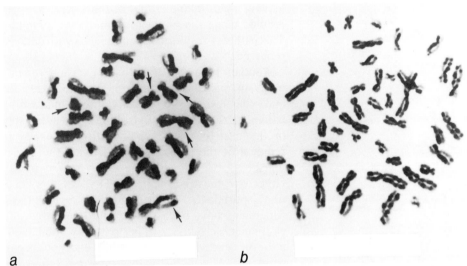

Fig. 6. Sister chromatid exchange assay of cell sensitivity. *(a)* **Undamaged normal cultured peripheral blood leukocytes have about 10 SCEs per metaphase.** *(b)* **Cultured peripheral blood leukocytes from a patient with Bloom's syndrome have a manyfold increase in spontaneous SCEs.** *(Reproduced from Chaganti et al [29], with permission.)*

an appropriate interval (usually 1 or more weeks). The emulsion is then developed. During the exposure interval the decay of tritium from the thymidine incorporated into the DNA exposes a small portion of the overlying emulsion. The tritium is revealed as a microscopic, dark grain in the developed emulsion located above the cellular location of the incorporated thymidine. This incorporation of thymidine occurs in phases of the cell cycle other than the S phase, in which DNA synthesis is normally scheduled. It is thus known

as unscheduled DNA synthesis (UDS). Figure 8 shows an example of measurement of UDS in cultured human fibroblasts. Figure 8a shows that, except for cells in S phase, there were very few grains over the nuclei of fibroblasts that received no UV radiation. Ultraviolet irradiation of normal fibroblasts resulted in a large increase in the number of grains over all the nuclei (Fig. 8b). In marked contrast, irradiation of the xeroderma pigmentosum fibroblasts resulted in very few grains over their nuclei (Fig. 8c). Counting the number

Fig. 7. Schematic diagram of DNA repair pathways in prokaryotes or eukaryotes. *(Modified from Kraemer [2].)*

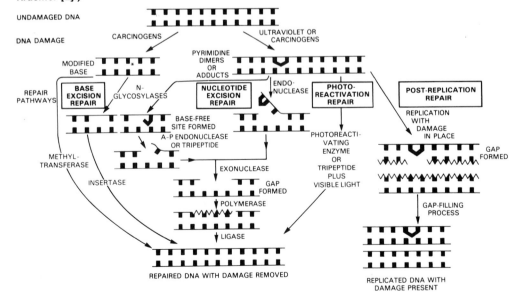

Table 3   Cellular damage induced by physical and chemical agents

Agent	Damage
Ultraviolet radiation	DNA: thymine dimers, thymine-cytosine dimers and adducts, cytosine-cytosine dimers and adducts, thymine glycols, DNA-protein cross-links
X-radiation	DNA strand breaks, altered bases (thymine glycols)
Psoralens plus UVA	DNA-psoralen monoadducts, DNA interstrand cross-links, psoralen-protein binding (high dose)
Mitomycin C	DNA interstrand cross-links
4-Nitroquinoline oxide (4NQO)	Binds to purines in DNA making bulky adducts
Acetoxyacetoaminofluorene (AAAF)	Binds to guanine in DNA making bulky adducts
Methylnitronitrosoguanidine (MNNG)	Methylates bases in DNA, binds to proteins

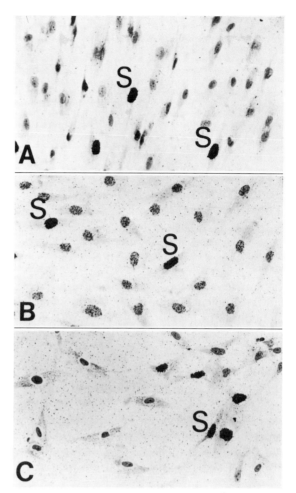

Fig. 8.   Unscheduled DNA synthesis assay of DNA repair. (A) No repair in unirradiated normal fibroblasts. S-phase cells are heavily labeled with radioactive thymidine. (B) Numerous autoradiographic grains overlie the nuclei of UV-irradiated normal fibroblasts, indicating the presence of unscheduled DNA synthesis. (C) Few autoradiographic grains overlie the nuclei of UV-irradiated xeroderma pigmentosum fibroblasts, indicating reduced unscheduled DNA synthesis.

of grains over the nuclei of irradiated cells provides a means of quantifying the extent of DNA excision repair.

A related assay of DNA excision repair in common use relies on hydroxyurea to selectively suppress S phase DNA synthesis while permitting DNA repair to continue. Damaged cells are incubated with hydroxyurea and tritiated thymidine. Thymidine incorporation into the culture is then determined by scintillation spectroscopy. This assay is thus much more rapid than autoradiography but cannot assess repair in individual cells.

Cell fusion studies have been utilized to determine whether cells with DNA repair defects have the same or different defects [1,2,36,37]. This technique involves treating a mixture of fibroblasts from two donors with an agent, such as inactivated Sendai virus or polyethylene glycol, which promotes syncitia formation (Fig. 9). The cell membranes fuse and the nuclei remain intact within the shared cytoplasm. A multinucleate cell with all the nuclei from one donor is termed a *homokaryon*. If at least one nucleus is from a different donor than the others, the multinucleated cell is termed a *heterokaryon*.

Fusion of fibroblasts from two xeroderma pigmentosum patients with DNA repair defects was followed by UV exposure and autoradiographic determination of unscheduled DNA synthesis (Fig. 10). The heterokaryons had a markedy increased amount of unscheduled DNA synthesis in comparison to the homokaryons or to the unfused mononuclear xeroderma pigmentosum cells. This

implies that the two fused xeroderma pigmentosum fibroblast strains had complementary DNA repair defects. Each strain supplied what the other was lacking. Such xeroderma pigmentosum fibroblasts are said to be in different DNA repair complementation groups. Heterokaryons resulting from xeroderma pigmentosum patients with the same DNA repair defect do not show an increase in post-UV unscheduled DNA synthesis. Such cells are said to be in the same complementation group.

In theory, such cell fusion testing can be applied to any two cell strains which have a measurable defect in the same assay in order to determine whether the defects are the same or different. Some systems may require nuclear fusion (hybrid

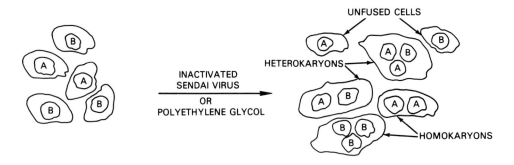

Fig. 9. Schematic diagram of cell fusion technique. Cocultured fibroblasts from two donors are treated with inactivated Sendai virus or polyethylene glycol to induce cell fusion.

formation) in addition to cytoplasmic fusion to manifest complementation. At present, complementation groups have been identified with fibroblasts from xeroderma pigmentosum and ataxia-telangiectasia patients.

Diseases with Cellular Hypersensitivity

The remainder of this chapter will present clinical features and laboratory abnormalities of the heritable diseases with cellular abnormalities listed on Table 4. The diseases will be discussed in terms

Fig. 10. Increased unscheduled DNA synthesis in complementing xeroderma pigmentosum heterokaryons. A mixed culture of fused xeroderma pigmentosum fibroblasts was exposed to UV irradiation, and unscheduled DNA synthesis was determined. The nuclei of S-phase cells (S) are heavily labeled with radioactive thymidine. The unfused mononuclear cells have the same low level of unscheduled DNA synthesis as the fused homokaryons (ho). The heterokaryons (arrows), containing nuclei from both xeroderma pigmentosum fibroblast strains, have increased unscheduled DNA synthesis, indicating mutual correction of their DNA repair defects.

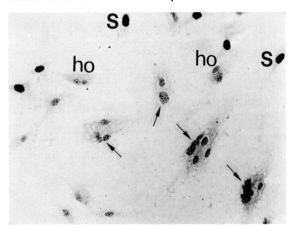

of the systems affected, the cellular hypersensitivity, and the relevance of the cellular abnormality to the clinical symptoms.

Xeroderma Pigmentosum

Definition. Xeroderma pigmentosum (XP) serves as the prototype heritable disease with cellular hypersensitivity [1–9]. Xeroderma pigmentosum is an autosomal recessive disease with sun sensitivity, photophobia, early onset of freckling, and subsequent neoplastic changes on sun-exposed surfaces. There is cellular hypersensitivity to UV radiation and certain chemicals in association with abnormal DNA repair. Some of the patients have progressive neurologic degeneration.

Frequency. XP has been estimated to occur with a frequency of 1:250,000 in the United States and to be more common in Japan [1]. Patients have been reported worldwide in all races. Consanguinity is common.

Clinical Features. Approximately half of xeroderma pigmentosum patients have a history of acute sunburn reaction on minimal UV radiation exposure. Continued sun exposure causes the patient's skin to become dry and parchment-like and hence the name *xeroderma* ("dry skin") (see Fig. 4a, color plate). Numerous freckle-like hyperpigmented macules appear, usually before 2 years of age (see Fig 4b, color plate). These are strikingly limited to sun-exposed areas. Premalignant actinic keratoses develop at an early age (see Fig. 4b, color plate). Basal cell and squamous cell carcinomas of the skin or eyes are present in most patients. The appearance of sun-exposed skin in children with xeroderma pigmentosum is similar

Table 4 Heritable diseases with cellular hypersensitivity

Disease	Clinical abnormalities					Cellular abnormalities	
	Cutaneous	Ocular	Nervous	Hematopoietic	Neoplasia	Type	Mechanism
Autosomal recessive							
Xeroderma pigmentosum	Sun sensitivity, atrophy, freckling	Photophobia, UV conjunctivitis, UV keratitis	Deafness, progressive mental deterioration	Normal	BCC, SCC, melanoma	UV-induced: cell killing, mutagenesis, chromosome breakage, SCE	Abnormal DNA repair
Ataxia-telangiectasia	Telangiectasia, x-ray sensitivity	Conjunctival telangiectasia Oculomotor dyspraxia	Progressive ataxia	Humoral and cellular immune defects	Lymphoreticular, GI	Spontaneous chromosome breakage; x-ray-induced: cell killing, chromosome breakage	Abnormal DNA repair (?)
Fanconi's anemia	Hyperpigmentation	Normal	Normal	Anemia	Leukemia, liver	Spontaneous chromosome breakage; mitomycin C–induced: cell killing, chromosome breakage	Abnormal DNA cross-link repair
Cockayne's syndrome	Sun sensitivity, hyperpigmentation	Retinal pigmentation	Progressive mental deterioration	Normal	None	UV-induced: cell killing, SCE	?
Bloom's syndrome	Telangiectasia, sun sensitivity	Normal	Normal	Defective immunity	Leukemia, GI	Spontaneous chromosome breakage, SCE	?
Chédiak-Higashi syndrome	Pigment dilution, gray hair	Hypopigmented irises	Normal	Defective immunity	?	UV-induced: cell killing	?
X-linked							
Dyskeratosis congenita	Poikiloderma, nail dystrophy	Stenosis of lacrimal duct	Normal	Anemia	GI	Psoralen-induced: SCE	?
Autosomal dominant							
Gardner's syndrome	Cysts, desmoids	Normal	Normal	Normal	Colon polyps and carcinoma	X-ray-induced: cell killing (some patients)	?
Basal cell nevus syndrome	Palmar pits, x-ray sensitivity	Cataract, coloboma	Mental retardation (some patients)	Normal	BCC, medulloblastoma, ovarian tumors	Spontaneous chromosome abnormalities (some patients)	?
Familial retinoblastoma	Normal	Retinoblastoma	Normal	Normal	Retinoblastoma Osteosarcoma	Chromosome deletion; x-ray-induced: cell killing	?
Tuberous sclerosis	White spots, shagreen patch, angiofibromas	Normal	Seizures	Normal	?	X-ray-induced: cell killing	?
Huntington's disease	Normal	Normal	Adult-onset mental deterioration	Normal	None	X-ray-induced: cell killing	?

to that occurring in farmers and sailors after many years of extreme sun exposure. Multiple primary melanomas may occur. More rarely, primary neoplasms of the oral cavity (especially the tip of the tongue) and the brain and leukemia have been reported.

Ocular abnormalities are almost as common as the cutaneous abnormalities and may be considered an important feature of xeroderma pigmentosum [2]. Photophobia is usually present and is associated with prominent conjunctival injection. Continued UV exposure of the eye may result in severe keratitis, (see Fig. 4c, color plate) and vascularization. The lids develop increased pigmentation and loss of lashes. Atrophy of the skin of the lids results in ectropion, entropion, or, in severe cases, complete loss of the lids. Benign conjunctival inflammatory masses or papillomas of the lids may be present. Epithelioma, squamous cell carcinoma, and melanoma of UV-exposed portions of the eye are common.

Progressive neurologic degeneration has been reported in approximately 40 percent of the patients [2]. Onset of neurologic abnormalities may be early in infancy or, in some patients, delayed until the second decade. The neurologic abnormalities may be mild (e.g., isolated hyporeflexia) or severe, with progressive mental retardation (see Fig. 4d, color plate), sensorineural deafness, spasticity, or seizures. The most severe form, known as the DeSanctis-Cacchione syndrome, involves the cutaneous and ocular manifestations of classic xeroderma pigmentosum plus additional neurologic and somatic abnormalities including microcephaly, progressive mental deterioration, low intelligence, hyporeflexia or areflexia, choreoathetosis, ataxia, spasticity, Achilles tendon shortening with eventual quadraparesis, markedly retarded growth, and immature sexual development. The complete DeSanctis-Cacchione syndrome has been recognized in very few patients; however, many xeroderma pigmentosum patients have one or more of its neurologic features. The predominant neuropathologic abnormality found at autopsy in patients with neurologic symptoms is loss (or absence) of neurons, particularly in the cerebrum and cerebellum.

Laboratory Abnormalities. There have been no consistent clinical-laboratory abnormalities in patients with xeroderma pigmentosum. Tests of cellular hypersensitivity, however, have shown uniformly abnormal results.

Cultured cells from xeroderma pigmentosum patients generally grow normally when not exposed to damaging agents. The population growth rate is reduced to a greater extent than normal, however, following exposure to UV radiation (Fig. 1) and cellular recovery is delayed. This delay in growth has been shown to be paralleled by a similar delay in recovery of the rate of DNA synthesis following UV radiation exposure [2].

Single-cell survival, as measured by colony-forming ability following UV radiation, is also reduced in xeroderma pigmentosum cells [1,2,19,24,38] (Fig. 2). A range of post-UV colony-forming abilities have been found with fibroblasts from patients, some having extremely low post-UV colony-forming ability and others having nearly normal survival.

Xeroderma pigmentosum fibroblasts are deficient in their ability to repair some UV-damaged viruses to a functionally active state [1,2,25]. This assay, known as host cell reactivation, has detected an abnormality in every form of xeroderma pigmentosum tested. Adenovirus 2 host cell reactivation is thus the most sensitive test for the xeroderma pigmentosum genetic defect.

Ultraviolet-irradiated xeroderma pigmentosum fibroblasts produce more mutations per survivor than normal fibroblasts [2]. This has been observed at several sites of mutation, including hypoxanthine-guanine phosphoribrose transferase (HGPRT) and diphtheria toxin resistance. If prevented from dividing for an interval after irradiation, normal cells apparently repair the damage induced, with resultant increased survival and fewer mutants per survivor. This phenomenon has been called *potentially lethal damage recovery* and is analogous to "liquid holding recovery" in bacteria. Xeroderma pigmentosum fibroblasts exhibit diminished or absent recovery from potentially lethal damage after UV irradiation, thereby indicating a defect in cellular recovery mechanisms.

Xeroderma pigmentosum cells generally are found to have a normal karyotype without excessive chromosome breakage or increased SCEs. Following exposure to UV radiation, however, an abnormally large increase in chromosome breakage and in SCEs has been observed [1,2,8,31]. The extent of this induced abnormality varies in different patients.

A number of DNA damaging agents other than UV radiation have been found to yield hypersensitive responses with xeroderma pigmentosum cells (Table 5) [2]. These hypersensitivities have been measured by studies of cell survival, host cell reactivation, mutagenesis, and chromosome integrity. These agents include drugs (psoralens, chlorpromazine), cancer chemotherapeutic

Table 5   Xeroderma pigmentosum: DNA damaging agents inducing cellular hypersensitivity

Drugs
  Psoralens plus long-wavelength UV radiation (PUVA)
  Chlorpromazine
  Nitrofurantoin
  Mitomycin C
  Anthramycin
  Platinum
  Bis(chloroethyl)nitrosourea (BCNU)
Carcinogens
  Aflatoxin
  Benzo[a]pyrene derivatives
  Nitroquinoline oxide derivatives (4NQ0)
  Acetoaminofluorene derivatives (AAF)
  Phenanthrene derivatives

agents [platinum, 1,3-bis-2,3-chloroethyl-1-nitrosourea (BCNU)], and chemical carcinogens (benzo[a]pyrene derivatives). Presumably, these agents induce DNA damage whose repair involves portions of the DNA repair pathways that are defective in xeroderma pigmentosum.

The hypersensitivity of cultured xeroderma pigmentosum cells to UV radiation damage was reported by Cleaver, in 1968 [39], to be the result of defective DNA repair. He found defective UV-induced repair replication, indicating a defect in the nucleotide excision repair system (Table 2). In 1970, Epstein et al. [33] demonstrated that the DNA repair defect was present in vivo as well by measurements of unscheduled DNA synthesis in the skin of patients. The fact that the xeroderma pigmentosum cells have a normal response to treatment with x-rays was interpreted as indicating that the UV DNA excision repair defect was at the level of endonuclease function. The other tests of nucleotide excision repair listed in Table 2 have shown abnormalities with most xeroderma pigmentosum cells and support the notion of the presence of defective UV endonuclease activity. However, up to 1982 no one has successfully isolated an UV endonuclease that is defective in xeroderma pigmentosum. The repair system is

probably more complex than indicated in Fig. 7. There is evidence that repair in xeroderma pigmentosum may involve defects in accessibility of the damaged DNA within its chromatin covering [2].

In 1972, investigators in the Netherlands, by using cell fusion techniques (Fig. 9), demonstrated genetic heterogeneity among the xeroderma pigmentosum DNA repair defects [36]. They fused cultured fibroblasts from two different patients and then measured UV-induced unscheduled DNA synthesis. The unfused cells had the typical low level of UV-induced unscheduled DNA synthesis seen in most xeroderma pigmentosum fibroblasts (Fig. 8). Fusion of cells from certain pairs of patients resulted in the presence of fused cells with nearly normal levels of unscheduled DNA synthesis (Fig. 10). In these heterokaryons each cell provides components that the other was lacking, resulting in enhanced DNA repair. These "complementing cells" thus have different DNA repair defects. Fibroblasts from patients with the same DNA repair defect do not correct each other when fused and are said to be in the same complementation group. In 1975, Kraemer et al. [37] reported that the first five complementation groups discovered had characteristic residual rates of UV-induced unscheduled DNA synthesis. They were thus named A through E, in order of increasing DNA repair activity. Groups F and G were discovered more recently [2]. Their rates of unscheduled DNA synthesis overlap with groups C and A, respectively. Thus, assignment of cells to complementation groups must be based on fusion studies, not on the rate of DNA repair. Up to 1982, seven such complementation groups have been identified (Table 6).

In 1971, Burk et al. [34] reported a patient with clinically severe xeroderma pigmentosum who had normal unscheduled DNA synthesis in his fibroblasts, lymphocytes, and even his tumor cells [1,2]. This patient subsequently was termed a xeroderma pigmentosum *variant*. Studies of cellular hyper-

Table 6   Xeroderma pigmentosum: Characteristics of DNA repair complementation groups

Complementation group	Skin cancer	Neurologic abnormalities	UDS, % of normal	Number of kindreds
A	+	+ and −	0.3–1.3	49
B	+	+	3–7	1
C	+	−	10–25	32
D	+	+	25–50	9
E	+	−	10–20	1
F	−	−	10–20	3
G	−	+	<5	2
Variant	+	−	100	21

sensitivity revealed a slightly increased sensitivity to UV-induced inhibition of cell growth and colony-forming ability, to adenovirus host-cell reactivation, and to UV-induced mutations in vitro [2,25]. DNA repair studies revealed the presence of a defect in a second DNA repair system [2,8], that of postreplication repair (Fig. 7). Cells from this patient had a delayed rate of increase of the molecular weight of newly replicating DNA following UV irradiation (Table 2). Further, these cells were especially sensitive to inhibition of this process by caffeine.

More recent studies have reported defective excision repair, due to altered AP endonuclease activity, and diminished photoreactivation repair in a few xeroderma pigmentosum cell strains [2]. These observations have not been confirmed by other laboratories. Synthesis of poly(ADP-ribose), a possible intracellular regulator, is much less stimulated by UV radiation treatment in xeroderma pigmentosum cells than in normal cells [40]. The significance of this finding is unclear at present.

Clinical-Laboratory Correlations. Patients with xeroderma pigmentosum are hypersensitive to UV radiation and so are their cultured cells. Cutaneous and ocular abnormalities are strikingly limited to UV-exposed areas and usually spare such UV-shielded locations as the axillae, buttocks, and retina.

At least eight different molecular defects are associated with the clinical abnormalities recognized as xeroderma pigmentosum, as indicated by the existence of seven complementation groups and the variant form. Complementation group A contains patients with the most severe neurologic and somatic abnormalities (the DeSanctis-Cacchione syndrome) as well as patients with minimal or no neurologic abnormalities. This form is seen in the United States, Europe, and the Middle East. It is the most common form of xeroderma pigmentosum in Japan [2].

Complementation group B at present is composed of a unique patient who had the cutaneous abnormalities characteristic of xeroderma pigmentosum (including neoplasms) in conjunction with neurologic and ocular abnormalities typical of Cockayne's syndrome. Her DNA repair defects were different from all the other patients tested to date [1,2,37].

Patients in complementation group C, with rare exceptions, have xeroderma pigmentosum with skin and ocular involvement without neurologic abnormalities. This is the most common group in the United States, Europe, and Egypt but has been found in one patient from Japan [1,2].

Patients in complementation group D may have late onset of neurologic abnormalities in their second decade of life [1,2,19,38].

Comlementation group E to date has been found in only one kindred in Europe. These two cousins had relatively mild cutaneous abnormalities without neurologic involvement. Their cultured cells had the unusual property of increasing their regional DNA repair rate with increasing UV exposure. Thus, at low doses the unscheduled DNA synthesis was very low while at high doses it was nearly normal [2].

Complementation group F patients have been found only in Japan. These three patients were free of neurologic abnormalities and had not had skin cancer [2].

Two patients in complementation group G have been identified in Europe. Both had neurologic abnormalities without skin cancer. Fibroblasts from one of the patients were found to be hypersensitive to killing by x-rays as well as to UV radiation [2].

Xeroderma pigmentosum variant cells have normal DNA nucleotide excision repair and thus do not fall in any of the complementation groups of cells with defective DNA excision repair. There is, however, defective postreplication repair (Fig. 7). Xeroderma pigmentosum variants have been identified in the United States, Europe, and Japan. None of the variants so far identified has neurologic abnormalities. The cutaneous and ocular abnormalities have been severe in some patients and mild in others. A family with four affected individuals was described in Germany; they had had extensive sun exposure and late onset of cutaneous cancers. These individuals had originally been thought to represent a separate disorder (pigmented xerodermoid) [41]. Recent cellular studies showed the findings typical of xeroderma pigmentosum variants.

The cutaneous and ocular changes in xeroderma pigmentosum patients are consistent with the notion that repeated insults by environmental agents, particularly UV radiation, produce continual DNA damage. Because of defective DNA repair, this damage results in cell death, diminished cell growth, or somatic cell mutations. Through mechanisms that are not understood, these cellular alterations lead to atrophy, hyper- and hypopigmentation, and telangiectasia, as well as benign and malignant neoplasms. Thus xeroderma pigmentosum provides strong support for the somatic mutation theory of carcinogenesis. Further, rigorous protection from UV radiation from early infancy in a few patients has been shown to prevent most of the serious cutaneous and ocular abnormalities.

Since cells from xeroderma pigmentosum patients are also hypersensitive to environmental mutagens (such as benzo[a]pyrene found in cigarette smoke) (Table 5), the question arises as to whether they have an increased susceptibility to developing internal neoplasms which may be carcinogen-induced. Review of the world literature has revealed a substantial number of cases of oral cavity neoplasms, particularly squamous cell carcinoma of the tip of the tongue [2]. It is unlikely that this site receives significant sun exposure. Leukemia and brain, lung, uterine, and testicular tumors have been reported in xeroderma pigmentosum patients. Studies are in progress to determine whether these represent a greater number than would be expected.

The neurologic abnormalities in xeroderma pigmentosum demonstrate the clinical features of progressive degeneration [1,2,19]. Severely affected patients lose their ability to walk and talk. Histologically, the picture is of loss (or absence) of neurons without evidence of vascular abnormality, deposition of abnormal material, or inflammatory reaction. It has been hypothesized, in analogy to the cutaneous degenerative changes, that the neurologic degeneration is a manifestation of unrepaired DNA damage. Since mature neurons do not divide, unrepaired DNA damage would lead to cell death without replacement by other neurons. This process would lead to progressive loss of neurologic function. The specific cause of such damage, whether by exogenous or endogenous agents, and the explanation of why some neurons are more severely affected than others is not known. The defects in xeroderma pigmentosum patients with associated neurologic disease have been shown to correlate with the UV sensitivity of their skin fibroblasts [2,19,38]. Post-UV colony-forming ability is diminished to the greatest extent in fibroblasts from patients with xeroderma pigmentosum who have severe neurologic abnormalities and to a much lesser extent in xeroderma pigmentosum patients without neurologic abnormalities, both within and among complementation groups. Thus, this is evidence that patients having xeroderma pigmentosum with neurologic abnormalities have a different defect in other tissues than patients without neurologic abnormalities.

Xeroderma pigmentosum heterozygotes (parents and some other relatives) are carriers of the gene for xeroderma pigmentosum but are clinically normal. There is some epidemiologic evidence to indicate that these people have an increased risk of developing skin cancer [42]. Most tests of cell function or DNA repair yield normal responses with cells from xeroderma pigmentosum heterozygotes. Unfortunately, up to 1981, there is no simple laboratory test that can reliably detect xeroderma pigmentosum heterozygotes. Until such a test is available, these epidemiologic data may not be justifiably applied to individual persons at risk of being heterozygotes.

Ataxia-Telangiectasia

Definition. Ataxia-telangiectasia is an autosomal recessive disease with progressive cerebellar ataxia, ocular and cutaneous telangiectasia, immune deficiency, and a high frequency of neoplasia [9,43,44]. There is clinical and laboratory evidence of x-ray hypersensitivity [3–15,21].

Frequency. Ataxia-telangiectasia is among the most common of the diseases described in this chapter. The frequency is approximately 1 patient (homozygote) per 40,000 births [43,45]. From this figure, one can estimate that the frequency of heterozygotes (carriers) would be on the order of 1 percent of the general population [45].

Clinical Features. The onset of ataxia-telangiectasia is usually in early childhood. Affected children develop progressive cerebellar ataxia resulting in loss of ability to coordinate movements. They have difficulty walking or using the upper extremities. Abnormal eye movements, called *oculomotor dyspraxia*, often develop. Intelligence is usually not affected. Deep tendon reflexes may be diminished or absent.

Frequent bacterial pulmonary or sinus infections may develop as a manifestation of immune deficiency. There is impairment of both humoral and delayed hypersensitivity. The thymus is rudimentary.

Cutaneous and ocular abnormalities usually occur after the onset of neurologic abnormalities. Telangiectasia of the bulbar conjunction may become prominent at 3 to 6 years of age, assisting in the differentiation of ataxia-telangiectasia from other forms of ataxia. Telangiectasia may be prominent on the pinnae, malar area, eyelids, neck, dorsa of the hands, and antecubital and popliteal fossae. The telangiectasia is not limited to sun-exposed sites. Vitiligo, café au lait spots, and other macular hyperpigmentation may be present. Acanthosis nigricans has been noted in ataxia-telangiectasia patients with occult and diagnosed neoplasms [9].

Insulin-resistant diabetes mellitus has been observed. Some of these patients have been found to have abnormal insulin receptors.

Approximately 10 percent of the patients develop neoplasms [9]. Eighty percent of the neoplasms develop before age 15. Lymphoproliferative disorders predominate, primarily lymphomas or lymphoblastic (not myeloid) leukemia. In a recent report from the Immunodeficiency Cancer Registery concerning 108 ataxia-telangiectasia patients with neoplasia, 48 had non-Hodgkin's lymphoma, 26 had leukemia, 12 had Hodgkin's disease, and 22 had carcinomas (involving stomach, brain, skin, ovary, liver, larynx, parotid gland, and breast) [46]. Several ataxia-telangiectasia patients have developed severe reactions to standard doses of radiotherapy for neoplasms. These reactions have included radionecrosis of the oropharynx and central nervous system deterioration leading to death. Thus, ataxia-telangiectasia patients have clinical hypersensitivity to ionizing radiation.

Epidemiologic studies of family members suggest that heterozygotes (parents and other carriers of the ataxia-telangiectasia genetic defect) who are clinically normal may have an increased risk of dying from neoplasms before age 45 [45]. The data suggest an increase in cancers of the ovary, stomach, and biliary tract. Since ataxia-telangiectasia heterozygotes may comprise 1 percent of the general population, they may comprise more than 5 percent of all persons dying from these cancers before age 45. Confirmation of this potentially very important observation awaits development of a reliable test for detection of ataxia-telangiectasia heterozgytes.

Laboratory Abnormalities. Clinical laboratory abnormalities primarily relate to humoral or cellular immune dysfunction. There is often decreased IgA (resulting from diminished IgA synthesis) and decreased IgE. An IgM macroglobin may be present. Other abnormalities include impaired delayed skin test reactivity, reduced ability to reject allogeneic skin grafts, reduced ability to be sensitized with dinitrochlorobenzene, reduced lymphocyte count, and poor lymphocyte mitogenic response to phytohemagglutinin, in vitro. There is also reduced helper T-cell function. Virtually 100 percent of the ataxia-telangiectasia patients have elevated α-fetoprotein, a finding that may sometimes be very useful in differential diagnosis.

Neurologic testing commonly shows reduced nerve conduction velocity and a neuropathic electromyogram. These findings point toward a primary neurologic degeneration [9].

Karyotypic analysis of peripheral blood leukocytes frequently shows a high frequency of "spontaneous" breaks, gaps, and translocations [9,26]. A common abnormality in ataxia-telangiectasia is a deletion or translocation involving a portion of chromosome 14. Several patients have been reported to have chromosomally distinct clones of abnormal circulating lymphocytes. In some patients those abnormal cells have been documented to increase in frequency and, in a few patients, to progress to leukemia. Increased spontaneous chromosome breakage has also been found in cultured skin fibroblasts, but, interestingly, not in lymphoblastoid cell lines.

Baseline SCE frequency is normal (Fig. 5). X-ray treatment of cultured ataxia-telangiectasia cells results in an abnormally large increase in chromosome breakage. However, there is a very small increase in SCEs following x-ray treatment in normal and ataxia-telangiectasia lymphocytes.

The observation of clinical x-ray hypersensitivity prompted the laboratory study of survival of ataxia-telangiectasia cells following x-irradiation. Cultured skin fibroblasts and lymphoblastoid cell lines (Fig. 1b) were found to be hypersensitive to killing by x-ray. Hypersensitivity to killing was found also to treatments with the chromotherapeutic agent bleomycin or with the carcinogen methylnitronitrosoguanidine (MNNG) (Table 3). These findings suggest that ataxia-telangiectasia cells may be an x-ray analogue of xeroderma pigmentosum [9]. There is one important difference, however: Ataxia-telangiectasia cells were found not to be hypermutable following x-ray.

The mechanism of the ataxia-telangiectasia hypersensitivity to x-rays and to certain chemicals is only partially understood. As measured by loss of endonuclease-sensitive sites, repair replication, and BND (benzylated naphthylated DEAE) cellulose chromatography (Table 2), some ataxia-telangiectasia cells have been shown to have defective DNA repair following x-ray or MNNG. Other ataxia-telangiectasia cell strains, equally as sensitive to killing by x-ray or MNNG, have no detectable DNA repair defects. Extracts of ataxia-telangiectasia cells have diminished ability to repair x-ray-damaged DNA to an extent that the DNA may function as a template for bacterial DNA polymerase in vitro. Cell fusion studies (Fig. 9) of x-ray-treated ataxia-telangiectasia cells using repair replication have indicated the existence of at least two complementation groups among repair-defective ataxia-telangiectasia strains [5,10].

A number of other abnormalities have recently been reported in ataxia-telangiectasia cells. Several laboratories independently discovered an apparent anomaly in that ataxia-telangiectasia cells fail to slow their rate of DNA synthesis following treatment with x-rays despite increased sensitivity to killing by x-rays. Normal cells do slow down DNA synthesis after x-ray injury. Probably this slowdown gives normal cells time to repair their damaged DNA before the next round of replication. The ataxia-telangiectasia cells would thus be more likely to suffer injury by x-rays when DNA synthesis continues at a rapid rate. This abnormal control of DNA synthesis may be mediated by a defective poly(ADP-ribose) control mechanism [47]. The relationship of these DNA synthesis abnormalities to the DNA repair pathways (Fig. 7) is not clear at present.

Other workers reported the presence of a "clastogenic factor" in serum and in medium from growing ataxia-telangiectasia cells [48]. This factor induces chromosome breaks in normal lymphocytes. The significance of these observations should be clarified in the future.

Clinical-Laboratory Correlations. Ataxia-telangiectasia, like xeroderma pigmentosum, has clinical features of progressive degeneration, particularly in the central nervous system [9]. Histopathologically, there is loss (or absence) of neurons without deposition or inflammation. In ataxia-telangiectasia, the major abnormalities are found in the cerebellum, particularly the loss of Purkinje cells. In contrast to xeroderma pigmentosum, there is relative sparing of the cerebrum. Consequently, in ataxia-telangiectasia cerebellar symptoms (ataxia, incoordination) predominate, while xeroderma pigmentosum patients with neurologic abnormalities may have early deterioration of intellectual functions and develop incoordination rather late. In both ataxia-telangiectasia and xeroderma pigmentosum, progressive loss of neurons may be the consequence of unrepaired DNA damage in cells that cannot be replaced by cell division [19]. The cause of the damage, whether from exogenous or endogenous factors, and the reason for the anatomic location of the affected cells is not known.

The clinical hypersensitivity to cancer-therapeutic doses of radiation is clearly correlated with the x-ray hypersensitivity of cultured cells. However, the role of x-radiation in the development of neoplasms is not as straightforward. One patient developed a carcinoma of the scalp 10 years after superficial radiation for tinea capitis [9]. However, the patient had a chronic radiodermatitis during the interval, which, in itself, might have induced the neoplasm. In contrast to xeroderma pigmentosum where cultured cells are hypermutable to UV radiation, cultured ataxia-telangiectasia cells have normal to low rates of x-ray-induced mutagenesis.

The lymphoreticular neoplasms (reticulum cell sarcoma, lymphoma, Hodgkin's disease) occurring in patients with ataxia-telangiectasia are unusual in their early age of onset (before 15 years in comparison to the median age of 55 to 59 years in the U.S. white population) and greatly increased occurrence (6 percent of patients vs. 13 per million annual incidence in the U.S. white population) [9,46]. The 2 percent prevalence of leukemia is also much greater than the 42 per million incidence in the U.S. white population. Particularly notable is the complete absence of acute or chronic myeloid leukemia. This distribution of types of neoplasms is different from that of children without ataxia-telangiectasia, where leukemia and central nervous system neoplasms are more common than lymphoma. The distribution of types of neoplasms seen in ataxia-telangiectasia patients is not that expected from radiation exposure. Neoplasms most commonly observed in populations receiving high doses of radiation are leukemia (myelogenous and lymphoid) and thyroid, breast, lung, bone, and gastrointestinal carcinomas without an increase in lymphoreticular neoplasms. The predominance of lymphoreticular neoplasms in ataxia-telangiectasia is similar to its predominance in other immunodeficiency diseases. Thus the immunodeficiency in ataxia-telangiectasia may be a more significant factor contributing to the high frequency of neoplasms than is the cellular hypersensitivity to ionizing radiation.

The relationship of the cellular hypersensitivity to the immune defects is at present speculative. Immune deficiency is often present in early childhood. There is no evidence of progression of immunologic defects as with the neurologic abnormalities. Rather than being the result of repeated postnatal insults (as may be the case for neurologic degeneration), both the immune deficiency and the cellular hypersensitivity may be the result of separate (or linked) developmental defects.

Fanconi's Anemia

Definition. Fanconi's anemia is an autosomal recessive disorder with anemia, developmental defects, and a high incidence of neoplasia. Approximately 200 patients have been reported in the literature [3–8,49–56].

Clinical Features. Hemopoietic manifestations usually have their onset before the age of 10 years. These consist of a hypocellular bone marrow with progressive decrease in the number of circulating platelets, granulocytes, and erythrocytes.

Sixty-six percent of 129 patients with Fanconi's anemia had skeletal malformations [53]. These included aplasia or hypoplasia of the thumb, metacarpals, or radius; less frequently, hip dislocation or scoliosis was reported. Sixty percent of the patients had short stature; most had low birth weight. Malformations of other organ systems were also observed. Twenty-eight percent of the patients had renal deformities, including renal aplasia and horseshoe kidney. Twenty-one percent had ocular abnormalities, including strabismus and microphthalmia; 20 percent of the patients had hypogonadism. Central nervous system abnormalities (hyperreflexia and mild mental retardation) were observed in less than 20 percent of the patients. Deafness due to deformities of the ear anatomy was present in less than 10 percent of the patients. Heart defects (patent ductus arteriosis, aortic stenosis, auricular septum defect) were observed in eight patients.

Cutaneous abnormalities were present in almost 80 percent of the patients. Hyperpigmentation was present from birth or early childhood. The hyperpigmentation was diffuse and accentuated over the neck, joints, and trunk. Café au lait spots and achromic lesions were present. Following repeated blood transfusions, hyperpigmentation due to iron overloading may be present.

Patients with Fanconi's anemia have a high incidence of neoplasia, particularly nonlymphatic leukemia [50]. In recent years hepatomas have been noted with increasing frequency. There is some suspicion that these hepatomas may be a late effect of the anabolic steroids used to treat the anemia.

The course is often progressively downhill with death from infection, hemorrhage, or neoplasia.

Laboratory Abnormalities. Clinical-laboratory abnormalities reflect the bone marrow failure. There is a hypocellular marrow with thrombocytoplasia, leukopenia, and anemia.

Fanconi's anemia is associated with a high frequency of spontaneous chromosomal abnormalities [50,55–57]. These include gaps, breaks, and translocations. With Fanconi's anemia cells the chromosomal abnormalities are increased to a greater extent than with normal cells following treatment with diepoxybutane, mitomycin C, psoralen plus UVA, or isonicotinic acid hydrazide (INH) [52,55–58].

The baseline frequency of SCEs is normal. However, following treatment with psoralen plus UVA the increase in SCEs in Fanconi's anemia lymphocytes is less than in normal fibroblasts.

Colony-forming ability of cultured fibroblasts is hypersensitive to inhibition by treatment with agents that form cross-links in DNA [4–8,49]. These include mitomycin C, busulfan, nitrogen mustard, and psoralen plus UVA (Table 3). Colony-forming ability has a normal response to killing by UV radiation. Some Fanconi's anemia fibroblast strains are slightly hypersensitive to killing by x-radiation, while others have a normal response [11].

The mechanism of the cellular hypersensitivity to DNA cross-linking agents is thought to involve defective DNA repair [49]. A detailed understanding of this defect has not yet been attained. Some Fanconi's anemia fibroblasts have been reported to have defective removal of an x-ray-induced thymidine analogue, thymine glycol (Table 3).

Cells from heterozygous carriers of Fanconi's anemia have a chromosomal response to damage with diepoxybutane [55] or with nitrogen mustard [56] intermediate between the homozygotes and normals.

Clinical-Laboratory Correlations. Fanconi's anemia is a progressive, degenerative disease with major involvement of the hematologic system. There is a high frequency of spontaneous chromosomal breakage in association with a high rate of neoplasia, particularly nonlymphatic leukemia. Immunodeficiency is not prominent. Cells are hypersensitive to killing and to induction of chromosome aberrations by DNA cross-linking agents. At present, incorporating these diverse observations into a unitary theory involves considerable speculation: The progressive nature of the disease is similar to xeroderma pigmentosum and ataxia-telangiectasia and suggests the presence of accumulated cellular damage. "Spontaneous" chromosomal breakage may be a manifestation of this damage. The neoplasia may be related to the chromosomal breakage. However, when considering two diseases with spontaneous chromosome breakage (Fanconi's anemia and ataxia-telangiectasia) lymphoid leukemia is absent in Fanconi's anemia and predominant in ataxia-telangiectasia. Nonlymphoid leukemia predominates in Fanconi's anemia and is absent in ataxia-telangiectasia. Thus other modifying factors, perhaps the immune defects in ataxia-telangiectasia, may be at work. The postulated damage may be caused by agents similar to the DNA cross-linking agents to which the Fanconi's anemia cells are hypersensitive. It should be noted that almost 40 percent of a recent series of neoplasms in Fanconi's anemia were hepatomas [50]. These had not been observed prior to 1959, when effective treatment of the anemia with exogenous androgens was introduced. It is possible that the prolonged life permitted expression of latent hepatomas or that the therapy induced hepatic neoplasia.

Clinical symptoms in Fanconi's anemia have been observed to vary from mild to severe and to be similar in multiple affected children within a family. Similarly, cells from different patients have shown different degrees of sensitivity to x-radiation damage and repair. This suggests that genetic heterogeneity may exist within Fanconi's anemia.

The chromosomal aberrations induced by diepoxybutane have been used successfully as a test for prenatal diagnosis of Fanconi's anemia [57]. Many more chromosome aberrations are induced by diepoxybutane in cultured amniotic fluid cells from Fanconi's anemia than from normal fetuses.

Cockayne's Syndrome

Definition. Cockayne's syndrome is an autosomal recessive degenerative disease with cutaneous, ocular, neurologic, and somatic abnormalities [3–8,59,60]. Fewer than 50 patients have been described in the literature.

Clinical Features. In 1936, Cockayne described a syndrome characterized by cachectic dwarfism, deafness, and pigmentary retinal degeneration with a characteristic "salt and pepper" appearance of the retina. The skin had photosensitivity and diffuse hyperpigmentation without the excessive pigmentary abnormalities seen in xeroderma pigmentosum. There was marked loss of subcutaneous fat resulting in a "wizened" appearance with typical "bird-headed" facies. Additional ocular findings included cataracts and optic atrophy.

Neurologic abnormalities, in addition to deafness, include peripheral neuropathy, normal pressure hydrocephalus, and microcephaly. Birth weight and early development are usually normal. The disease onset is most often in the second year of life, with slowly progressive neurologic degeneration. Intellectual deterioration may be nonuniform with some functions preserved better than others.

X-ray examination may show thickened skull. Bone age is usually normal. Height and weight are usually well below the third percentile for the age.

Cockayne's syndrome is not associated with an increased incidence of neoplasia.

Laboratory Abnormalities. Clinical laboratory testing often shows sensorineural deafness, neuropathic electromyogram, and slow motor nerve conduction velocity [59]. The electroencephalogram may be abnormal. Computerized tomography may be diagnostically useful in the detection of normal pressure hydrocephalus [59].

As with xeroderma pigmentosum, cultured cells (fibroblasts or lymphocytes) from Cockayne's syndrome patients are hypersensitive to UV-induced inhibition of growth and colony-forming ability [3–8,21,61–63]. They are also hypersensitive to killing by the carcinogen 4-nitroquinoline oxide (4NQO) (Table 3).

Host cell reactivation of UV-damaged adenovirus (Table 1) is reduced, although generally to a lesser extent than in xeroderma pigmentosum [25]. Studies of induced mutations in Cockayne's syndrome cells have not been published.

Chromosome karyotype and SCE frequency is generally normal in untreated cells. Ultraviolet treatment of Cockayne's syndrome cells results in a greater than normal increase in SCEs [38,64].

These cellular abnormalities are similar to those of xeroderma pigmentosum. However, the Cockayne's syndrome cells do not have the same DNA repair defects as in xeroderma pigmentosum. There is, however, a prolonged decrease in the rate of DNA synthesis following UV irradiation [62]. Despite investigation in a number of laboratories, no mechanism has been found for the cellular abnormalities in Cockayne's syndrome.

Clinical-Laboratory Correlation. Cockayne's syndrome, like xeroderma pigmentosum and ataxia-telangiectasia, is a disease of progressive neurologic degeneration. Pathologically there is loss (or absence) of neurons without inflammatory reaction or deposition of material. This is consistent with the theory that the neurons are damaged repeatedly but do not recover fully and die [1,19]. Since mature neurons cannot divide, the dead neurons are not replaced, resulting in progressive loss of neurologic functioning. As in xeroderma pigmentosum and ataxia-telangiectasia, the cause of this damage and the reason for the precise anatomic location of the damage is not known.

Despite similar UV radiation hypersensitivity to cell killing in Cockayne's syndrome as in xeroderma pigmentosum, patients with Cockayne's syndrome do not have an increased frequency of cutaneous (or internal) neoplasia. The only Cockayne's syndrome patient in the literature with multiple skin cancers also had xeroderma pigmentosum [1,59]. This unusual patient also had a unique DNA repair defect and is the only patient in complementation group B (Table 6) [37]. Thus cellular hypersensitivity, in the absence of a documented DNA repair defect, does not necessarily result in increased neoplasia.

Bloom's Syndrome

Definition. Bloom's syndrome is an autosomal recessive disease characterized by sun sensitivity, facial telangiectasia, short stature, and a high frequency of neoplasia [3–8,30,50,65,66]. The Bloom's Syndrome Registry has documented 99 cases worldwide. Bloom's syndrome is most frequent among Ashkenazi Jews where the carrier rate has been estimated as 1:120 [67].

Clinical Features. Facial erythema and telangiectasia superficially resembling lupus erythematosus often is present within the first few weeks after birth in the malar area, on the nose, and around the ears [65,66]. Sun exposure accentuates these abnormalities and may induce bullae with bleeding and crusting of the lips and eyelids. The telangiectatic lesions often involve the ears and dorsa of the hands but characteristically spare the trunk, buttocks, and lower extremities. The intensity of the facial lesions may vary from minimal telangiectasia around the lips to severe erythema of the malar area, cheeks and nose (see Fig. 5, color plate). Café au lait spots are common, at times accompanied by adjacent depigmented areas.

Affected children are generally born at full term but are of low birth weight, averaging approximately 2000 g. Patients are well-proportioned but small. Adult height is usually under 150 cm. Patients have a long, narrow head, with a characteristic facies consisting of a narrow prominent nose, relatively hypoplastic malar areas, and a receding chin. Major skeletal abnormalities are unusual. Neurologic abnormalities are uncommon and intelligence is generally normal.

Bloom's syndrome patients are predisposed to multiple severe infections of the respiratory or gastrointestinal tracts. There is a tendency for the frequency of infections to decrease with advancing age. There is immune dysfunction [68].

Sexual development generally appears to be normal but male infertility due to defective sperm is the rule [69].

Approximately 20 percent of Bloom's syndrome patients develop neoplasms—half occur before the age of 20 years [50,67]. These neoplasms have included lymphatic and nonlymphatic leukemias, lymphosarcoma, lymphoma, and carcinomas of the gastrointestinal tract. Bloom's syndrome patients have at least a 100-fold increase in the risk of dying from cancer.

Laboratory Abnormalities. Laboratory studies of immunity have shown diminished immunoglobulin levels, reduced cellular proliferative response to mitogens, and decreased proliferation in the mixed leukocyte reaction [68].

Studies of gonadal function in males revealed azoospermia and a high follicle-stimulating hormone (FSH) response to leuteinizing hormone–releasing hormone (LHRH) [69]. The studies indicated primary hypogonadism mainly affecting the tubular element of the testis. There was relative sparing of the androgen-secreting Leydig cells, resulting in puberty within normal limits.

Cytogenetic abnormalities are found in cultured cells from virtually all patients with Bloom's syndrome [3–8,26–30,65,70,71]; these include a high frequency of chromosomal breakage and rearrangements, including isochromatid gaps and breaks, transverse breakage at centromeres, dicentric chromosomes, and acentric fragments. The most characteristic of these aberrations, the quadriradial configuration, was found in 0.5 to 14.0 percent of all dividing PHA-stimulated lymphocytes from Bloom's syndrome patients (Fig. 4) [30]. Quadriradials are believed to be the result of a rearrangement before the onset of mitosis, resulting from the exchange of chromatid segments of two homologous chromosomes. The quadriradial is almost never found in cells from normal individuals. There is also a markedly elevated rate of spontaneous SCEs in Bloom's syndrome cells (Fig. 6). Increased SCEs and the presence of quadriradials are considered essential for the diagnosis of Bloom's syndrome.

The carcinogen, ethylmethane sulfonate, induces a greater increase in SCEs in Bloom's syndrome lymphocytes than in lymphocytes from normals [30]. Bloom's syndrome cells show a normal increase in chromosome aberrations when treated with x-rays in G_1 phase of the cell cycle but show a greater than normal increase when irradiated in G_2.

Fusion (Fig. 9) of Bloom's syndrome fibroblasts

with rodent cells, or with normal human fibroblasts, results in a normal rate of SCEs in the fused cells [70]. This result implies that the defect in Bloom's syndrome cells is the consequence of the loss of a normal function rather than the acquisition of a new abnormal function.

Some Bloom's syndrome fibroblasts have been reported to be hypersensitive to killing by UV radiation. Other Bloom's syndrome strains have a normal response to UV radiation. Cells from three Japanese Bloom's syndrome patients were hypersensitive to killing by mitomycin C (Table 3). Recently Bloom's syndrome fibroblasts were reported to have an eight- to tenfold increase in the spontaneous mutation rate [72].

The molecular basis for these abnormalities remains elusive. No consistent DNA repair abnormalities have been documented. The rate of DNA chain elongation was found to be significantly slower than with normal fibroblasts [71]. Other studies found a markedly increased rate of interchange of DNA between newly synthesized and older DNA strands consistent with the observed increase in SCEs.

Clinical-Laboratory Correlations. The clinical diagnosis of Bloom's syndrome is confirmed by the findings of increased SCE and increased chromosome breakage, including the presence of quadriradials.

The high frequency of neoplasia in Bloom's syndrome may be related to the chromosome breakage or the immune deficiency (or both), as in ataxia-telangiectasia. The observation of increased spontaneous mutation rate in cultured cells suggests that somatic mutations may play a role in the neoplasia. Homologous chromosome exchange (as in quadriradials) may be a mechanism whereby heterozygous (recessive) traits become homozygous within somatic cells and thereby result in mutation or neoplasia.

Variable UV radiation hypersensitivity among cell lines suggests the possibility of different defects in different patients with Bloom's syndrome.

Dyskeratosis Congenita

Definition. Dyskeratosis congenita, the Zinsser-Engman-Cole syndrome, is an X-linked multisystem disease with cutaneous, mucosal, ocular, gastrointestinal, and hematologic abnormalities and an increased incidence of cancer. Approximately 70 cases are recorded in the literature, including some female cases [3–8,73–75].

Clinical Features. The most common features are hyperpigmentation, dystrophic nails, and leukoplakia [73]. During the first decade of life patients develop reticulated poikiloderma of sun-exposed areas, with hyperpigmentation and occasionally bullae. Nail dystrophy is present in virtually all patients, beginning at approximately age 2 to 5 years. The nails initially split easily and then develop longitudinal ridging with irregular free edges. Eventually the nails become smaller, resulting in rudiments remaining. The fingernails are usually involved before the toenails. Other skin abnormalities include atrophic, wrinkled skin over the dorsa of hands and feet and hyperhydrosis and hyperkeratosis of the palms and soles with disappearance of dermal ridges (absence of fingerprints).

Leukoplakia may be present in any mucosal site [73]. The oral mucosa is the most frequent, but leukoplakia has also been found in the urethra, glans penis, vagina, and rectum. Mucosal surfaces such as the esophagus, urethra, and lacrimal duct may become constricted and stenotic, resulting in dysphagia, dysuria, and epiphora. Multiple dental caries and early loss of teeth are common. Approximately half of the patients have had subnormal intelligence. Patients may have multiple infections.

There is an increased incidence of neoplasia, particularly squamous cell carcinoma of the mouth, rectum, cervix, vagina, esophagus, and skin. Several patients have had multiple primary neoplasms. Most neoplasms occurred in the third or fourth decade. None of the patients had leukemia. Half of the patients developed anemia secondary to bone marrow failure in the second or third decade. Leukopenia and thrombocytopenia may also be present, resulting in a hematologic picture similar to Fanconi's anemia.

Laboratory Abnormalities. Immune function was studied in only a small number of patients. Defects in immunoglobulin levels and in cell-mediated immunity were found in some patients.

Chromosomes are usually normal in untreated cells. There is a report of one patient with elevated spontaneous SCEs [75]. Treatment of peripheral blood leukocytes from two patients with psoralens plus UV radiation in vitro induced abnormally large increases in SCEs [74]. Up to 1981, cell survival studies were not reported.

Clinical-Laboratory Correlation. Dyskeratosis congenita, like Fanconi's anemia, is associated with anemia and increased incidence of neoplasia. However, patients with dyskeratosis congenita do not have the developmental malformations or spontaneous chromosomal breakage seen in Fanconi's anemia. In both disorders, however, there is a suggestion of an abnormal chromosomal response to the DNA cross-linking induced by psoralens. In dyskeratosis congenita, abnormally large increases in numbers of SCEs were induced in lymphocytes [74], while in Fanconi's anemia there was an abnormally small increase.

Like ataxia-telangiectasia, dyskeratosis congenita has an increased incidence of neoplasia and immune deficiency. However, the types of neoplasia most commonly seen in ataxia-telangiectasia, lymphoma and leukemia, have not been reported in dyskeratosis congenita. The mechanism and the extent of cellular abnormalities in dyskeratosis congenita are presently not understood.

Gardner's Syndrome

Definition. Gardner's syndrome is an autosomal dominant form of familial adenomatous polyposis of the colon associated with multiple osteomas and soft tissue tumors. Patients have a high frequency of colonic carcinoma. Gardner's syndrome has been estimated to occur with a frequency of 1 in 14,000 persons [76].

Clinical Features. The cutaneous and osseous abnormalities usually precede recognition of colonic polyps in patients with Gardner's syndrome. Cutaneous lesions consist of cystic lesions (sebaceous or epidermal inclusion cysts) which may occur all over the body surface but have a predilection for the scalp and face. They often occur with increasing frequency in children and stabilize later in life. Subcutaneous fibromas may be present.

Desmoid tumors may occur, particularly in surgical scars along the abdominal wall. They are believed to arise from the connective tissue of muscle. The desmoid tumors may be locally invasive, destroying muscle or occasionally forming massive "mesenteric fibromatosis." Histologically they may be mistaken for low-grade fibrosarcomas.

Bony abnormalities are found in at least half of the patients, mostly involving membranous bone of the calvaria and face [76]. They may be true osteomas or irregular cortical thickenings. They include odontomas, rudimentary or supernumerary teeth, osteodontomas, dentigerous cysts, and unerupted teeth. Dentures at an early age are common. Scoliosis is frequent.

The intestinal polyposis occurs mainly in the colon but may occasionally be present in the duodenum and elsewhere in the gastrointestinal tract. The adenomatous polyps are identical to those in familial multiple polyposis without extraintestinal involvement. At least half of the patients have polyps by the end of the third decade of life. There is a very high frequency of malignant degeneration of the polyps. In a recent series of patients with familial polyposis and colon cancer, approximately 60 percent had developed colon cancer by age 40 years [76]. This is at least 30 years earlier in life than the age of a comparable proportion of the colon cancer patients in the U.S. population. Other tumors reported in patients with Gardner's syndrome include adrenal carcinoma, thyroid carcinoma, ovarian tumors, melanoma, carcinoid tumors, and leiomyomas of the gastrointestinal tract and retroperitoneum.

Laboratory Abnormalities. Abnormalities in routine laboratory tests relate to the bony alterations detected on x-ray examination and the polyps of the colon. There may be anemia associated with bleeding from the gastrointestinal tract.

Analysis of chromosomes from cultured fibroblasts from patients in two families with Gardner's syndrome showed an increased percentage of cells with a tetraploid number of chromosomes (11 to 35 percent in patients vs. 0 to 4 percent in normal controls) [77]. Other studies of growth of cultured Gardner's syndrome fibroblasts showed a lack of contact inhibition and a decreased serum requirement for growth [78]. The cells had a greatly increased susceptability to transformation by the Kirsten murine sarcoma virus.

Studies of cell survival showed an increased sensitivity to inhibition of colony-forming ability by x-radiation, UV radiation, and mitomycin C in fibroblast cultures from an affected father and daughter [79]. The mechanism of this sensitivity was not determined.

Clinical-Laboratory Correlations. Patients with Gardner's syndrome have progressive degenerative changes in the colon and to a lesser extent in skin and bones. Exuberant muscle connective tissue fibroblast proliferation following surgery leads to desmoid formation. Skin fibroblasts grow very well in culture, often growing in criss-crossed layers, a property rarely seen with normal fibroblasts. They were readily transformed by murine sarcoma virus. Chromosomal tetraploidy was present. These cellular abnormalities may reflect the abnormal cell growth in vivo. The hypersensitivity to radiation, and, indeed, most of the other cellular abnormalities, have been described in very few affected individuals. A more complete explanation will require further studies.

Basal Cell Nevus Syndrome

Definition. Basal cell nevus syndrome is a progressive degenerative multisystem disorder characterized by early onset of mandibular cysts and basal cell carcinomas. Inheritance is autosomal dominant with variable penetrance. There may be a high spontaneous mutation rate. The frequency of the basal cell nevus syndrome is not known but the disease is not rare [80,81].

Clinical Features. The early features of the basal cell nevus syndrome usually do not involve the skin (Table 7). Patients may be born with congenital blindness (due to coloboma, cataracts, or glaucoma) or hydrocephalus. Multiple cysts of the mandible or maxilla with keratinized lining (keratocysts) may occur early in the disease. Patients have a characteristic facies with broad nasal root, frontal bossing, well-developed supraorbital ridges, hypertelorism, and mild mandibular prognathism. There may be lateral displacement of the inner canthi (dystopia canthorum).

The most common cutaneous abnormality is the presence of multiple basal cell carcinomas. These may occur early in life in sites shielded from sunlight as well as in sites exposed to sunlight. Patients may have a few to dozens or hundreds of basal cell carcinomas. The term *nevus* in basal cell nevus syndrome is an old medical term referring to any circumscribed lesion believed to arise under genetic influence. It referred to vascular or nonvascular growths and not just nevus cell nevi, or "moles," as in the terminology of today. The *nevi* in the basal cell nevus syndrome are true basal cell carcinomas.

Approximately 50 percent of the patients have minute pits (epidermal defects in keratin production) of the palms and soles. There may be few to hundreds of these pits. They are more numerous on the lateral surfaces of the palms, soles, and fingers. Other cutaneous lesions include milia, multiple cysts, lipomas, and fibromas or desmoids.

The keratocysts of the jaws are lined with squamous epithelium. They have extensive keratinization and walls of connective tissue. They may range in size from a few millimeters to several centimeters in diameter. Recurrences after surgery are common. Teeth may be carious, misshapen, or in abnormal locations. Ameloblastomas, an oral analogue of the basal cell carcinoma, may occur.

Brachymetacarpalism (Albright's sign) consists of a short fourth metacarpal [82]. It is easily seen by examining the knuckles on the dorsum of a clenched fist and verified by hand x-ray (Fig. 11*a*). In addition to the basal cell nevus syndrome, the Albright's sign is seen in pseudohypoparathyroidism, Turner's syndrome, and pseudopseudohypoparathyroidism. Rib or vertebral abnormalities are common. Lamellar calcification or the falx is often a valuable diagnostic sign (Fig. 11*b*).

Mental retardation is present in a minority of the patients. The electroencephalogram may show nonspecific abnormalities. Congenital abnormalities include agenesis of the corpus callosum and congenital hydrocephalus.

Other abnormalities in some patients include male hypogonadism with absent or undescended testes, infantile external genitalia, female pubic hair pattern, and scanty facial hair. Ovarian fibromas and pelvic calcification may be present. Lymphatic mesenteric cysts may necessitate laparotomy [80].

Patients with the basal cell nevus syndrome are subject to internal neoplasms as well as to cutaneous basal cell carcinomas. These include ameloblastomas of the oral cavity, fibrosarcoma of the jaw, ovarian fibromas, teratomas, or cystadenomas. Medulloblastoma of the brain has been present in several patients. Treatment of the medulloblastoma with standard dosage of radio-

---

Table 7   Basal cell nevus syndrome: Clinical features

Cutaneous abnormalities
  Multiple basal cell carcinomas
  Pits in palms and soles
  Benign lesions: milia, cysts, lipomas, fibromas
Characteristic facies
  Broad nasal root
  Frontal bossing
  Hypertelorism
Osseous abnormalities
  Oral: jaw cysts, defective dentition, ameloblastoma
  Ribs: bifid, splayed, pectus excavatum
  Brachymetacarpalism
Ocular abnormalities
  Hypertelorism
  Dystopia canthorum
  Strabismus
  Congenital blindness: cataracts, coloboma, glaucoma
Neurologic abnormalities
  Mental retardation
  Calcification of the dura
  Congenital hydrocephalus
  Medulloblastoma
Endocrine abnormalities
  Male hypogonadism: absent or undescended testes
  Female: ovarian fibromas

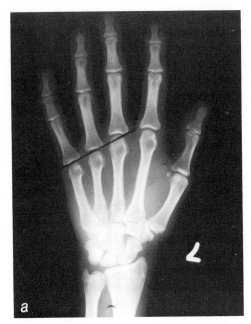 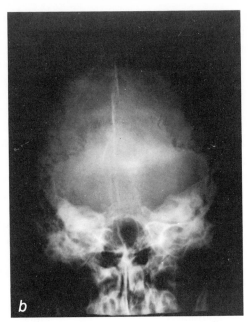

Fig. 11.   Basal cell nevus syndrome. *(a)* **Short fourth metacarpal (Albright's sign). A line drawn through the distal ends of the fifth and fourth metacarpals intersects the third metacarpal proximal to its end.** *(b)* **Lamellar calcification of the falx.**

therapy has resulted in a remarkable phenomenon: Numerous basal cell carcinomas appeared in the skin within 4 years; these were strikingly limited to the portions of skin which were exposed in the radiotherapy field [83].

Laboratory Abnormalities. Most standard clinical laboratory tests are normal in patients with basal cell nevus syndrome. Chromosome abnormalities have been found in a small number of patients [84]. Two patients in one family had an unusual group F chromosome (a "marker chromosome") with an unusually long pair of secondary constrictions in one pair of arms. Other cells from these patients showed deletions of portions of these chromosomes. In another study, two basal cell nevus syndrome patients had increased rates of chromosome breakage and rearrangement in cultured fibroblasts. Studies of induced breakage or of SCEs have not been published.

The clinical observation of the induction of numerous basal cell carcinomas in skin in the path of radiotherapy for treatment of central nervous system neoplasms prompted the study of x-ray sensitivity of cultured cells from patients with basal cell nevus syndrome. Studies of dermal fibroblasts have shown normal survival response following x-ray [4].

Clinical-Laboratory Correlations. Patients with basal cell nevus syndrome have features of progressive degeneration with occurrence of multiple jaw cysts and basal cell carcinomas. A few patients have chromosomal abnormalities, but this has not been studied systematically in a large series of patients.

There is striking clinical x-ray induction of basal cell carcinomas. However, a corresponding cellular radiohypersensitivity has not been demonstrated. Perhaps the defect is limited to the epidermal basal cells and not found in the dermal fibroblasts that are usually cultured.

Retinoblastoma

Definition. Retinoblastoma is a childhood tumor of the retina. It occurs with a frequency of approximately 1 per 20,000 live births in an hereditary and a nonhereditary form [7,85–88].

Clinical Features. Retinoblastoma is diagnosed most frequently in children between 2 and 6 years of age. Approximately 10 percent of patients are diagnosed at birth. About 60 percent of the cases are nonhereditary. Forty percent are hereditary, inherited in an autosomal dominant manner from an affected survivor or a nonaffected latent gene carrier, or due to a new germinal mutation in a healthy patient. Retinoblastoma is equally frequent in the left and right eyes and is bilateral in about 25 percent of cases. Rarely the pineal gland is also involved (so-called trilateral retinoblastoma). Overall, about 94 percent of all retinoblastoma cases, both hereditary and nonhereditary, are sporadic. All cases with bilateral retinoblastoma are hereditary and about 10 to 15 percent of the unilateral cases are sporadic, but due to a new germinal mutation. Approximately 25 percent of infants with 13q$^-$ chromosome deletion syndrome have retinoblastoma [85].

The most frequent presenting symptom is the amaurotic "cat's eye" (Fig. 12) [85]. This results from a growing retinal tumor filling the vitreous humor and producing a white pupillary reflex (leukocoria) in the normally black pupillary opening. Another sign is turning the face toward the side of the diseased eye when reading or looking at something in detail. This sign may be misinterpreted as a "tic" or torticollis. It results from use of the normal eye to compensate for deficient vision in the affected eye. Retinoblastoma may be associated with heterochromia of the iris with the affected eye having the darker iris. Early lesions may present as decreased vision or strabismus.

The clinical diagnosis is made by fundoscopic examination. Early tumors may appear as one or more white, elevated retinal masses with indistinct borders. Tumor progression may involve the vitreous or the choroid, producing retinal detachment and a white pupillary reflex. Continued tumor growth may result in secondary glaucoma, photophobia, or hemorrhage.

Diagnosis of localized retinoblastoma may be suggested by fluorescein angiography. Masses may be localized by ultrasonography. Intraocular calcifications in children are highly suggestive of retinoblastoma.

The tumor most often metastasizes to subcutaneous tissue of the head and preauricular lymph nodes. Distant metastases may occur. The most common cause of death is brain metastasis.

Treatment consists mainly of surgical enucleation of the affected eye and/or local x-radiation. The 5-year cure rate in the United States is above 80 percent, one of the highest for any childhood neoplams [85].

Survivors of retinoblastoma have an increased risk of developing a second neoplasm, particularly osteosarcomas [89,90]. Osteosarcomas have occurred in sites not treated with radiation as well as in sites in the field of radiation therapy. Other second neoplasms have included rhabdomyosarcoma, leukemia, thyroid adenocarcinoma, and melanoma. In the hereditary form of retinoblastoma the risk of developing nonradiogenic osteosarcoma was increased 230-fold in carriers of the retinoblastoma gene (whether clinically affected or not) [90].

Laboratory Abnormalities. Chromosome studies of cultured cells from some patients with retinoblas-

Fig. 12.   Retinoblastoma. Amaurotic "cat's eye" in a child with retinoblastoma of the left eye. *(Photograph courtesy of Jerry S. Shields.)*

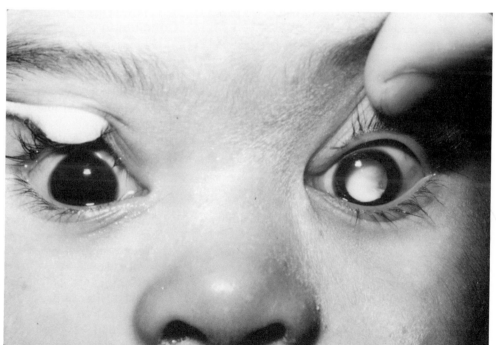

toma have shown a specific defect: deletion of the q14 band on the long arm of chromosome 13. A few patients with congenital abnormalities, including retinal lesions but without retinoblastoma, were found to have deletions in chromosome 13 not including the q14 region. Thus this region is suspected of containing genetic material responsible for prevention of development of retinoblastoma.

Cultured fibroblasts from patients with retinoblastoma and deletion of a portion of chromosome 13 were found to be hypersensitive to inhibition of colony forming by x-radiation [14,15]. Fibroblasts from patients with hereditary retinoblastoma without chromosome deletion were mildly hypersensitive to x-ray-induced killing. Fibroblasts from patients with sporadic retinoblastoma had normal x-ray survival. Studies of x-ray-induced chromosome abnormalities or mutagenesis have not been published. The basis for the x-ray hypersensitivity in cultured cells from patients with hereditary retinoblastoma has been postulated to involve abnormal DNA repair. However, no DNA repair defect has yet been reported in these cells.

Clinical-Laboratory Correlation. The hereditary forms of retinoblastoma are unusually susceptible to development of multiple primary tumors in one retina, to bilateral retinoblastomas, and to other primary neoplasms at distant sites. These occur in sites receiving radiation as well as in nonradiated sites. Cells from patients with hereditary retinoblastoma are hypersensitive to killing by x-radiation. These observations have been cited as supporting a "two hit" model of carcinogenesis, as proposed by Knudson et al. [91]. According to this theory, cancer is the result of two distinct mutations, each occurring with a frequency of about 1 in 1 million. Both mutations would thus occur by chance with a frequency of 1 in 10^{12}, an exceedingly rare event. Patients with hereditary retinoblastoma are assumed to have inherited the first mutation. This mutation is thus present in all their cells. Their cells thus need only be subjected to a single mutation to develop cancer. Patients with hereditary retinoblastoma do develop retinoblastoma at a younger age than do patients with the spontaneous form. The x-ray hypersensitivity of all their cells may further predispose to the development of the second mutation in ocular and other tissues.

Other Disorders

Investigations of a number of other disorders have led to publications describing cellular hypersensitivity (Table 4). Generally, each paper described abnormalities in a small number of affected individuals.

Fibroblasts from two tuberous sclerosis patients (of three tested) showed increased sensitivity to inhibition of colony-forming ability by hypoxic gamma radiation [10].

Lymphoblastoid cell lines from four patients with Huntington's disease were abnormally sensitive to x-ray inhibition of cell growth [92].

Lymphoblastoid cell lines from two patients with Chédiak-Higashi syndrome [93,94] were abnormally sensitive to growth inhibition by UV radiation and by treatment with the carcinogen 4-nitroquinoline oxide [95]. No defect in DNA repair was detected to explain this hypersensitivity.

Fibroblasts from a patient with extreme sun sensitivity and dwarfism were found to be hypersensitive to inhibition of colony-forming ability by 254- and 310-nm UV radiation [96]. These fibroblasts differed from xeroderma pigmentosum in that they were hypersensitive to inhibition of colony formation by the carcinogen ethylmethane sulfonate and had normal survival following treatment with n-hydroxyacetoaminofluorene (Table 3). No DNA repair defects have been identified in this cell line.

Fibroblasts from a patient with juvenile dermatomyositis who developed a basal cell carcinoma of the eyelid at age 16 years were found to be hypersensitive to x-ray and to 313-nm UV radiation [97]. No DNA repair defect was found.

Conclusion

Increased sensitivity to some physical and chemical agents has been recognized in a small number of heritable diseases in recent years (Table 4). Clinical hypersensitivity to sunlight or to radiotherapy has been shown to be manifested by a corresponding cellular hypersensitivity in xeroderma pigmentosum, Cockayne's syndrome, and ataxia-telangiectasia. In xeroderma pigmentosum and in some patients with ataxia-telangiectasia the cellular hypersensitivity has been shown to be related to defective DNA repair.

Spontaneous chromosomal breakage is a feature of ataxia-telangiectasia, Bloom's syndrome, and Fanconi's anemia. As with most of these disorders, the molecular mechanisms involved in the chromosomal abnormalities are just beginning to be understood.

Recognition of the hypersensitivity in these disorders has significance for diagnosis of several of them. Diagnosis of Bloom's syndrome, Fanconi's anemia, and xeroderma pigmentosum may be facilitated by examining chromosomal abnormalities or DNA repair. Prenatal diagnosis has been accomplished in xeroderma pigmentosum and Fanconi's anemia on the basis of cellular hypersensitivity to UV radiation [35] and to diepoxybutane [57], respectively.

Although these heritable diseases are rare, carriers of the affected genes can be calculated to comprise several percent of the general population. These individuals are usually free of clinical symptoms. However, epidemiologic studies have suggested that they may have an increased risk of neoplasia. In particular, heterozygous carriers of ataxia-telangiectasia may have a fivefold increased risk of dying from ovarian, stomach, or biliary tract cancer before age 45 [45]. Since they may comprise 1 percent of the general population, they may thus represent 5 percent of the persons dying from these cancers before age 45 years. There is a similar suggestion that persons heterozygous for xeroderma pigmentosum have an increased risk of developing skin cancer [42]. Asymptomatic carriers of the retinoblastoma genetic defect have a 200-fold increased risk of developing osteosarcoma [90]. Many of these individuals may be at an increased risk from exposure to environmental agents. There are thus implications for cancer control, preventive medicine, and occupational medicine. At present, however, there is no laboratory test that can reliably detect the asymptomatic carriers of most of these disorders.

There is a tantalizing link between these cellular abnormalities and certain common clinical features such as neoplasia, neurologic degeneration, and immune deficiency. Progressive cutaneous, neoplastic, or neurologic degeneration (as in xeroderma pigmentosum, ataxia-telangiectasia, Cockayne's syndrome, dyskeratosis congenita, basal cell nevus syndrome, retinoblastoma, Gardner's syndrome, or Huntington's disease) may be the result of impaired survival of cells subjected to damage by exogenous or endogenous physical or chemical agents. Immune deficiency is seen in ataxia-telangiectasia, Bloom's syndrome, Chédiak-Higashi syndrome, and dyskeratosis congenita. The immune deficiency may be related to in utero damage, to defective DNA processing at a crucial stage of embryonic development, or to other, not presently identified, defects. A better understanding of the relationship between these clinical abnormalities and the cellular defects in these patients will undoubtedly provide insights to disease in normal individuals.

Appendix

In order to gather quantitative information on clinical abnormalities in several of these rare disorders and to provide insights into etiology, four registries have been established:

1. Patients with xeroderma pigmentosum should be reported to:
   Xeroderma Pigmentosum Registry
   c/o Department of Pathology
   Medical Science Building, Room C520
   CMDNJ—New Jersey Medical School
   100 Bergen Street
   Newark, NJ 07103
2. Patients with Bloom's syndrome should be reported to:
   Bloom's Syndrome Registry
   c/o Laboratory of Human Genetics
   The New York Blood Center
   310 East 67 Street
   New York, NY 10021
3. Patients with immunodeficiency (e.g., ataxia-telangiectasia) and cancer should be reported to:
   Immunodeficiency—Cancer Registry
   Box 609 Mayo
   University of Minnesota
   Minneapolis, MN 55455
4. Patients with Gardner's syndrome should be reported to:
   Familial Polyposis and Gardner's
       Syndrome Registry
   c/o Dr. Martin Lipkin
   Memorial Hospital for Cancer Research
   1275 York Avenue
   New York, NY 10021

References

* 1. Robbins JH et al: Xeroderma pigmentosum: an inherited disease with sun sensitivity, multiple cutaneous neoplasms, and abnormal DNA repair. *Ann Intern Med* **80**:221–248, 1974
* 2. Kraemer KH: Xeroderma pigmentosum, in *Clinical Dermatology*, vol 4. Edited by DJ Demis et al. Harper & Row, Hagerstown, 1980, pp 1–33
* 3. Setlow RB: Repair deficient human disorders and cancer. *Nature* **271**:713–717, 1978.
* 4. Arlett CF, Lehmann AR: Human disorders showing increased sensitivity to the induction of genetic damage. *Ann Rev Genet* **12**:95–115, 1978
* 5. Paterson MC: Environmental carcinogenesis and imperfect repair of damaged DNA in *Homo sapiens:* causal

* Indicates general references.

relation revealed by rare hereditary disorders, in *Carcinogens: Identification and Mechanisms of Action*. Edited by AC Griffin, CR Shaw. Raven, New York, 1979, pp 251–276

* 6. Friedberg EC et al: Human diseases associated with defective DNA repair. *Adv Radiat Biol* 8:85–174, 1979

* 7. Gianelli F: DNA repair in human diseases. *Clin Exp Dermatol* 5:119–138, 1980

* 8. Lehmann AR, Karran P: DNA repair. *Int Rev Cytol* 72:101–146, 1981

* 9. Kraemer KH: Progressive degenerative diseases associated with defective DNA repair: xeroderma pigmentosum and ataxia telangiectasia, in *DNA Repair Processes*. Edited by WW Nichols, DG Murphy. Symposium Specialists, Miami, 1977, pp 37–71

*10. Paterson MC et al: Gamma ray hypersensitivity and faulty DNA repair in cultured cells from humans exhibiting familial cancer proneness, in *Radiation Research*. Edited by S Okada et al. Toppan, Tokyo, 1979, pp 484–495

 11. Arlett CF, Harcourt SA: Survey of radiosensitivity in a variety of human cell strains. *Cancer Res* 40:926–932, 1980

 12. Smith PJ, Paterson MC: Abnormal responses to mid-ultraviolet light of cultured fibroblasts from patients with disorders featuring sunlight sensitivity. *Cancer Res* 41:511–518, 1981

*13. Paterson MC, Smith PJ: Ataxia telangiectasia: an inherited human disorder involving hypersensitivity to ionizing radiation and related DNA-damaging chemicals. *Ann Rev Genet* 13:291–318, 1979

 14. Weichselbaum RR, Little JB: Familial retinoblastoma and ataxia telangiectasia: human models for the study of DNA damage and repair. *Cancer* 45:775–779, 1980

 15. Weichselbaum RR et al: X-ray sensitivity of fifty-three human diploid fibroblast cell strains from patients with characterized genetic disorders. *Cancer Res* 40:920–925, 1980

*16. Mulvihill JJ: Genetic repertory of human neoplasia, in *Genetics of Human Cancer*. Edited by JJ Mulvihill et al. Raven, New York, 1977, pp 137–144

*17. Reed WB: Congenital and genetic skin disorders with tumor formation. *Australas J Dermatol* 16:95–108, 1975

*18. Lynch HT, Frichot BC: Skin, heredity and cancer. *Semin Oncol* 5:67–84, 1978

*19. Robbins JH: Significance of repair of human DNA: evidence from studies of xeroderma pigmentosum. *J Natl Cancer Inst* 61:645–656, 1978

*20. Paul J: *Cell and Tissue Culture*. Churchill Livingstone, London, 1973, 430 pp

 21. Henderson EE, Ribecky R: DNA repair in lymphoblastoid cell lines established from human genetic disorders. *Chem Biol Interact* 33:63–81, 1980

*22. Friedberg EC, Hanawalt PC (Eds): *DNA Repair: A Laboratory Manual of Research Procedures*. Marcel Dekker, New York, 1981, 637 pp

 23. Kraemer KH et al: Survival of human lymphoblastoid cells after DNA damage measured by growth in microtiter wells. *Mutat Res* 72:285–294, 1980

 24. Kraemer KH et al: Colony-forming ability of ultraviolet-irradiated xeroderma pigmentosum fibroblasts from different DNA repair complementation groups. *Biochim Biophys Acta* 442:147–153, 1976

*25. Day RS: Human adenoviruses as DNA repair probes, in *DNA Repair Processes*. Edited by WW Nichols, DG Murphy. Symposium Specialists, Miami, 1977, pp 119–145

*26. Harnden DG, Taylor AMR: Chromosomes and neoplasia. *Ann Hum Genet* 9:1–70, 1979

*27. Shiraishi Y, Sandberg AA: Sister chromatid exchange in human chromosomes, including observations in neoplasia. *Cancer Genet Cytogenet* 1:363–380, 1980

*28. Latt SA, Schreck RR: Sister chromatid exchange analysis. *Am J Hum Genet* 32:297–313, 1980

 29. Chaganti RSK et al: A manyfold increase in sister chromatid exchanges in Bloom's syndrome lymphocytes. *Proc Natl Acad Sci USA* 71:4508–4512, 1974

 30. German J, Schonberg S: Bloom's syndrome. IX. Review of cytological and biochemical aspects, in *Genetic and Environmental Factors in Experimental and Human Cancer*. Edited by HV Gelboin et al. Japan Scientific Societies Press, Tokyo, 1980, pp 175–186

 31. Chang WS et al: Ultraviolet light-induced sister chromatid exchanges in xeroderma pigmentosum and in Cockayne's syndrome lymphocyte cell lines. *Cancer Res* 38:1601–1609, 1978

*32. Laval J, Laval F: Enzymology of DNA repair, in *Molecular and Cellular Aspects of Carcinogen Screening Tests*. Edited by R Montesano et al. IARC Scientific Publications, Lyon, 1980, No 27, pp 55–73

 33. Epstein JH et al: Defect in DNA synthesis in skin of patients with xeroderma pigmentosum demonstrated in vivo. *Science* 168:1477–1478, 1970

 34. Burk PG et al: Ultraviolet stimulated thymidine incorporation in xeroderma pigmentosum lymphocytes. *J Lab Clin Med* 77:759–767, 1971

 35. Ramsay CA et al: Prenatal diagnosis of xeroderma pigmentosum: report of the first successful case. *Lancet* 2:1109–1112, 1974

 36. De Weerd-Kastelein EA et al: Genetic heterogeneity of xeroderma pigmentosum demonstrated by somatic cell hybridization. *Nature* 238:80–83, 1972

 37. Kraemer KH et al: Genetic heterogeneity in xeroderma pigmentosum: complementation groups and their relationship to DNA repair rates. *Proc Natl Acad Sci USA* 72:59–63, 1975

 38. Robbins JH, Moshell AN: DNA repair processes protect human beings from premature solar skin damage: evidence from studies of xeroderma pigmentosum. *J Invest Dermatol* 73:102–107, 1979

 39. Cleaver JE: Defective repair replication of DNA in xeroderma pigmentosum. *Nature* 218:652–656, 1968

 40. Berger NA et al: Defective poly(adenosine diphosphoribose) synthesis in xeroderma pigmentosum. *Biochemistry* 19:289–293, 1980

 41. Hofmann H et al: Pigmented xerodermoid: first report of a family. *Bull Cancer (Paris)* 63:347–350, 1978

 42. Swift M, Chase C: Cancer in families with xeroderma pigmentosum. *J Natl Cancer Inst* 62:1415–1421, 1979

*43. Sedgwick RP, Boder E: Ataxia telangiectasia, in *Handbook of Clinical Neurology*, vol 14. Edited by PJ Vinken, GW Bruyn. North-Holland, Amsterdam, 1972, pp 267–339

*44. McFarlin DE et al: Ataxia telangiectasia. *Medicine (Baltimore)* 51:281–314, 1972

 45. Swift M et al: Malignant neoplasms in the families of patients with ataxia telangiectasis. *Cancer Res* 36:209–215, 1976

 46. Spector BD et al: Epidemiology of cancer in ataxia-telangiectasia, in *Ataxia-Telangiectasia—A Cellular and Molecular Link Between Cancer Neuropathy and Immune Deficiency*. Edited by BA Bridges, DG Harnden. Wiley, New York, 1982, pp 103–138

47. Edwards MJ, Taylor AMR: Unusual levels of (ADP-ribose)$_n$ and DNA synthesis in ataxia telangiectasia cells following gamma-ray irradiation. *Nature* **287**:745–747, 1980

48. Shaham M et al: A diffusable clastogenic factor in ataxia telangiectasia. *Cytogenet Cell Genet* **27**:155–161, 1980

49. Fujiwara Y et al: Cross-link repair in human cells and its possible defect in Fanconi's anemia cells. *J Mol Biol* **113**:635–649, 1977

50. German JG: The cancers in chromosome-breakage syndromes, in *Radiation Research*. Edited by S Okada et al. Toppan, Tokyo, 1979, pp 496–505

*51. Nilsson LR: Chronic pancytopenia with multiple congenital abnormalities (Fanconi's anemia). *Acta Paediatr Scand* **49**:518–529, 1960

52. Sasaki M, Tonomura A: A high susceptibility of Fanconi's anemia to chromosome breakage by DNA cross-linking agents. *Cancer Res* **33**:1829–1836, 1973

*53. Gmyrek D, Syllm-Rapoport I: Fanconi's anemia: analysis of 129 described cases. *Z Kinderheilkd* **91**:294–337, 1964

*54. Schroeder TM et al: Formal genetics of Fanconi's anemia. *Hum Genet* **32**:257–288, 1976

*55. Auerbach AD, Wolman SR: Carcinogen-induced chromosome breakage in chromosome instability syndromes. *Cancer Genet Cytogenet* **1**:21–28, 1979

56. Berger R et al: Sister chromatid exchanges induced by nitrogen mustard in Fanconi's anemia: application to the detection of heterozygotes and interpretation of the results. *Cancer Genet Cytogenet* **2**:259–267, 1980

57. Auerbach AD et al: Pre-and postnatal diagnosis and carrier detection of Fanconi anemia by cytogenetic method. *Pediatrics* **67**:128–135, 1981

58. Schroeder TM, Stahl-Mauge C: Mutagenic effects of isonicotinic acid hydracide in Fanconi's anemia. *Hum Genet* **52**:309–321, 1979

59. Brumback RA et al: Normal pressure hydrocephalus: recognition and relationship to neurological abnormalities in Cockayne's syndrome. *Arch Neurol* **35**:337–345, 1978

60. Riggs W, Seibert J: Cockayne's syndrome: roentgen findings. *Am J Roentgenol* **116**:623–633, 1972

61. Wade MH, Chu EHY: Effects of DNA damaging agents of cultured fibroblasts derived from patients with Cockayne's syndrome. *Mutat Res* **59**:49–60, 1979

62. Lehmann AR et al: Abnormal kinetics of DNA synthesis in ultraviolet light-irradiated cells from patients with Cockayne's syndrome. *Cancer Res* **39**:4237–4241, 1979

63. Andrews AD et al: Cockayne's syndrome fibroblasts have increased sensitivity to ultraviolet light but normal rates of unscheduled DNA synthesis. *J Invest Dermatol* **70**:237–239, 1978

64. Marshall RR et al: Increased sensitivity of cell strains from Cockayne's syndrome to sister chromatid exchange induction and cell killing by UV light. *Mutat Res* **69**:107–112, 1980

*65. German J: Bloom's syndrome. II. The prototype of human genetic disorders predisposing to chromosome instability and cancer, in *Chromosomes and Cancer*. Edited by J German. Wiley, New York, 1974, pp 601–617

66. Bloom D: Congenital telangiectatic erythema resembling lupus erythematosus in dwarfs. *Am J Dis Child* **88**:754–758, 1954

67. German J et al: Bloom's syndrome. VII. Progress report for 1978. *Clin Genet* **15**:361–367, 1979

68. Weemaes CMR et al: Immune responses in four patients with Bloom syndrome. *Clin Immunol Immunopathol* **12**:12–19, 1979

69. Kauli R et al: Gonadal function in Bloom's syndrome. *Clin Endocrinol* **6**:285–289, 1977

70. Alhadeff B et al: High rate of sister chromatid exchanges of Bloom's syndrome is corrected in rodent human somatic cell hybrids. *Cytogenet Cell Genet* **27**:8–23, 1980

71. Hand R, German J: Bloom's syndrome: DNA replication in cultured fibroblasts and lymphocytes. *Hum Genet* **38**:297–306, 1977

72. Gupta RS, Goldstein S: Diphtheria toxin resistance in human fibroblast cell strains from normal and cancer-prone individuals, *Mutat Res* **73**:331–338, 1980

73. Sirnavin C, Trowbridge AA: Dyskeratosis congenita: clinical features and genetic aspects. Report of a family and review of the literature. *J Med Genet* **12**:339–354, 1975

74. Carter DM et al: Psoralen-DNA cross-linking photoadducts in dyskeratosis congenita: delay in excision and promotion of sister chromatid exchange. *J Invest Dermatol* **73**:97–101, 1979

75. Burgdorf W et al: Sister chromatid exchange in dyskeratosis congenita. *J Med Genet* **14**:256–257, 1977

*76. Lipkin M et al: Memorial Hospital registry of population groups at high risk for cancer of the large intestine: age of onset of neoplasms. *Prev Med* **9**:335–345, 1980

77. Danes BS: The Gardner syndrome: increased tetraploidy in cultured skin fibroblast. *J Med Genet* **13**:52–56, 1976

78. Kopelovich L: Phenotypic markers in human skin fibroblasts as possible diagnostic indices of hereditary adenomatosis of the colon and rectum. *Cancer* **40**:2534–2541, 1977

79. Little JB et al: Abnormal sensitivity of diploid skin fibroblasts from a family with Gardner's syndrome to the lethal effects of x-irradiation, ultraviolet light, and mitomycin C. *Mutat Res* **70**:241–250, 1980

*80. Berlin NI et al: Basal cell nevus syndrome. *Ann Intern Med* **64**:403–421, 1966

*81. Dunnick NR et al: Nevoid basal cell carcinoma syndrome: radiographic manifestations including cystlike lesions of the phalanges. *Radiology* **127**:331–334, 1978

82. Slater S: An evaluation of the metacarpal sign (short fourth metacarpal). *Pediatrics* **46**:468–471, 1970

83. Strong LC: Theories of pathogenesis: mutation and cancer, in *Genetics of Cancer*. Edited by JJ Mulvihill et al. Raven, New York, 1977, pp 401–416

84. Happle R, Hoehn H: Cytogenetic studies on cultured fibroblast-like cells derived from basal cell carcinoma tissue. *Clin Genet* **4**:17–24, 1973

*85. Shields JA, Augsburger JJ: Current approaches to the diagnosis and management of retinoblastoma. *Surv Ophthalmol* **25**:347–372, 1981

*86. Francois J: Costenbader Memorial Lecture: Genesis and genetics of retinoblastoma. *Adv Ophthalmol* **39**:181–209, 1979

87. Gaitan-Yanguas M: Retinoblastoma: analysis of 235 cases. *Int J Radiat Oncol Biol Phys* **4**:359–365, 1978

*88. Vogel F: Genetics of retinoblastoma. *Hum Genet* **52**:1–54, 1979

*89. Meadows AT et al: Patterns of second malignant neoplasms in children. *Cancer* **40**:1903–1911, 1977

90. Matsunaga E: Hereditary retinoblastoma: host resistance and second primary tumors. *J Natl Cancer Inst* **65**:47–51, 1980

91. Knudson AG et al: Mutation and childhood cancer: a probabilistic model for the incidence of retinoblastoma. *Proc Natl Acad Sci USA* **72**:5116–5120, 1975

92. Moschell AN et al: Radiosensitivity in Huntington's

disease: implications for pathogenesis and presymptomatic diagnosis. *Lancet* **1:**9–11, 1980

*93. Blume RS, Wolff SM: The Chédiak-Higashi syndrome: studies in four patients and a review of the literature. *Medicine (Baltimore)* **51:**247–280, 1972

*94. Wolff SM et al: The Chédiak-Higashi syndrome: studies of host defenses. *Ann Intern Med* **76:**293–306, 1972

95. Tanaka H, Orii T: High sensitivity but normal DNA-repair activity after UV irradiation in Epstein-Barr virus-transformed lymphoblastoid cell lines from Chédiak-Higashi syndrome. *Mutat Res* **72:**143–150, 1980

96. Arlett CF et al: A human subject with a new defect in repair of ultraviolet damage. *J Invest Dermatol* **70:**173–178, 1978

97. Smith PJ et al: In vitro radiosensitivity in a patient with dermatomyositis and cancer. *Lancet* **1:**216–217, 1981

CUTANEOUS T-CELL LYMPHOMA (MYCOSIS FUNGOIDES, SÉZARY SYNDROME, AND RELATED PRESENTATIONS)

Richard L. Edelson

With the evolution of cellular immunology, hematooncology entered a new phase. Lymphoreticular malignancies, previously classified solely by morphologic criteria, could now be characterized on the basis of distinguishing immunologic features. The effects on our understanding of cutaneous lymphoma have been particularly profound and are the subjects of this chapter.

During the early part of the past decade, it became apparent that the only lymphomatous malignancies of adults that could regularly be shown to be of T-cell origin were those exhibiting prominent skin involvement [1] (Figs. 1–4). This group included the leukemic exfoliative erythroderma commonly referred to as the *Sézary syndrome* and the nonleukemic process known as *mycosis fungoides*. Whereas the relationship between those two processes had long been suspected [2], it was surprising that other clinical and histopathologic presentations of skin lymphoma often described as "reticulum-cell sarcoma," "lymphoma cutis," "histiocytic lymphoma," etc., were also found to be T-cell neoplasms [3].

Because of the distinguishing clinical and cellular denominators of the primary cutaneous lymphomas, they were united in 1975 under the designation *cutaneous T-cell lymphoma* (CTCL), replacing the descriptive and eponymic nomenclature that had previously been used to identify subgroups of this spectrum of disease [4]. In 1978 the National Cancer Institute Workshop on the subject concluded that the term *cutaneous T-cell lymphoma*

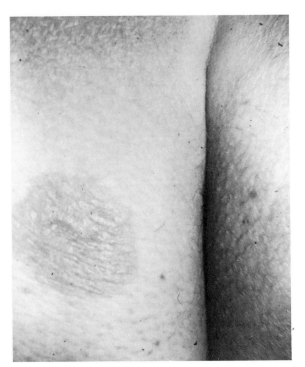

Fig. 1.   Single, laterally extending plaque of epidermotropic CTCL.

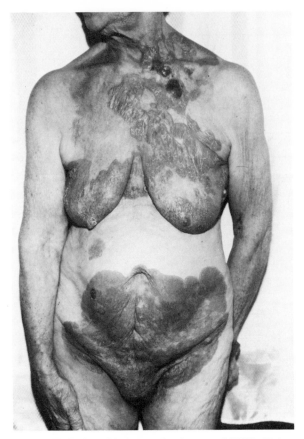

Fig. 2.   Multiple epidermotropic plaques of CTCL. Note tumor formation by subclone(s) in region proximal to left clavicle.

should be adopted [5], and CTCL has subsequently received wide usage. This review will highlight the clinically relevant advances made in the understanding of this disorder during the past decade.

Historical Perspective

Until the 1970s, the large majority of contributions to the understanding of cutaneous lymphomas came from careful morphologic and clinical descriptions. The resulting nomenclature, which implied the presence of numerous distinct lymphoproliferative processes originating in the skin, was descriptive and controversial.

Alibert [6] introduced the term *mycosis fungoides* to characterize a single case in which tumors resembling mushrooms evolved from a desquamating rash. Bazin [7] suggested an orderly natural progression from an undiagnosable "premycotic" phase to discrete plaque lesions and then to tumors. Vidal and Brocq [8] recognized a *d'emblée* variant characterized by rapidly developing tumors, without progression through premycotic and plaque phases, and Besnier and Hallopeau [9] identified an erythrodermic phase. In 1938, Sézary and Bouvrain [2] reported the triad of erythroderma, leukemia composed of large mononuclear cells with redundantly folded **nuclei,** and enlarged pe-

ripheral lymph nodes infiltrated by the same characteristic abnormal cells as were found in the blood. This "Sézary syndrome" was first formally recognized in the American medical literature 23 years later by Taswell and Winkelmann, who reported several similar cases from the Mayo Clinic [10]. In 1968, Lutzner and Jordan extended Sézary's original light microscopic analysis of the circulating abnormal cells by using electron microscopy to visualize a "serpentine," or highly convoluted, nucleus [11].

However, a sharp distinction between the Sézary syndrome and mycosis fungoides was not universally accepted. A more unified concept was suggested by Clendenning et al. [12], who noted significant percentages of atypical circulating lymphocytes in patients with plaque and tumor lesions of mycosis fungoides.

Demonstration that these clinical presentations represented neoplasms of lymphocytes, rather than of monocytes, as had initially been suggested, came from studies using cytogenetics and cellular immunology. First, Crossen et al. [13] and Lutzner et al. [14] performed karyotype analysis to dem-

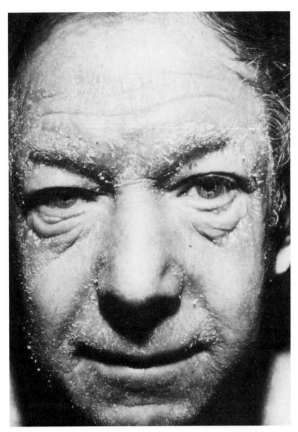

Fig. 3.   Exfoliative erythroderma secondary to leukemic epidermotropic CTCL (Sézary syndrome).

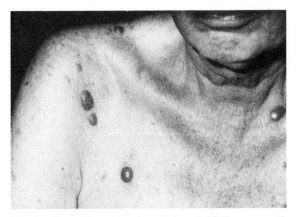

Fig. 4.   Nonepidermotropic nodules of CTCL, apparently secondary to miliary spread of aggressive clone.

onstrate that Sézary cells could occasionally proliferate in response to the lymphocyte mitogen phytohemagglutinin. The demonstration that the neoplastic cells of the Sézary syndrome [15,16] and mycosis fungoides [1] exhibit membrane features characteristic of T lymphocytes provided more definitive evidence that these disorders are malignancies of T cells.

The relationship between these cutaneous lymphoproliferative processes and the often-associated internal lymphomas was clarified when Epstein et al. [17] reported a natural progression of mycosis fungoides from a localized skin form to one characterized by widely disseminated visceral infiltration involving virtually all internal tissues. Subsequently, it became clear that extracutaneous lymphoma resulted from the dissemination of the original malignant T cells [1]. Finally, two independent histopathologic studies of autopsy material suggested that even the visceral disease retained a microscopic appearance characteristic of mycosis fungoides [18,19]. These cumulative data indicated that the Sézary syndrome and mycosis fungoides were T-cell malignancies which clini-

cally first involved the integument and subsequently became widely disseminated.

During the 1970s, immunologic techniques were applied to the study of those lymphoreticular malignancies distinguished by apparent primary cutaneous involvement. The studies indicated that, with remarkable regularity, these disorders are malignancies of T lymphocytes with phenotypic features of helper T cells [20]. CTCL, therefore, constitutes a spectrum of disease, which includes not only mycosis fungoides and Sézary syndrome but other lymphoreticular neoplasms distinguished by apparent primary skin infiltration by neoplastic helper T cells. In order to facilitate the transition from old to new nomenclature, periodic reference will be made in this review to classical mycosis fungoides and Sézary syndrome as epidermotropic variants of CTCL and to reticulum-cell sarcoma and lymphoma cutis as nonepidermotropic variants of CTCL. (Fig. 5).

Clinical Features

Accurate determination of the natural course of untreated CTCL may never be possible because it is not ethical to withhold palliative or potentially curative therapy from patients having a debilitating and life-threatening disease. An additional problem in the interpretation of most clinical studies is that the patients have been selected to conform to predetermined concepts of disease. In this manner, dermatology groups have concentrated efforts on the epidermotropic variants (mycosis fungoides and the Sézary syndrome), while hematooncology groups have concentrated on the more disseminated, nonepidermotropic phases of the disease. In short, most dermatologic series of cutaneous

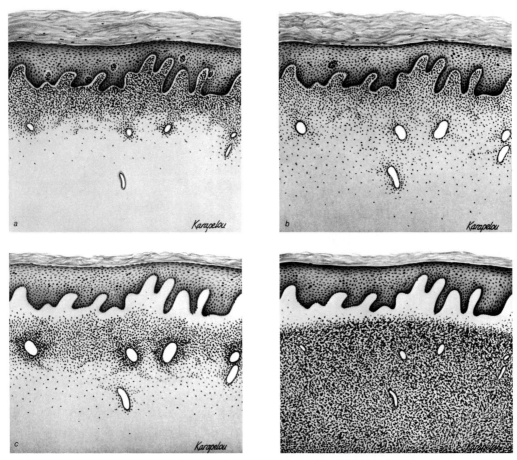

Fig. 5. Microscopic appearance of skin lesions of cutaneous T-cell lymphoma. Lesions can generally be divided into one of the following four categories: (*a*) Epidermotropic cutaneous plaque composed of a dense mononuclear cell infiltrate in the papillary dermis abutting directly on the epidermis. Single cells and Pautrier's microabscess are found within the epidermis. (*b*) Epidermotropic erythroderma composed of dermal infiltrate containing fewer cells and having a poorly defined lower border. Exocytosis of atypical mononuclear cells into the epidermis is apparent but less prominent than in the epidermotropic cutaneous plaque. (*c*) Nonepidermotropic erythroderma composed of dense infiltration in upper part of the dermis. The papillary dermis is largely spared, and scattered intraepidermal accumulations of these cells are less prominent than in the epidermotropic forms. (*d*) Nonepidermotropic papules, nodules, and tumors composed of massive infiltration of the dermis by atypical mononuclear cells. The papillary dermis subjacent to the epidermis is largely spared. Infrequent atypical mononuclear cells can be identified in the epidermis.

lymphoma patients include only those conforming to preconceived histopathologic and clinical criteria of mycosis fungoides, which is now appreciated to represent less than half of the entire spectrum of CTCL.

Nevertheless, three separate studies of large populations of patients have yielded valuable information. Epstein et al. [17] retrospectively analyzed 144 patients, hospitalized at the National Cancer Institute over a 15-year period, who had cutaneous histopathology characteristic of classical mycosis fungoides. None of those patients had been lost to follow-up, and extensive autopsy information was obtained on many. Several important prognostic indicators were established.

First, the mean survival was 8.8 years from the onset of skin lesions, and less than 5 years from standard histologic diagnosis. Second, presence of either palpable adenopathy or cutaneous tumors was associated with a mean survival of only 2.5 years. When the patients with palpable lymphadenopathy were subdivided on the basis of histopathology, those with microscopic evidence of lymph node involvement had a mean survival of 18 months, compared with 34 months for those with simple dermatopathic changes. Patients with clinically evident spleno- or hepatomegaly had mean survivals of only 3 months.

Rappaport and Thomas [18] made two particularly significant observations from a detailed histopathologic study of autopsies of 45 of the patients in the series of Epstein et al. First, mycosis fungoides differed from Hodgkin's disease by not progressing in orderly fashion from one set of lymph nodes to another. In essence, once the malignancy clinically escaped the confines of the skin, the local peripheral lymph nodes did not appear to slow generalized dissemination to viscera. That observation has important clinical implications, since it indicates that once clear microscopic involvement of peripheral lymph nodes occurs, widespread dissemination throughout other tissues can be expected. Therefore, further microscopic staging of other tissues may not be required to fully establish the necessity of systemic therapy. Second, extension to visceral organs did not indicate development of a second lymphoma, since cytologically the picture remained clearly representative of CTCL, rather than of some other type of lymphoma.

Three more recent studies have the advantage of being prospective in design. First, certain prognostic indicators have already emerged from the studies of the Mycosis Fungoides Cooperative Group [21]. Lamberg et al. established that prognosis worsens as plaques, papules, or eczematous patches become more extensive to cover greater than 10 percent of the body; when cutaneous tumors emerge; or when generalized erythroderma supervenes.

Second, 36 consecutively presenting CTCL patients were investigated at Columbia-Presbyterian Medical Center [3]. Subjects were preselected on the basis that their lymphoma presented initially in the skin, that they had received no prior systemic therapy, and that they presented directly to physicians associated with that medical center rather than through referral. In that manner it was possible to compare the frequency of various clinical presentations of CTCL with those of other types of lymphoproliferative disorders. Surprisingly, the epidermotropic forms (mycosis fungoides and Sézary syndrome) together constituted only 36 percent of the patients. Five of the 13 patients who initially had epidermotropic disease developed nonepidermotropic skin lesions during the short follow-up period of that study, while only a single patient who was undergoing chemotherapy had skin lesions that evolved from nonepidermotropic to epidermotropic. These data suggested a natural progression from epidermotropic to nonepidermotropic T-cell lymphoma. Furthermore, loss and/or absence of epidermotropism by the malignant T cells was frequently associated with systemic dissemination of CTCL. During the observation

period, CTCL as a cumulative diagnosis was noted more frequently than Hodgkin's disease in the same cachement area and, indeed, was the most common type of lymphoma identified.

A high frequency of extracutaneous dissemination of CTCL is also indicated by the prospective studies of Bunn et al. at the National Cancer Institute [22]. Of 49 consecutively studied patients who had not yet received systemic therapy, extracutaneous lymphoma was identified by light microscopy in 51 percent and by special procedures (cytogenetics, electron microscopy, T-cell cytology) in 88 percent. Those findings suggested that by the time standard histologic diagnosis can be made, the malignant T cells have usually already disseminated via the circulation to extracutaneous sites. Cytogenetics was the most sensitive of the special studies for detecting peripheral blood involvement. Previous impressions that lymph node involvement is frequently underdiagnosed were confirmed by the observation that 81 percent of nondiagnostic nodes were positive by the special studies. Lymphangiograms and gallium scans did not appear to be sensitive tests for extracutaneous disease. A close correlation between lymph node and blood involvement was recognized; whereas 19 of 23 patients with circulating malignant cells had positive lymph node biopsies, only 3 of 21 patients without identified blood involvement had diagnosable lymph node involvement. These findings extended previous observations and strongly indicated that CTCL disseminated early via the circulation rather than by secondary extension along contiguous lymph nodes as in Hodgkin's disease.

Considering the documented extracutaneous involvement at autopsy of CTCL patients (Table 1)

Table 1 Extracutaneous involvement at autopsy in CTCL patients

Reference	Autopsies, no.	Extracutaneous involvement, no.
Epstein et al. [17]	86	75
Cyr et al. [23]	23	13
Block et al. [24]	17	14
Fuks et al. [25]	56	30
Farber et al. [26]	7	6
Long and Mihm [19]	15	15
Rappaport and Thomas [18]	45	32
Cawley et al. [27]	10	8
Berman [28]	18	16
Heita and Socha [29]	54	51
Gall [30]	41	19
Allen [31]	21	3
Clendenning et al. [12]	13	12
Total	406	294 (72%)

and the varied sites of dissemination in those patients (Table 2), it is not surprising that symptomatic disease has been identified in vivo in virtually every organ system (Table 3). The liver may be the most frequently involved internal organ [22], but clinical evaluation such as physical examination, liver chemistries, and liver-spleen scans do not appear to be diagnostically helpful in early disease.

Pathogenesis

Advances in the understanding of cellular immunology have permitted refined characterization of the various lymphoproliferative diseases. Since normal lymphocytes can be divided into two developmentally and functionally distinct groups (T and B cells), new classifications of these malignancies have been based on cytoplasmic and membrane markers of the malignant cells [66]. In this manner, CTCL can be distinguished from all other neoplastic processes by the regularity with which its malignant cells are shown to have the phenotypic or functional properties of helper T cells [2]. Regardless of whether the clinical presentation is that of localized epidermotropic disease (mycosis fungoides or Sézary's syndrome) or nonepidermotropic cutaneous disease (reticulum-cell sarcoma, etc.), immunologic studies of the malignant cells of CTCL have unified the varying clinical presentations. Therefore, in the same manner that malignant melanoma constitutes a recognized spectrum of disease all secondary to malignant proliferation of melanocytes, CTCL indicates a malignancy of helper T cells. By further analogy with malignant melanoma, differences in the types

of clinical presentations should not be obscured, since they reflect differences of the biologic behavior of the malignant cells and are indicators of different prognoses.

The only group of lymphoproliferative disorders regularly demonstrated to be neoplasms of helper T cells is CTCL [2], suggesting that at least some malignant helper T cells have a particular affinity for the skin. The propensity that these cells have to infiltrate the skin is in marked contrast to the abnormal cells of the two most common B-cell leukemias of adults, chronic lymphocytic leukemia and lymphosarcoma cell leukemia [66].

Functional and membrane properties of the neoplastic cells of CTCL have been investigated. Like their normal helper T-cell counterparts, the malignant cells from approximately half of the patients studied have the functional property of facilitating normal B-cell differentiation into immunoglobulin-secreting plasma cells [67,68]. Monoclonal antibodies specifically reactive with the differentiation antigens of helper T cells react with the malignant cells of nearly all studied individuals with CTCL [20].

The tissue distribution of extracutaneous spread of CTCL probably reflects the T-cell properties of the malignant cells. The limited or often absent bone marrow infiltration, sometimes even in the presence of extreme lymphocytosis in the leukemic state, probably results from the extramedullary proliferation of malignant, as well as normal, thymus-derived cells and their circulatory pathway through the body (tending to spare the bone marrow). Therefore, in contrast to the situation in B-cell (bone marrow–derived) malignancies, bone marrow production of normal myeloid elements is

Table 2   Sites of dissemination of CTCL in autopsy studies

Reference	Lymph nodes	Spleen	Liver	Lungs	Bone marrow	Gastrointestinal tract	Kidneys	Heart	Central nervous system
Cawley et al. [29]	7/10	4/10	2/10	2/10	5/10	—	2/10	4/10	—
Cyr et al [23]	4/23	6/23	5/23	4/23	—	2/23	5/23	2/23	—
Farber et al. [26]	4/7	6/7	6/7	—	0/7	2/7	2/7	2/7	—
Epstein et al. [17]	51/86	43/86	35/86	37/86	23/86	30/86	23/86	15/86	17/86
Rappaport and Thomas [18]	24/32	19/32	17/32	21/32	12/31	—	14/32	12/32	4/28
Long and Mihm [19]	15/15	12/15	13/15	8/15	7/15	6/15	2/15	1/15	—
Total	105/173 (61%)	90/173 (52%)	78/173 (42%)	72/166 (43%)	47/149 (32%)	40/131 (31%)	48/173 (28%)	36/173 (21%)	21/114 (18%)

Table 3   Extracutaneous manifestations of CTCL

Organ system	Manifestation	Reference
Pulmonary	Parenchymal nodules	32–34
	Pulmonary infiltrates	32–35
	Pleural effusion	35
	Mediastinal and/or hilar adenopathy	35
Ocular	Intraocular disease—optic nerve, retina, choroid	36–38
	Extraocular disease—lid, conjunctiva, cornea	39, 40
Skeletal	Solitary or numerous osteolytic lesions	41–44*
	Diffuse osteoporosis	*
	Arthritis	45
Oral	Infiltrated lesions, manifested as raised or eroded areas, on lips, buccal mucosa, tongue, larynx	46–49
Nervous	Intracerebral tumor mass	50, 51
	Leptomeningeal disease	52–54
	Peripheral neuropathy	55, 56
	Cerebral hemorrhage	57
	Progressive multifocal leukoencephalopathy	58
Gastro-intestinal	Diarrhea	59
	Ascites	60
	Hemorrhage	61
Cardio-vascular	Congestive cardiac failure	24, 62
	Cardiac arrhythmias	24, 62
Renal	Progressive renal failure	24
Hematologic	Eosinophilia	23
	Monocytosis	23
	Monoclonal paraproteinemia	63, 64
	Cryoglobulinemia	65

* PA Bunn, Jr., personal communication.

preserved until late in the course of CTCL when a blast crisis may occur [69]. Initial lymph node and spleen infiltration involves the localization of clusters of the abnormal T cells in the T-cell paracortex and periarteriolar sheath, respectively [18], rather than in the B-cell follicles (Fig. 6). As the disease progresses, normal T cells may be displaced from those locations, thereby compromising normal T-cell interactions with other cells. The propensity of normal T cells to recirculate rapidly through soft tissues may also explain why, in CTCL, lymph nodes do not appear to be barriers to the systemic dissemination of the disease once the malignancy has escaped the confines of the skin [18].

The residual functional capacity of the malignant T cells probably has significance on the immunologic competence of the affected patient, particularly when the disorder has reached an advanced state in which the abnormal cells constitute a large percentage of the total body pool of mononuclear leukocytes (Fig. 7). Since the malignant T cells are incapable of specific response to microbial antigens [4], disseminated disease is often associated with serious secondary infections. At least in the leukemic state, the malignant T cells frequently produce macrophage inhibitory factor [70], which impedes monocyte mobilization to peripheral sites and further compromises the immunologic defenses of the patient. The observation that CTCL is a malignancy of helper T cells may explain the frequent elevation of serum immunoglobulins, particularly of the T cell–dependent classes IgG, IgE, and IgA [71]. This observation is again in contrast with the situation in the B-cell malignancies, in which hypogammaglobulinemia is a regular phenomenom [66]. This elevation of serum immunoglobulins in CTCL is sometimes associated with monoclonal gammopathies and autoantibodies [68].

Substantial evidence has recently accumulated to indicate that disseminated CTCL arises from expansion of a single malignant clone of helper T cells [72] (Fig. 8). First, cytogenetic determinations using chromosome banding patterns have revealed common structural chromosomal aberrations in the malignant cells infiltrating distinct tissue sites in individual patients. No single chromosomal alteration appears to be distinctive of this disease, since the abnormalities noted in each patient were distinctive for that individual. Second, phenotypic markers of the malignant cells of CTCL, from use of monoclonal antibodies, have also been most consistent with a clonal evolution of the disorder [20]. In those studies, cells from individual patients express distinctive patterns of reactivity, further suggesting that the abnormal cells arose from a clonal expansion of a single T cell. Together, these two sets of studies provide convincing evidence of the monoclonality of CTCL and have significant implications for the staging of patients with the disorder.

Since it now appears that CTCL is a monoclonal process, noncontiguous skin lesions can occur only following hematogenous spread. Therefore, multiple discrete lesions indicate dissemination of the process beyond the confines of the skin. These observations are extended by the studies of Berger et al. [73], who have produced two monoclonal antibodies that appear to react preferentially with the neoplastic cells of CTCL. Preliminary observations with those antibodies indicated that most patients with CTCL have substantial populations of reactive circulating lymphocytes, even when

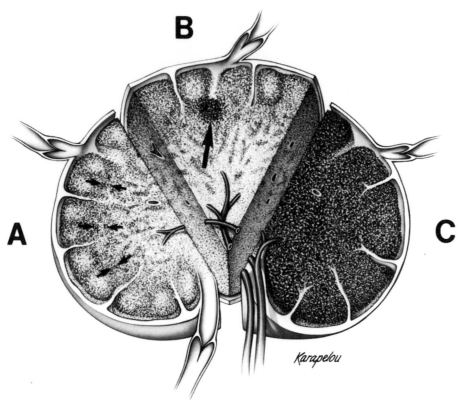

Fig. 6. A schematic of lymph node involvement in cutaneous T-cell lymphoma. (a) The dermatopathic phase: Subjacent to the follicles, melanin from the inflamed skin has been deposited (small arrows). (b) Early cellular involvement: Focal accumulations of neoplastic cells are found immediately outside remnant of a follicle (large arrow). (c) Late stage: A homogeneous accumulation of malignant T cells completely effaces the normal lymphoid architecture.

the total blood lymphocyte count is within normal limits.

In summary, currently available information is most consistent with CTCL representing a monoclonal expansion of a population of helper T cells, which initially have a strong affinity for the epidermis (Fig. 6). The disease may initially involve a confined region of the skin with subsequent progressive formation of subclones composed of cells that have decreased affinity for the epidermis and increased propensity for hematogenous spread to visceral and noncontiguous cutaneous sites. The gross and microscopic morphology of individual skin lesions appears to reflect the growth pattern and level of differentiation of the malignant cells: Plaques indicate lateral extension of relatively differentiated malignant cells; tumors represent a vertical growth pattern by more malignant subclones exhibiting less affinity for the epidermis; and widespread skin disease appears to be a direct reflection of hematogenous spread. The worst prognosis is portended by disseminated nodular nonepidermotopic lesions, possibly because their presence results from miliary metastasis by the neoplastic cells, accompanied by particularly aggressive local growth at sites where they settle.

Diagnosis and Evaluation

The advances in recent years in identifying patients with CTCL have been largely secondary to the application of special techniques. The limitations of light microscopic diagnostic criteria are underscored by the observation that a mean of 3.8 years was noted between the onset of skin lesions and the occurrence of diagnostic histopathology in the study of Epstein et al. [17]. The cumulative data from the Stanford clinical trial of electron-beam radiotherapy [74] and from the Temple experience with topical Mustargen [75] indicate that the best chance for a long-term clinical response in CTCL is obtained from skin-directed therapy during the early phases of the disease. It is likely that the frequent failure of these therapeutic modalities reflects intervention at a time too late in the evolution of the disease.

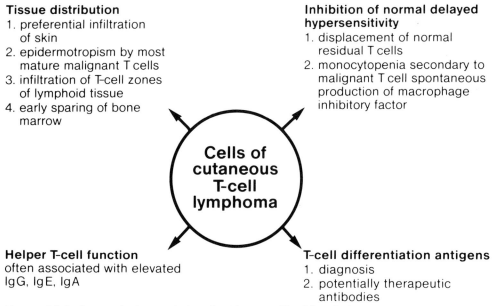

Tissue distribution
1. preferential infiltration of skin
2. epidermotropism by most mature malignant T cells
3. infiltration of T-cell zones of lymphoid tissue
4. early sparing of bone marrow

Inhibition of normal delayed hypersensitivity
1. displacement of normal residual T cells
2. monocytopenia secondary to malignant T cell spontaneous production of macrophage inhibitory factor

Cells of cutaneous T-cell lymphoma

Helper T-cell function
often associated with elevated IgG, IgE, IgA

T-cell differentiation antigens
1. diagnosis
2. potentially therapeutic antibodies

Fig. 7.   Clinicoimmunologic correlations in cutaneous T-cell lymphoma.

Because of the referral system in Great Britain, Samman [76] was able to collect a large series of cases of parapsoriasis en plaques. On the basis of the morphology of the skin lesions, the patients were divided into two diagnostic categories: "chronic superficial dermatitis" histologically resembling mild eczematous dermatitis, and "prereticulotic poikiloderma" histologically characterized by a bandlike subepidermal infiltrate. Although no individuals in the first group developed lesions characteristic of lymphoma, 9 percent of those in the poikiloderma group died of lymphoma during the period of observation and 70 percent had persistent and often progressive skin disease. Those findings, therefore, suggested that prereticulotic poikiloderma should be distinguished from the other form of parapsoriasis en plaques and be treated as an early stage of cutaneous T-cell lymphoma.

Although the initial malignant event probably occurs in a single T cell, which subsequently proliferates to form a malignant clone, the earliest stages in the development of cutaneous T-cell lymphoma involve cellular alterations currently too subtle to permit their identification. Generally, as a malignancy evolves, progressively more abnormal and aggressive subclones develop, which ultimately overwhelm the host. In the process of becoming increasingly aggressive, malignant cells often begin to have increasing difficulty with the mechanics of normal mitosis.

Abnormalities of chromosome replication and segregation then occur during metaphase, leading to gross structural changes, such as abnormally high or low numbers of chromosomes in the malignant cells, chromosome breaks, or translocation of the material from one chromosome to another. Despite the likelihood that these struc-

Fig. 8.   Schema of subclone formation and spread from a unifocal origin. The neoplastic event apparently occurs in a single mature T cell, which then proliferates to form a clone of malignant T cells that may still have an affinity for epidermis. With progressive evolution of malignant subclones, the malignant cells lose affinity for epidermis and disseminate widely to lymph nodes, dermis, viscera, and blood.

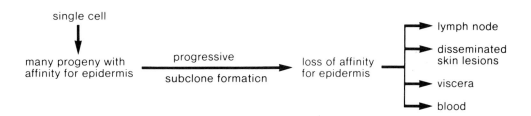

single cell

many progeny with affinity for epidermis → progressive subclone formation → loss of affinity for epidermis → lymph node / disseminated skin lesions / viscera / blood

tural chromosomal changes occur late in the evolution of populations of malignant cells, they currently represent one of our most sensitive tests for the presence of CTCL.

Van Vloten et al. [77] reported that quantitation of DNA content in mononuclear cells that have infiltrated the skin permitted identification of abnormal amounts of DNA content in the malignant T cells in situ. While each of 21 DNA plots (histograms) from overt CTCL lesions revealed abnormalities in DNA content, each of 12 individuals with a clinical diagnosis of parapsoriasis but with normal DNA histograms had a benign course. Of greatest significance, the individuals with parapsoriasis-like lesions and abnormal histograms had a poor prognosis: Ten of these 12 individuals subsequently developed overt cutaneous lymphoma. This method, referred to as *cytophotometry,* is a promising diagnostic test but is less precise than karyotype analysis, which requires mitotic figures. DNA histograms are not as sensitive as karyotype analysis since additions or deletions of DNA must be at least 10 percent of the normal diploid content to permit recognition of abnormality. In addition, karyotype analysis permits identification of far more subtle structural changes in the chromosomes (Fig. 9). The disadvantage of karyotype analysis is that it requires that the abnormal cells enter mitosis during the test period.

Bunn et al. [22] compared cytogenetics (karyotype analysis) with electron microscopy and T-cell cytology as special diagnostic techniques. The most sensitive test for identification of blood or lymph node involvement was karyotype analysis, with 64 percent of patients with normal blood smears being positive and 81 percent of histologically negative lymph nodes also being positive. Although the cytology in cytocentrifuge preparations of sheep erythrocyte-rosetted T cells and electron microscopy also were more sensitive than standard examination of blood and tissue, cytogenetic analysis was the most useful test. Since it can be readily performed in service laboratories at most large medical centers, it has great potential applicability.

The morphology of infiltrating mononuclear cells in cutaneous lesions presents difficulties as a diagnostic test. Whereas deeply indented nuclei are often characteristic of infiltrating malignant T cells in skin [78] and blood [11], normal T cells can also be stimulated by mitogens or by soluble antigens to develop deeply redundant or folded nuclei closely resembling those of typical Sézary cells [79]. Second, quantitation of nuclear contour in-

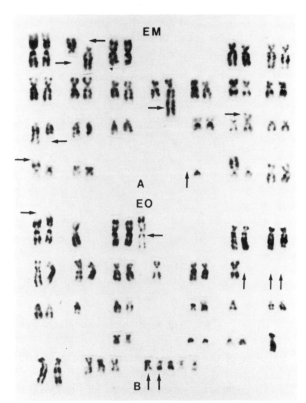

Fig. 9. Karyotypes from two CTCL patients (EM and EO). Arrows indicate physically altered chromosomes in the neoplastic cells, including additions, deletions, and marker chromosomes. These karyotypes strongly support the diagnosis of malignancy and also represent "cellular fingerprints" of the particular population of neoplastic cells.

dices by planimetry indicates that lesions of lichen planus (clearly a benign disorder) contain as high a percentage of infiltrating cells with deeply infolded nuclei, as do lesions of CTCL [80]. Hence, it seems that abnormal nuclear morphology may be indicative of "activation" of T cells but not necessarily pathognomonic for malignancy. Efforts by Meier et al. (C. J. L. M. Meier, personal communication) to combine nuclear contour indices with computerized statistical analysis are encouraging but preliminary.

Application of the new technology of monoclonal antibodies to tissue diagnosis is most promising. Antibodies, which appear to react preferentially with malignant rather than benign infiltrating T cells, can be directly conjugated with peroxidase and then used to identify malignant cells in situ [81] (Fig. 10). However, these observations are extremely preliminary and numerous benign skin disorders need to be evaluated in parallel before a conclusion about this technology can be reached.

The cutaneous T cell–lymphoma workshop

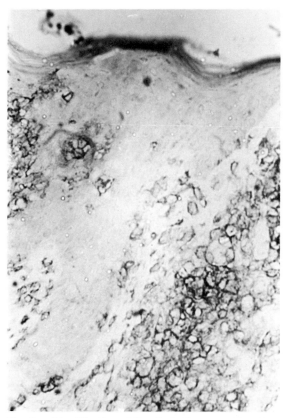

Fig. 10.   Identification of T cells in tissue section. Perox-idase-conjugated monoclonal anti-T-cell antibody specifi-cally binds to infiltrating T cells in the dermis and epidermis, highlighting the cytoplasmic membranes of positive cells.

sponsored by the National Cancer Institute [5] suggested a system for staging and classification of the disease (Table 4). Since large numbers of patients are currently being staged and followed using these criteria, it is advisable for all subjects to be characterized in the same manner. Recommendations for patient evaluation or presentation are summarized in Table 5.

Treatment

Once a diagnosis of CTCL has been established, the physician must discover whether the disease is confined to the skin, has extended to visceral tissue, has an associated overt leukemic component, or has entered a phase of rapid cellular proliferation. Identification of the extent and nature of the lymphoma will then allow appropriate selection of therapy. Presence of peripheral lymph node infiltration and blood involvement correlate well with presence of extracutaneous spread [22], indicating that sampling of these tissues may ob-

viate the requirement for other surgical staging procedures.

For CTCL clinically limited to the skin, both electron-beam and topical chemotherapy can be efficacious. Photochemotherapy combining 8-methoxypsoralen and ultraviolet-A (PUVA) also appears to be a valuable modality in such clinical situations.

The malignant cells of CTCL, like their normal counterparts, are extremely radiosensitive [82]. The primary problem with x-irradiation in CTCL is toxicity to normal lymphocytes rather than resistance of the malignant cell population. For example, total-body x-irradiation when delivered in fractionated doses of 30 to 50 rads/week for the treatment of lymphoma results in severe lympho-penia after cumulative radiation of only 100 to 150 rads [83]. The efficacy of x-irradiation must, therefore, be balanced against the side effects.

Orthovoltage x-irradiation has regularly been demonstrated to be palliative [84]. Small-field or "spot" orthovoltage radiotherapy using soft x-rays (60 to 100 kV with half-value layers with 1 to 1.5 mm of Al) fractionated to doses of 75 to 500 rads and total doses of 800 to 1500 rads generally can eliminate individual plaques or tumors. "Total-skin x-ray bath" tested by Sommerville [85] at fractionated doses of 10 rads per day to cumulative doses of 200 to 900 rads was effective but resulted in severe complications such as agranulocytosis, severe radiation dermatitis, and death. More recently, Le Bourgeois et al. [86] suggested use of total body-surface orthovoltage x-ray delivered by a fixed 55-kV generator to a moving couch, allowing high radiation doses distributed homogeneously over the skin surface with low penetration to deeper tissues. This complicated technique has yielded encouraging short-term responses with only limited complications in the first 25 treated patients.

Attention has been directed to electron-beam radiotherapy of CTCL largely because of both the clinical response to and the toxicity from total-skin x-ray bath. Since 2.5-meV electrons have a limited penetration and deposit all energy in superficial tissues, with the depth of penetration dependent on the energy, the total body surface can be efficiently irradiated without exposing deep tissues [87]. A 4-meV electron beam has been recommended by the Stanford University group, since the 50 percent depth dose of that energy is 11.4 mm and the 5 percent depth dose is limited to less than 20 mm [88]. This energy is therefore sufficient to adequately treat most lymphomas localized to the epidermis and dermis while avoid-

Table 4   Staging of cutaneous T-cell lymphoma

Classification	Description
T: Skin	
T_0	Clinically and/or histopathologically suggestive lesions
T_1	Limited plaques, papules, or eczematous patches covering $< 10\%$ of the skin surface
T_2	Generalized plaques, papules, or erythematous patches covering $\geq 10\%$ of the skin surface
T_3	Tumors (≥ 1)
T_4	Generalized erythroderma
N: Lymph nodes	
N_0	No palpable adenopathy, lymph node pathology negative for CTCL
N_1	Palpable adenopathy, lymph node pathology negative for CTCL
N_2	No palpable adenopathy, lymph node pathology positive for CTCL
N_3	Palpable adenopathy, lymph node pathology positive for CTCL
B: Peripheral blood	
B_0	Atypical circulating cells not present ($< 5\%$)
B_1	Atypical circulating cells present ($> 5\%$); record total WBC and total lymphocyte counts and number of atypical cells/100 lymphocytes
M: Visceral organs	
M_0	No visceral organ involvement
M_1	Visceral involvement (must have pathology confirmation and organ involved should be specified)

ing deeper tissues. A total dose of 4500 rads delivered in fractions of 200 rads over a period of 8 to 9 weeks is well tolerated by most patients [89], but larger individual doses can be associated with severe chronic radiation dermatitis.

Nearly all patients receiving total-body electron-beam therapy experience severe dryness of the skin and variable scaling. A minority of patients will also experience erythema, desquamation, or frank bullae. These acute sequelae usually resolve following cessation of therapy, and their resolution generally can be accelerated by a short course of systemic corticosteroids. Sweat gland impairment leading to transient anhidrosis and associated temporary skin dryness usually resolves with the recovery of eccrine function in 6 to 9 months [90].

Table 5   Patient evaluation

I. Diagnosis
  A. Complete history and physical examination, including whole body mapping of skin lesions
  B. CBC with determination of absolute lymphocyte counts and percentage of atypical convoluted lymphocytes
  C. Serum chemistries, including liver and renal function tests, uric acid, lactic dehydrogenase isoenzymes, quantitative immunoglobulins
  D. Multiple skin biopsies (routine paraffin-embedded and 1-mm Epon-embedded sections reviewed by light microscopy)

II. Extent of disease
  A. Lymph node biopsy, studies as in Ic and cytogenetically (karyotyping)
  B. Further evaluation of specific organ systems when involvement is suggested by history or examination
  C. In vivo and in vitro response to microbial antigens, to estimate level of T-cell competence

Epilation is to be expected following the course of treatment, but unless hair follicles have been destroyed by the cutaneous lymphoma, hair regenerates in 4 to 6 months. Following a single course of electron-beam therapy that has been appropriately fractionated, chronic radiodermatitis is rare, although repeated courses of electron-beam therapy, inadequate fractionation of dose, or superimposition on prior orthovoltage radiation or extensive topical chemotherapy can produce such changes [91]. Squamous carcinomas of the skin infrequently occur in radiated sites [92].

Encouraging results with electron-beam therapy have been obtained by Fuks et al. [93], who were able to induce cutaneous remission in 94 percent of individuals receiving 3000 to 3600 rads. Long-term remissions occurred in approximately half of those patients with limited skin disease and in a quarter of those with generalized plaques, but not in any individuals with skin tumors. Lymphadenopathy, even in the absence of overt histologic evidence of infiltration by malignant cells, indicated a poor prognosis, with more than 33 percent of those individuals developing extracutaneous lymphoma during the follow-up period. Nisce and Safai [94] obtained similar results. Spittle [95] found lower doses (1600 to 2600 rads) of electron-beam radiotherapy to be less efficacious.

Vonderheid et al. [96] have achieved similar results in their extensive experience with topical nitrogen mustard (mechlorethamine hydrochloride). Their 5-year survival rates with topical nitrogen mustard for limited plaque, generalized plaque, tumor stage, and generalized erythema were 85, 75, 42, and 50 percent, respectively.

These results closely resemble those of electron-beam therapy (88, 60, 11, and 54 percent, respectively), revealing that the approaches are of approximately equal benefit at comparable stages of disease. However, the topical nitrogen mustard therapy has the comparative disadvantages of being a topical allergen in many patients with limited CTCL and requiring continuation of application for indefinite periods of time.

Nevertheless, the observations of Vonderheid et al. [97] that 90 percent of 67 patients with limited disease (no tumors, lymphadenopathy, or clinically apparent visceral involvement) were placed in remission by topical nitrogen mustard therapy and that 67 percent were maintained at a disease-free state for the short follow-up period are encouraging. It is difficult to determine whether induction of delayed hypersensitivity to this agent improves clinical response, since hyporesponsiveness to topical allergens is, by itself, an indicator of advanced disease. Because Vonderheid et al. continue to apply nitrogen mustard to the entire skin surface even following achievement of complete remission, clear evidence of cure with this regimen is not available.

Since the nitrosourea BCNU does not cross-react with nitrogen mustard, it can be topically applied to patients allergic to mechlorethamine. Zackheim et al. [98] used topical BCNU to treat 40 patients with CTCL. Each of three patients with minimally infiltrated plaques and 16 of 21 patients with moderately infiltrated plaques cleared with this approach, although long-term benefit is not fully established. The observed side effects included contact hypersensitivity (10 percent), posttreatment telangiectasia (35 percent), severe erythema (33 percent), and mild bone marrow depression (30 percent). BCNU, therefore, may be an appropriate alternative to topical nitrogen mustard in the treatment of patients with CTCL limited to the skin.

Gilchrest [99] reported that PUVA treatment can produce a definite clinical response in CTCL. Of 11 patients, 7 completely cleared and 3 others showed marked improvement. Four patients remained clear of recurrent disease for more than 3 years while receiving maintenance therapy. In contrast, all six individuals whose PUVA therapy was discontinued developed recurrent progressive CTCL. Results from the clinical trial of Roenigk [100] also suggest that maintenance therapy may be required. In that study, remission persisted in 10 of 12 patients receiving continuous PUVA therapy. Eight patients with parapsoriasis en plaques and 35 patients with overt CTCL also cleared

while receiving PUVA therapy, but the postremission follow-up was for shorter periods in these two groups.

Treatment of CTCL with overt visceral involvement has been less successful. Palliation has been obtained with single-agent chemotherapy [101], but improved longevity has not been noted [17]. Although several prospective clinical trials with combinations of different chemotherapeutic agents are currently being performed at several medical centers, substantiated evidence of long-term remissions following cessation of therapy has not yet been achieved in significant numbers of patients. A combination of cyclophosphamide, vincristine, prednisone, and bleomycin produced a median duration of remission of 47 weeks in those patients who had achieved an initial complete remission in the study of the Southwest Oncology Group [102], but only 29 percent of the patients achieved such a complete remission. The median survival of all groups with extracutaneous disease in that study was 95 weeks or less. Promising short-term results have been obtained by Griem et al. [103], who combined whole-body electron-beam therapy with combination chemotherapy in patients, yielding better results than either the electron-beam or chemotherapy alone in advanced disease. Bunn et al. [104] combined a rotating course of multidrug therapy with electron-beam radiotherapy and achieved several apparent complete remissions of varying duration in 8 of 24 patients with palpable lymphadenopathy and/or visceral involvement. Similar short-term results were achieved by the Columbia University group using the Price-Hill chemotherapeutic regimen [105], with significant beneficial response induced in all seven treated patients and temporary remission in four. In short, various combinations of chemotherapeutic agents are capable of inducing substantial but variable clinical response in most patients with histologically apparent extracutaneous CTCL. However, no single regimen has been shown to be curative of advanced disease.

Two experimental modalities merit brief mention. First, leukopheresis can produce a clinically relevant tumor mass reduction in selected patients experiencing the leukemic phase of CTCL [105]. Marked palliation and maintenance for up to 3 years were accomplished in clinical situations distinguished by limited bone marrow involvement, marked lymphocytosis (more than 30,000/mm^3), and low rates of leukemic cell renewal [106]. Second, intravenously administered heterologous antithymocyte globulin, produced by immunizing horses with normal human thymocytes, induced marked clinical responses in three of four patients with advanced CTCL [107]. More specific and potent monclonal anti-T-cell antibodies are now available, and it is possible that this form of therapy may become an important part of combination chemotherapeutic regimens. It is important to emphasize that even though current therapies for extracutaneous disease do not appear to be curative in significant numbers of patients, palliation of this disfiguring and debilitating disorder is in itself meritorious.

Conclusion

Application of the relatively new discipline of cellular immunology to the study of lymphomas has permitted recognition of the entity *cutaneous T-cell lymphoma* and unification of an artificially splintered group of disorders. Substantial progress has been made toward an understanding of the natural evolution of the process, and it now appears that the cumulative incidence of CTCL approximates that of Hodgkin's disease. Correlations between clinical and immunologic findings have been established, and improved chemotherapeutic regimens have been devised for extracutaneous involvement. Production of monoclonal antibodies with increased specificity for the malignant T cells should facilitate in situ diagnosis of CTCL and earlier initiation of potentially curative therapy.

CTCL appears to be a neoplastic amplification of a normal population of helper T cells with an affinity for the skin. Identification of the mechanisms that underly the normal T cell–epidermis interaction, determination of the tissues of origin of the neoplastic T cells, and recognition of tumor-specific membrane antigens represent the most important challenges for the near future. The new techniques of in vitro growth of differentiating human epidermis and the production of monoclonal antibodies for the first time permit rational optimism about the opportunity of solving these mysteries. It seems likely that the actual basis of CTCL will be fully uncovered only when the underlying nature of the normal T cell–epidermis interaction is fully elucidated.

References

1. Edelson RL et al: Preferential cutaneous infiltration by neoplastic thymus-derived lymphocytes. *Ann Intern Med* **80**:685–692, 1974

2. Sézary A, Bouvrain Y: Erythrodermie avec présence de cellules monstrueuses dans le derme et le sang circulant. *Bull Soc Fr Dermatol Syphiligr* **45**:254–260, 1938

3. Edelson RL: Cutaneous T cell lymphoma: mycosis fungoides, Sézary syndrome, and other variants. *J Am Acad Dermatol* **2**:89–106, 1980

4. Edelson RL: Cutaneous T-cell lymphomas. *Perspect Ann Intern Med* **83**:548–552, 1975

5. Lamberg SI, Bunn PA Jr (Eds): Proceedings of the workshop on cutaneous T cell lymphomas (mycosis fungoides and Sézary syndrome). *Cancer Treat Rep* **63**:561–736, 1979

6. Alibert JL: *Descriptions des Maladies de la Peau; Observées à l'Hôpital St. Louis et Exposition des Meilleures Méthodes Suivies pour leur Traitement.* Barrois l'Aine et Fils, Paris, 1806, p 157

7. Bazin E: *Lecons sur le Traitement des Maladies Chroniques en Général Affections de la Peau en Particulier par l'Emploi Comparé des Eaux Minérales de l'Hydrothérapie et des Moyens Pharmaceutiques.* Adrien Delahaye, Paris, 1870, p 425

8. Vidal E, Brocq L: Etude sur le mycosis fungoide. *France Medical* **2**:946, 969, 993, 1005, 1019, 1885

9. Besnier E, Hallopeau H: On the erythrodermia of mycosis fungoides. *J Cutan Genito Urin Dis* **10**:453, 1892

10. Taswell HF, Winkelmann RK: Sézary syndrome—a malignant reticulemic erythroderma. *JAMA* **177**:465–472, 1961

11. Lutzner MA, Jordan HW: The ultrastructure of an abnormal cell in Sézary's syndrome. *Blood* **31**:719–726, 1968

12. Clendenning WE et al: Mycosis fungoides. Relationship to malignant cutaneous reticulosis and the Sézary syndrome. *Arch Dermatol* **89**:785–792, 1964

13. Crossen PE et al: The Sézary syndrome. Cytogenetic studies and identification of the Sézary cell as an abnormal lymphocyte. *Am J Med* **50**:25–34, 1971

14. Lutzner MA et al: Cytogenetic, cytophotometric, and ultrastructural study of large cerebriform cells of the Sézary syndrome and description of a small-cell variant. *J Natl Cancer Inst* **50**:1145–1162, 1973

15. Broome JD et al: Leukemic cells with membrane properties of thymus-derived (T) lymphocytes in a case of Sézary's syndrome: morphologic and immunologic studies. *Clin Immunol Immunopathol* **1**:319–329, 1973

16. Brouet J-C et al: Indications of the thymus-derived nature of the proliferating cells in six patients with Sézary's syndrome. *N Engl J Med* **289**:341–344, 1973

17. Epstein EH Jr et al: Mycosis fungoides. Survival, prognostic features, response to therapy, and autopsy findings. *Medicine (Baltimore)* **51**:61–72, 1972

18. Rappaport H, Thomas LB: Mycosis fungoides: the pathology of extracutaneous involvement. *Cancer* **34**:1198–1229, 1974

19. Long JC, Mihm MC: Mycosis fungoides with extracutaneous dissemination: a distinct clinicopathologic entity. *Cancer* **34**:1745–1755, 1974

20. Kung PC et al: Cutaneous T cell lymphoma: characterization by monoclonal antibodies. *Blood* **57**:261–266, 1981

21. Lamberg SI et al: Mycosis fungoides cooperative study. *Arch Dermatol* **111**:457–459, 1975

22. Bunn PA et al: Prospective staging evaluation of patients with cutaneous T cell lymphomas. *Ann Intern Med* **93**:223–230, 1980

23. Cyr DP et al: Mycosis fungoides. Hematologic findings and terminal course. *Arch Dermatol* **94**:558–573, 1966

24. Block JG et al: Mycosis fungoides. Natural history and

aspects of its relationship to other malignant lymphomas. *Am J Med* **34:**228–235, 1963

25. Fuks ZY et al: Prognostic signs and the management of the mycosis fungoides. *Cancer* **32:**1385–1395, 1973

26. Farber EM et al: The natural history of mycosis fungoides. *Calif Med* **87:**225–230, 1957

27. Cawley EP et al: Is mycosis fungoides a reticuloendothelial neoplastic entity? *Arch Dermatol Syphilol* **64:**255–272, 1951

28. Berman L: Pathologic nature of mycosis fungoides. *Arch Pathol* **29:**530–540, 1940

29. Heite JH, Socha P: Häufigkeitsanalytische untersuchungen zur Symptomologies der Mycosis fungoides. *Arch Dermatol (Berlin)* **193:**118–142, 1951

30. Gall EA: Enigmas in lymphoma: reticulum cell sarcoma and mycosis fungoides. *Minn Med* **38:**674–681, 1955

31. Allen AC: Mycosis fungoides in the skin, in *The Skin— A Clinicopathological Treatise*. Mosby, St Louis, 1954, pp 1010–1019

32. Bluefarb SM, Steinberg HS: Pulmonary manifestations of mycosis fungoides. *Ann Intern Med* **36:**625–639, 1952

33. Reinhard EH et al: Mycosis fungoides with pulmonary and neurologic complications. *Am J Med* **42:**128–138, 1967

34. Marglin SI et al: Mycosis fungoides. Radiographic manifestations of extracutaneous intrathoracic involvement. *Radiology* **130:**35–37, 1979

35. Israel RH: Mycosis fungoides with rapidly progressive pulmonary infiltration. *Radiology* **125:**10, 1977

36. Pariser DM: Mycosis fungoides involving the brain and optic nerves. *Arch Dermatol* **114:**397–399, 1978

37. Keltner JL et al: Mycosis fungoides. Intraocular and central nervous system involvement. *Arch Ophthalmol* **95:**645–650, 1977

38. Foerster HC: Mycosis fungoides with intraocular involvement. *Trans Am Acad Ophthalmol Otolaryngol* **64:**308–313, 1960

39. Kitchen CK: Mycosis fungoides keratitis. *Am J Ophthalmol* **55:**758–761, 1963

40. Wolter JR et al: Corneal involvement in mycosis fungoides. *Am J Ophthalmol* **55:**317–322, 1963

41. Poulsen A: On mycosis fungoides. *Acta Derm Venereol (Stockh)* **21:**365–400, 1940

42. Greer KE et al: Multiple osteolytic lesions in a patient with mycosis fungoides. *Arch Dermatol* **113:**1242–1244, 1977

43. O'Reilly GV et al: Skeletal involvement in mycosis fungoides. *Am J Roentgenol* **129:**741–743, 1977

44. Moschella SL et al: Case 52–1971. *N Engl J Med* **285:**1526–1532, 1971

45. Gottlieb M et al: Arthritis in a patient with mycosis fungoides. Complete remission after radiotherapy. *Arthritis Rheum* **22:**424–425, 1979

46. Laskaris GC et al: Mycosis fungoides with oral manifestations. *Oral Surg* **46:**40–42, 1978

47. Hood AF et al: Laryngeal mycosis fungoides. *Cancer* **43:**1527–1532, 1979

48. Calhoun NR, Johnson CC: Oral manifestation of mycosis fungoides. *Oral Surg, Oral Med, Oral Pathol* **22:**261–264, 1966

49. Cohn AM et al: Mycosis fungoides with involvement of the oral cavity. *Arch Otolaryngol* **93:**330–333, 1971

50. Gerstenbrand F et al: Cerebrale Beteilung bei Sézary Syndrom. *J Neurol* **212:**55–64, 1976

51. Weber MB, McGavran MH: Mycosis fungoides involving the brain. *Arch Neurol* **16:**645–650, 1967

52. Lundberg WB et al: Leptomeningeal mycosis fungoides. *Cancer* **38:**2149–2153, 1976

53. Hauch TW et al: Meningeal mycosis fungoides: clinical and cellular characteristics. *Ann Intern Med* **82:**499–505, 1975

54. Gold JH et al: Meningeal mycosis fungoides: cytologic and ultrastructural aspects. *Acta Cytol (Baltimore)* **20:**349–355, 1976

55. Peress NS et al: Combined myelopathy and radiculoneuropathy with malignant lymphoproliferative disease. *Arch Neurol* **36:**311–313, 1979

56. Bargman H, Coupe RL: Sézary's syndrome. Report of a case showing peripheral neuropathy and bone marrow fibrosis. *Arch Dermatol* **114:**1360–1362, 1978

57. Azzarelli B, Roessmann U: A morphologic study of intracerebral hemorrhage in a case of acute leukemia. *Arch Pathol Lab Med* **102:**43–45, 1978

58. Caldwell I, Dyan AD: Mycosis fungoides and progressive multifocal leukoencephalopathy. *Br J Dermatol* **82:**176–181, 1970

59. Cohen MI et al: Gastrointestinal involvement in the Sézary syndrome. *Gastroenterology* **73:**145–149, 1977

60. Vernon SE, Rosenthal DL: Sézary cells in ascitic fluid. *Acta Cytol (Baltimore)* **23:**408–411, 1979

61. Edgcomb J et al: Mycosis fungoides, in The First International Conference on the Biology of Cutaneous Cancer, April 6–11, 1962, Philadelphia. Edited by F Urbach. *Natl Cancer Inst Monogr* **10:**275–280, 1963

62. Roberts WC et al: Heart in malignant lymphoma (Hodgkin's disease, lymphosarcoma, reticulum cell sarcoma and mycosis fungoides). A study of 196 autopsy cases. *Am J Cardiol* **22:**85–107, 1968

63. Broder S et al: The Sézary syndrome. A malignant proliferation of helper T cells. *J Clin Invest* **58:**1297–1306, 1976

64. Kövary PM et al: Paraproteinaemia in Sézary syndrome. *Dermatologica* **154:**138–146, 1977

65. Joyner MV et al: Cutaneous T-cell lymphoma in association with a monoclonal gammopathy. *Arch Dermatol* **115:**326–328, 1979

66. Shevach EM et al: Receptors for complement and immunoglobulin on human animal lymphoid cells. *Transplant Rev* **16:**3–41, 1973

67. Broder S et al: The Sézary syndrome. A malignant proliferation of helper T cells. *J Clin Invest* **58:**1297–1306, 1976

68. Berger CL et al: Cutaneous T cell lymphoma: neoplasm of T cells with helper activity. *Blood* **53:**642–651, 1979

69. Edelson RL et al: Antithymocyte globulin in the management of cutaneous T cell lymphoma. *Cancer Treat Rep* **63:**675–680, 1979

70. Yoshida T et al: Migration inhibitory in serum and cell supernatants in patients with Sézary syndrome. *J Immunol* **114:**914–918, 1975

71. Blaylock WK et al: Normal immunologic reactivity in patients with the lymphoma mycosis fungoides. *Cancer* **19:**223–236, 1966

72. Edelson RL et al: Karyotype studies of cutaneous T cell lymphoma: evidence for clonal origin. *J Invest Dermatol* **73:**548–550, 1979

73. Berger CL et al: Production of monoclonal antibodies reactive with the neoplastic lymphocytes of cutaneous T cell lymphoma. *Clin Res* **29:**558A, 1981

74. Hoppe RT et al: Radiation therapy in the management of cutaneous T-cell lymphomas. *Cancer Treat Rep* **63:**625–632, 1979

75. Vonderheid EC et al: Topical chemotherapy and immunotherapy of mycosis fungoides. *Arch Dermatol* **113:**454–462, 1977

76. Samman PD: Chronic superficial dermatitis and poikiloderma. *Bull Cancer (Paris)* **64:**177–186, 1977

77. Van Vloten WA et al: Cytophotometric studies on mycosis fungoides and other cutaneous reticuloses. *Bull Cancer (Paris)* **64:**249–258, 1977

78. Lutzner MA et al: Ultrastructure of abnormal cells in Sézary syndrome, mycosis fungoides, and parapsoriasis en plaques. *Arch Dermatol* **103:**375–386, 1971

79. Yeckley JA et al: Production of Sézary-like cells from normal lymphocytes. *Arch Dermatol* **111:**29–32, 1975

80. Schneiderman P et al: Lymphomatoid papulosis: immunologic and ultrastructural studies. *Clin Res* **23:**455A, 1975

81. Chu A et al: Dermal Langerhans cells in cutaneous lymphoma: an *in situ* study using monoclonal antibodies. *Clin Res* **29:**590A, 1981

82. Trowel OA: The sensitivity of lymphocytes to ionizing irradiation. *J Pathol Bacteriol* **64:**687–704, 1952

83. Qasim MM: Blood and bone marrow response following total body irradiation in patients with lymphosarcomas. *Eur J Cancer* **13:**483–487, 1977

84. Levin OL, Behrman HT: Roentgen ray therapy of mycosis fungoides. *Arch Dermatol Syphilol* **21:**307, 1945

85. Sommerville J: Mycosis fungoides treated with general x-ray bath. *Br J Dermatol* **51:**323–324, 1939

86. Le Bourgeois J-P et al: Whole cutaneous irradiation in mycosis fungoides with 55 Kv x-rays. *Bull Cancer (Paris)* **64:**322, 1977

87. Trump JG et al: High energy electrons for the treatment of extensive superficial malignant lesions. *Am J Roentgenol* **69:**623–629, 1963

88. Hoppe RT et al: Radiation therapy in the management of cutaneous T-cell lymphomas. *Cancer Treat Rep* **63:**625–632, 1979

89. Hoppe RT et al: The rationale for curative therapy in mycosis fungoides. *Int J Radiat Oncol Biol Phys* **2:**843–851, 1977

90. Price NM: Cited in Ref 88

91. Price NM: Radiation dermatitis following electron beam therapy. An evaluation of patients ten years after total skin irradiation for mycosis fungoides. *Arch Dermatol* **114:**63–66, 1978

92. Grollman JH et al: Total skin electron beam therapy of lymphoma cutis and generalized psoriasis—clinical experience and adverse reactions. *Radiology* **87:**908–915, 1966

93. Fuks Z et al: The role of total skin irradiation with electrons in the management of mycosis fungoides. *Bull Cancer (Paris)* **64:**291–304, 1977

94. Nisce LZ, Safai B: Once weekly total-skin electron-beam therapy for mycosis fungoides: 7 years' experience. *Cancer Treat Rep* **63:**633–638, 1979

95. Spittle MF: Electron-beam therapy in England. *Cancer Treat Rep* **63:**639–641, 1979

96. Vonderheid EC et al: A 10-year experience with topical mechlorethamine for mycosis fungoides: comparison with patients treated by total-skin electron-beam therapy. *Cancer Treat Rep* **63:**681–689, 1979

97. Vonderheid EC et al: Topical chemotherapy and immunotherapy of mycosis fungoides. *Arch Dermatol* **113:**454–462, 1977

98. Zackheim HS et al: Treatment of mycosis fungoides with topical BCNU. *Cancer Treat Rep* **63:**623, 1979

99. Gilchrest BA: Methoxsalen photochemotherapy for mycosis fungoides. *Cancer Treat Rep* **63:**663–667, 1979

100. Roenigk HH Jr: Photochemotherapy for mycosis fungoides: long-term followup study. *Cancer Treat Rep* **63:**669–673, 1979

101. Moschella SL: The present status of chemotherapy in dermatology. *Med Clin North Am* **56:**725–745, 1972

102. Grozea PN et al: Combination chemotherapy for mycosis fungoides: a Southwest Oncology Group study. *Cancer Treat Rep* **63:**647–653, 1979

103. Griem ML et al: Combined therapy for patients with mycosis fungoides. *Cancer Treat Rep* **63:**655–657, 1979

104. Bunn PA Jr et al: Combined modality therapy with electron-beam irradiation and systemic chemotherapy for cutaneous T-cell lymphomas. *Cancer Treat Rep* **63:**713–717, 1979

105. Edelson RL et al: Successful management of the Sézary syndrome: mobilization and removal of extravascular neoplastic T cells by leukopheresis. *N Engl J Med* **291:**293–294, 1974

106. Edelson RL: Efficacy of leukopheresis procedures in the management of cutaneous T cell lymphoma-leukemic phase. *Proceedings of the Fourth Advanced Blood Components Seminar* **4:**1–7, 1977

107. Edelson RL et al: Antithymocyte globulin in the management of cutaneous T cell lymphoma. *Cancer Treat Rep* **63:**675–680, 1979

EPIDERMAL DIFFERENTIATION AND KERATINIZATION

Irwin M. Freedberg

Many of the major breakthroughs in scientific inquiry have been made by those who believe Robert Herrick's seventeenth century dictum—"Nothing's so hard but search will find it out."—but a phrase from Shakespeare—"There is a time for all things."—makes the statement much more applicable. There are no limits to the search as long as it is carried out at the appropriate time. As is apparent from much of the material presented in this volume, questions can and should be posed when techniques have been developed that are adequate for their resolution. At some time in the future, the history of our knowledge in the areas of keratinization and epidermal differentiation will be written, and it seems certain that our immediate past, the present, and the short-term future will be recorded as years in which major breakthroughs in our knowledge of these areas were made. The reasons for this are not that new questions have been formulated, but that the techniques to obtain answers to many long-standing problems have become available. These techniques include our abilities to propagate epidermal cells in vitro from a variety of sources, to prepare extremely specific antibodies to a number of surface and intracellular epidermal constituents, and to dissect the pathways of cellular metabolism in epidermal as well as all other cells.

Supported in part by grants from the National Institute of Arthritis, Metabolic, Digestive and Kidney Diseases (AM-21358) and Estee Lauder Inc.

In this chapter we shall summarize the new information that has arisen from studies in this area and relate the results to problems of clinical cutaneous disease in humans. The data themselves have arisen from work in multiple laboratories throughout the world, and the investigators have been biochemists, cell biologists, electron microscopists, immunologists, as well as clinicians with a focused interest in the skin.

Epidermal Cell Culture

It has been known since the beginning of the twentieth century that human skin may be kept alive in vitro for relatively prolonged periods and that this tissue will grow following reimplantation on a donor site. The techniques used for such experiments 80 years ago were similar to the procedures used at the present time for studies of explanted epidermis, although there have been improvements in media, culture dishes, and incubators. Major progress has been made since a reproducible technique for the culture of dispersed mammalian keratinizing epithelial cells was described several years ago by Rheinwald and Green [1]; however, the older explant procedures remain important and useful.

Starting with relatively small pieces of skin (several square millimeters), a medium which contains a buffered salt solution, appropriate antibiotics, fetal calf serum, and the growth factors discussed below, large numbers of cells may be obtained within a period of 1 to several weeks. The procedures that are most applicable to such studies have been reviewed recently by the workers in Slaga's laboratory at Oak Ridge [2]. Tissue from newborns (foreskin) or adults (punch or excision biopsy) may be used; within a few days following placement on a culture dish, outgrowth of epithelial cells occurs. Although the original tissue consists of epidermis and a thin layer of dermis, dermal outgrowth is inhibited in early cultures by the process of epiboly in which the epithelial cells grow down the side of the tissue sample and onto the surface of the culture dish. The connective tissue is essentially sealed in by this phenomenon. If the tissue is placed in the culture dish in such a way that attachment of the connective tissue layer to the surface is not adequate, epiboly may result in the epithelium growing around the entire tissue block rather than out onto the dish. However, fibroblast outgrowth eventually becomes a problem in almost all long-term, explant cultures.

Once the epidermal outgrowth begins in early explants, stratification occurs and the epidermis matures by a process similar to that which takes place in vivo. Cell division is found in the lowest layers and the more superficial cells show evidence of membrane thickening and loss of intracellular organelles (nuclei, ribosomes, mitochondria) characteristic of normal differentiation. The original sample can be cut out of the center of the explant and the outgrowth will continue to migrate, divide, and stratify until it fills the culture dish. Until very recently, one of the major disadvantages to the explant technique has been that the cells from such epidermal cultures could not be passaged. As soon as the epithelial sheets were dispersed, removed from the original culture vessel, and placed in a new in vitro environment, growth stopped.

Much recent effort has been expended to define the conditions that effect the growth of these explants so that they can be used to study the effects of genes, disease, pharmacologic agents, and environmental factors such as carcinogens upon epidermal growth and differentiation. It has been found that fetal calf serum at a concentration of approximately 10% is required for optimal growth and that hydrocortisone and epidermal growth factor (EGF) enhance outgrowth while insulin over a broad concentration range inhibits the cultures. Human epidermal outgrowth is maximum at 37°C, although mouse epidermis grows best at an incubation temperature of 31°C. The oxygen tension, pH, and age of donor (tissue from young donors grows better than that from older subjects) have also been found to be important variables [2]. Price and his coworkers [3] have described a new medium containing horse serum (10%) in which human epidermal outgrowth is enhanced. Although EGF and hydrocortisone have no effect in the horse serum–containing medium, the authors report the successful subculture of human epidermal cells without feeder cells to the sixth culture generation.

As we have already noted, a change in the field of epidermal cell culture occurred in 1975 when Rheinwald and Green described the successful serial subculture of epithelial cells derived from a mouse teratoma [1] and from human newborn foreskin [4]. Although dissociated mouse epidermal cells inoculated at extremely high density had been shown to multiply and differentiate for limited periods of time [5], long-term experiments had not been possible previously. The new technique required the addition of lethally irradiated 3T3 fibroblasts as a feeder layer, and the procedure has subsequently been applied with minor modifications equally successfully to other epithelia [6,7]. The initial plating efficiency was low (0.1 to 1.0 percent), but on subsequent transfers it rose to 1.5 percent. The cells could be propagated for 20 to 50 generations but a finite limit remained and permanent cell lines were not obtained. Rheinwald and Green found, in agreement with older explant studies, that growth was better and culture lifetime longer when tissue was obtained from newborns as compared to older donors. The 3T3 cells, whose multiplication could be stopped with mitomycin C as effectively as with x-ray exposure [6], are required since they condition the medium and inhibit the outgrowth of human fibroblasts that contaminate the original sample. Without 3T3 cells, the human fibroblasts rapidly overgrow the culture dish.

Within several days of culture the centers of the inocula begin to become stratified into a structure that resembles epidermis. Cell division occurs in the motile cells of the basal layer and the cells in the more superficial layers become larger in size, accumulate protein, and form the cornified envelope characteristic of terminal epidermal differentiation [8]. Differentiation is not identical to that in vivo, however, for the cells of the superficial layers in the cultures retain their nuclei and, as will be discussed more completely subsequently, the keratin polypeptides characteristic of normal stratum corneum are not synthesized. Terminal differentiation of epidermal cells grown in this way can be initiated by suspending the cells in a semisolid methylcellulose medium rather than in the usual liquid environment [8].

A number of the variables involved in such epidermal cultures have been studied by Rheinwald, Green, and their associates [9] as well as by others [10,11]. The technique can yield over 100 million epidermal cells from a single foreskin in 2 weeks so adequate tissue may be obtained for a number of biochemical, immunologic, and, as will be discussed subsequently, clinical purposes. The cells may be removed from the culture dishes and stored in liquid nitrogen with very good subsequent recovery of colony-forming capacity. Hydrocortisone is required if the keratinocyte colonies are to develop normal morphology early in their growth, and EGF increases the colony-forming ability of the cells. In the presence of EGF, keratinocytes from newborns will survive up to 150 generations [12]. If the keratinocytes are cultured in a vessel which had previously supported a confluent 3T3 monolayer, they will grow without 3T3 cells if fibroblast-conditioned medium and hydrocortisone

are used. Colony-forming ability is significantly decreased, however, and the requirements for hydrocortisone and conditioned medium are absolute. EGF in nanogram quantities has also been found to increase the rate of proliferation and effect the differentiation of epithelial cells from other species as well [13].

Yuspa, Hennings, and their associates have published a series of studies [11,14,15] in which they have emphasized the importance of the calcium concentration on the growth and differentiation of epidermal cells. If the cells are grown in a low-calcium medium, (0.05 to 0.1 mM), they continue to proliferate and synthesize protein, but they do not stratify, differentiate, or form desmosomes. When the calcium concentration is elevated (1.2 mM), desmosomes form within 2 hr, DNA synthesis begins to decrease within less than 12 hr, the cells stratify in several days, and terminal differentiation begins. The biochemical mechanism by which this calcium switch occurs has not yet been clarified but it probably involves a posttranslation modification of a previously synthesized macromolecule (see below). Cells that have undergone malignant transformation are not subject to the same controls [16].

Recent studies of the epidermal cell culture system have focused upon attempts to eliminate the 3T3 cells so that interpretation of results would not require consideration of fibroblast contamination. Liu, Eaton, and Karasek [17] have used a collagen surface and have shown that keratinocytes from newborn foreskin may be subcultured in this way with high efficiency for three subpassages in the presence of hydrocortisone and EGF. Fibronectin-coated plates [18] support the growth of human keratinocytes even in the absence of serum, and, if the medium composition, pH, temperature, calcium concentration, cell density, and hormonal additions are carefully controlled, prolonged subculture is possible [19–22] in the absence of feeder layers.

These culture techniques with dissociated cells have been used for a number of the studies which we shall discuss subsequently, but one of the most interesting recent biologic applications has come from the work of Doran, Vidrich, and Sun [23], who used tissue from rabbit epidermis, esophagus, and corneal epithelium to determine whether intrinsic or extrinsic influences are involved in epithelial differentiation. All three tissues behaved quite similarly when they were cultured in vitro with 3T3 feeders. When the cells that had propogated were removed from the culture and placed subcutaneously in athymic mice, which did not have the immunocapacity to mount a rejection reaction against the rabbit cells, multiplication occurred and nodules were formed which resembled the tissue of origin. The epidermis formed an orthokeratinized nodule, the esophagus a parakeratinized one, and the corneal epithelium remained nonkeratinized. Since there were no specific dermal influences involved, the conclusion of the studies was that the intrinsic differentiation program of these cell lines was more significant than was extrinsic modulation. If the culture techniques had not been available, these studies would not have been possible even though the significance of the questions approached has been recognized for many decades. A similar conclusion will be evident in the subsequent discussions of differentiation and keratinization. Herrick and Shakespeare considered together are correct.

The Epidermal Cytoskeleton

Keratin—The Structure

Soon after tissues were first examined with the electron microscope, it became apparent that they contained a complex, heterogeneous, intracellular system of filaments. The initial components of this system that were recognized included actin, myosin, and tubulin, whose diameters were calculated to average approximately 60, 150 and 250 Å, respectively. In addition, other intracytoplasmic filaments were noted, and since the diameter of these latter structures was found to be between 70 and 110 Å, they were called intermediate filaments. They are also commonly referred to as 100 Å or 10-nM filaments. Although they were first believed to be breakdown products of either myosin or tubulin, overwhelming evidence has been presented that the structures are unique and heterogeneous. They form a major part of the cytoskeleton of most cells and probably fulfill a variety of functions [24] related to cell shape, spatial organization, and perhaps informational transfer. The

nucleus contains structures that are similar to intermediate filaments [25], but most studies have focused upon those in the cytoplasm. It is known that many intracellular structures including polyribosomes [26], mitochondria, nucleic acids [27], enzymes and mediators such as creatinine phosphokinase [28], and the cyclic nucleotides are attached to the cytoskeleton. Recent evidence indicates that components of the network may be directly synthesized in situ [26].

Based upon their biochemical and antigenic heterogeneity, a number of classes of intermediate filaments in different cell types can be recognized [29]. They are summarized in Table 1.

Antibodies to the several intermediate filaments have been prepared and these may be complexed with appropriate indicators for use in immunofluorescent studies. Figure 1 is an example of the structures that are seen when cultured epidermal cells are stained with such a complex. The keratin filaments form a cytoskeletal array throughout the cytoplasm of the cell running from the membrane, where electron microscopic studies indicate that they insert into the desmosomal complexes, to the deeper portions of the cell, where they appear to form a basketlike structure surrounding the nucleus [30].

In order to determine the relationship between keratin filaments and the other types of intermediate filaments, antibodies prepared to keratin have been used to stain a variety of cultured cells and tissue sections. The results of these studies, which have been undertaken predominantly by Sun, Green, and their colleagues in Boston and Baltimore [31] and by Franke, Weber, Osborn, and their co-workers in Heidelberg [32], indicate that, rather than being limited to epidermis and epidermal appendages, keratin filaments form a major portion of the cytoskeleton of all cells of epithelial origin. The results of such tissue staining are summarized in Table 2 and Fig. 2. When cells from many of these tissues were cultured using procedures similar to those discussed above, a pattern of intermediate filaments equivalent to that displayed in

Table 1   Characteristics of intermediate filaments

Intermediate filament (synonym)	Polypeptide (approximate molecular weight)	Predominant localization
Keratin	42,000–68,000 (multiple)	Epithelial cells
Vimentin (decamin) (Greek — wavy)	52,000	Mesenchymal cells
Desmin (skeletin) (Greek — bond)	50,000	Muscle cells
Glial filaments	50,000	Glial cells
Neurofilaments	200,000, 150,000, 68,000	Neurons

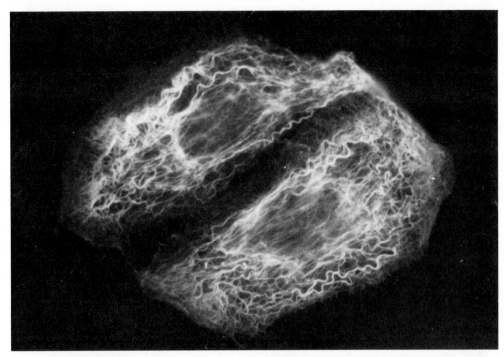

Fig. 1.   Cultured human epidermal cells stained with fluorescent antikeratin antiserum. X ≃ 300. (*Courtesy of T. T. Sun.*)

Fig. 1 was seen. Keratin filaments also were identified in a number of cell lines of epithelial origin including HeLa and Me180 cells, originally derived from humans, and PtK2 cells from rat kangaroo kidney.

When antibodies were raised to the other intermediate filament polypeptides and used to stain many of these same tissues and cell lines, it was found that more than one type of intermediate filament may occur in any given cell. For example, both vimentin and keratin are present in HeLa and PtK2, and when such cells are treated with colcemid, the vimentin component of the cytoskeleton

Table 2   Localization of keratin intermediate filaments

Predominant	Present
Epidermis	Bile ducts
Sweat gland (duct, secretory, and myoepithelial cells)	Pancreatic ducts
	Intestinal mucosa
Hair follicle	Tracheal and bronchial epithelium
Tongue epithelium	Uterine epithelium
Mammary gland epithelium	Oviduct cells (ciliated)
Salivary glands (ducts)	Urinary tract epithelium
Hassall's corpuscle and reticuloepithelial cells of thymus	Renal collecting ducts
Corneal epithelium	
Conjunctival epithelium	
Vaginal epithelium	
Esophageal epithelium	
Anal mucosa	

collapses into a perinuclear whorl, while the keratin structure is unaffected [33]. When cells containing both vimentin and keratin undergo mitosis, the vimentin filaments become involved in formation and orientation of the mitotic spindle. At the same time the keratin components are relatively unchanged, continuing to subserve a cytoskeleton function [34].

Embryologic studies have indicated that the several cell types may be distinguished by staining for intermediate filament components early in development [35]. The keratin filaments actually are recognized before other cytoskeletal components in the trophectoderm cells of the mouse blastocyst [36].

Thus, keratin as a cytoskeletal component is one of the first such structures that develops embryologically and, from a developmental point of view, it is also one of the oldest cytoskeletal components. The epidermis of the lamprey eel, which evolved at least 100 million years ago and has probably not changed significantly since that time, contains keratin intermediate filaments. The problem that remains, however, is that the biologic function of the structural cytokeratin filaments remains unknown save for the general role discussed above. No specific cytokeratin-associated proteins have been identified, and nothing is known of the control of keratin filament organization in the cell. Specific functional data may arise from

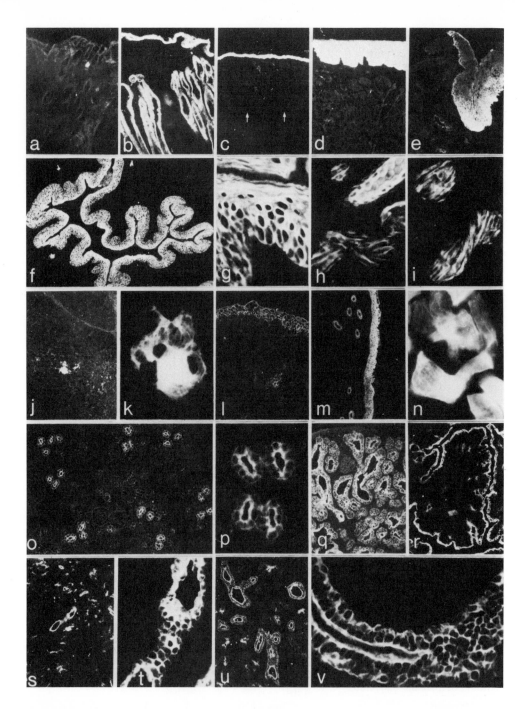

Fig. 2   Immunofluorescent staining of frozen sections of tissues by antiserum to human epidermal keratins. Frozen sections (5 μm) were stained with rabbit antiserum and fluorescein isothiocyanate—conjugated goat antirabbit IgG. Except for the human eccrine sweat glands (h,i) and intestine (n), all tissues are from rabbit. (a) Skin. Preimmune serum control. (b) Skin. Note the staining of epidermis and hair follicles. (c) Cornea. Note staining of epithelium. Arrows mark the endothelial layer. (d) Tongue (inferior surface). (e) Anorectal junction. Rectal epithelium stained much more weakly than anal epithelium. (f) and (g) Esophagus. (h) Eccrine sweat gland. Ductal portion at top right. Several groups of myoepithelial cells of the secretory portion can also be seen. (i) Groups of myoepithelial cells of eccrine sweat gland. (j) Thymus. Note the staining of a Hassall's corpuscle. (k) Hassall's corpuscle of the thymus. (l) Bladder. Note staining of transitional epithelium. (m) Trachea, tangential section. Note staining of the epithelium and ducts of the tracheal glands. (n) Small intestine. Desquamated epithelial cells obtained from human autopsy. Note the fibrous distribution of the stain in some cells. (o) and (p) Kidney. Note the staining of collecting ducts. (q) Cervix. Note staining of endocervical glands. (r) Uterus. Note staining of uterine epithelium. (s) and (t) Pancreas. Note staining of ducts. (u) and (v) Submaxillary gland. Note staining of ducts. Magnification for (n) is X 1080; for (g), (h), (i), (k), (p), (t), and (v), X 430; and for all others, X 70. (From Sun et al [31], with permission.)

biochemical studies similar to those described below or through use of some of the newer morphologic procedures currently being developed to permit three-dimensional analysis of these intracellular components [37,38].

Keratin—The Protein Family

In parallel with the studies we have already described of keratin as a component of the cytoskeleton, a number of investigators have initiated analysis of keratin as a protein molecule, and the new knowledge in this area during the past several years has become equally extensive and important.

Keratin was originally defined on the basis of its solubility characteristics. It was considered to be a protein, insoluble in dilute aqueous buffers, which could be solubilized in the presence of concentrated denaturants (urea or sodium dodecyl sulfate) with or without reducing agents such as mercaptoethanol or dithiothreitol. Although it has been found, subsequently, that keratin is not a single species, these solubility characteristics describe each of the members of the keratin family. The data in Table 1 indicate that there are several keratin polypeptides, which vary in molecular weight between approximately 42,000 and 68,000 daltons. Keratins are actually more complex than any of the other intermediate filament proteins.

The keratin polypeptides may be separated from each other by electrophoretic or chromatographic procedures and they are found to be immunologically distinct although biochemically closely related. The amino acid composition of the polypeptides (high glycine, glutamic acid, serine, aspartic acid; low-sulfur amino acids) is similar, the NH_2-terminal serine and the COOH-terminal glycine are common, and the percentage helix is the same in all [39]. If the denaturing agents used to solubilize the molecules are removed by dialysis, the keratin polypeptide mixtures will repolymerize to form filaments basically identical to those of the original structures. As will be discussed below, such in vitro polymerization will occur only if more than one of the keratin polypeptides is present in the solution. The reason for this is not apparent. X-ray analysis of the original extracted material or of the repolymerized filaments indicates that keratin is a triple-chain, coiled-coil, helical structure.

Although a number of workers have published studies indicating the keratin is composed of more than a single polypeptide [40–43], the major contributions in this area have been made by Baden [44], Steinert [45], and their coworkers during their analyses of the composition of bovine snout and hoof epidermis. These studies indicated that, based upon solubility criteria, there were up to eight keratin polypeptides that could be extracted from the tissues. Four or five of the polypeptides were predominant, but when the two tissues were compared, there were distinct differences between the proteins themselves and their peptide digestion products, although the species of origin was the same. This multiplicity of keratin proteins and their heterogeneity could not be attributed to proteolytic activity or preparative artifacts.

As described above, if the denaturants used to solubilize keratin are removed by dialysis, the subunits will polymerize in vitro to form filaments with the same general structure (as determined by electron microscopy or x-ray analysis) as the original keratin filaments. Steinert and his coworkers [46] have shown that this repolymerization will occur only if more than one subunit is present. The subunit relationship of the three-chain keratin molecule is stoichiometric since the polypeptides are found in either a 1:2 (2 component) or a 1:1:1 (3 component) ratio in the product. As noted previously, the reason for this requirement is not yet apparent.

Similar biochemical heterogeneity of keratin occurs in humans as well as in experimental animals, and there are further differences in the polypeptides of epidermis and hair, which have been described recently [47]. The relative proportions of the polypeptides can be altered by exogenous, environmental influences [48] and there are changes that occur in a programmed manner during growth and development of the epidermis. These developmental changes became apparent when the keratin polypeptides of cells cultured in vitro were analyzed. Sun and Green [49] noted that there were abundant proteins present in cultured human epidermal cells which resembled the keratins of stratum corneum in their insolubility, overall polypeptide composition, capacity to form filaments, and immunologic reactivity. There were differences, however, related to the fact that the keratins synthesized in the culture were not cross-linked by intermolecular disulfide bonds and the largest keratin species (MW~63,000 to 65,000) was not produced by the cultured cells. Fuchs and Green [50] extended the studies by performing amino acid analysis and preparing peptide maps from the keratins of the cultured cells and of normal stratum corneum. They showed that major relationships exist among the several members of the family and they raised the possibility that there was a repeating subunit among all the keratins. This possibility has since been extended to many of the other intermediate filament proteins as well, although the subunit has not yet been isolated.

Two types of immunologic analysis have been undertaken to further define the developmental pathways and heterogeneity of keratin polypeptides in human epidermis. In the first type, the keratins have been isolated, separated, and used to prepare antibodies by either classical procedures [51] or by the recently developed hybridoma technique [52]. The second procedure depends upon the use of autoantibodies produced by patients with diseases such as lupus erythematosus [53] or undergoing a graft-versus-host reaction following bone marrow transplantation [54]. These studies have shown that there are some keratin polypeptides which can be recognized only in the basal cell layer (MW = ~46,000) and others, which are of higher molecular weight (~62,000 to 67,000), that appear first in the spinous and granular layers. Other keratin polypeptides are found in all epidermal cells. It is currently assumed that the species limited to the basal layer are modified in some way as the cells migrate to the surface and undergo further differentiation. This is an area that is currently under active study, and one that will progress rapidly as new sources of antibodies become available.

Even with this evidence of heterogeneity among the several keratins, the bulk of the evidence indicates that there are strong relationships among the keratins as well as among all members of the intermediate filament family. Steinert, Idler, and Goldman [55] analyzed the keratin filaments from bovine hoof and the intermediate filaments from baby hamster kidney cells propagated in vitro and found similar, linear, three-chain units containing regions of coiled-coil α-helix interspersed with areas of non-α-helix. The α-helical sections were of the same size while the adjoining non-α-helical domains were of variable size; the investigators concluded that the similarities among the molecules could be attributed to the helical areas while the differences in solubility, antigenicity, and other properties were due to the nonhelical regions. A model of the structure proposed is reproduced in Fig. 3, and, although the analogy to the constant and variable regions of immunoglobulins proposed by several authors [24,56] may be an oversimplification, it explains many of the structural similarities and biochemical differences that have been noted. Isolation of the common subunit, if it exists, is now required.

Keratin Synthesis

The past several years have witnessed progress in our understanding of the pathways and controls of keratin synthesis in epidermis and epidermal appendages which is essentially equal to the progress already discussed in the areas of keratin structure and biochemistry. Major contributions have come from the laboratories of Rogers and

Fig. 3. Model of the three-chain structural unit of keratin. The two three-chain coiled-coil α-helical segments (~ 180 Å long) are separated by a region (~ 40 Å) of non-α-helix. (*Redrawn by Steinert from [55], with permission.*)

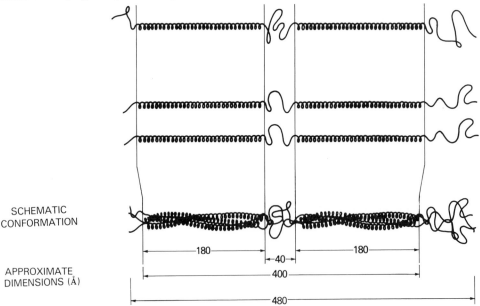

SCHEMATIC
CONFORMATION

APPROXIMATE
DIMENSIONS (Å)

his colleagues in Australia [57], Bernstein and his coworkers in Michigan [43], Freedberg et al. in Boston and Baltimore [58], and, within the past 5 years, Green and his associates at the Massachusetts Institute of Technology [59].

In addition to the experiments directed specifically at the synthesis of fibrous, keratin-like proteins, some data are available concerning the specific synthesis of nonkeratinous proteins such as the components of the keratohyaline granules. Those studies evolved from the earlier experiments of Fukuyama et al. [60,61], who showed that radiolabeled arginine, cystine, histidine, and serine were incorporated into proteins in the cells of the granular layer. Electron microscopic autoradiography indicated further that the subcellular sites for histidine and cystine incorporation were different. Histidine was incorporated first outside of the granules and within 6 hr of injection into experimental animals it concentrated in the granules themselves, while cystine was localized to the "dense deposits" at the edge of the keratohyaline granules [62]. The granules are apparently composed of at least two components one of which contains histidine in relatively large amounts while the other contains significant amounts of cystine. It has been concluded that the cystine-rich material is probably the protein previously studied by Matoltsy and Matoltsy [63] and the histidine-rich component is related to the perchloric acid–soluble protein, high in glycine and histidine, which was isolated from newborn rat epidermis by Hoober and Bernstein [64]. An exquisitely controlled process of protein synthesis must exist in the granular layer cells so that the final steps of epidermal differentiation can occur. The actual synthesis of these proteins has been studied recently in a number of other laboratories. Balmain and his associates [65] proved that a histidine-rich protein of molecular weight 27,000 was synthesized in fetal rodent epidermis at the same time that keratohyaline granules were produced. In vitro studies of the same tissue [66] indicated that several histidine-rich proteins of molecular weight 70,000 to 120,000 were rapidly synthesized. One of these proteins was produced at a stage before the appearance of keratohyaline granules and could represent a precursor material. Freinkel and Weir [67] also noted histidine incorporation into fetal epidermis at a period before the appearance of mature keratohyaline granules.

Ball and his coworkers in Bernstein's laboratory [68] have extended the studies of the production of histidine-rich proteins in newborn epidermis and have developed an hypothesis which states that the actual product of translation (a species they label HRP_0) is rapidly polymerized to a heterogeneous molecule (HRP_I) which then is processed to a smaller molecule (HRP_{II}) as the granular cells move to the stratum corneum. Parallel studies have come from Dale and her associates [69,70] indicating that a basic protein equivalent to the histidine-rich protein can be isolated from the stratum corneum of newborn rat skin. This material, whose molecular weight is approximately 50,000, interacts with isolated keratin polypeptides to form macrofibrils, whose structure resembles the keratin pattern of stratum corneum cells [71]. A precursor of the basic protein can be purified from an epidermal extract and the precursor was found to contain up to 15 to 20 mol of phosphate per mole of protein while the product is nonphosphorylated [72]. It has not yet been determined what the role of this phosphate actually is.

During the past several years much of the work by investigators analyzing the pathways and controls of protein synthesis in epidermis and epidermal appendages has been directed specifically at keratin messenger RNA. The feather keratin messenger was the first one analyzed in experiments carried out by Rogers and his associates in Australia [73]. The messenger was isolated and its accumulation in the cytoplasm was found to be the rate-limiting step in feather keratin synthesis [74]. It was shown subsequently that although there were between 100 and 240 feather genes, large areas of the messenger were not translated [57,75]. The messenger itself consisted of some unique and some repetitive sequences. The significance of the duplication and the nontranslated areas has not been clarified, although it has been recognized as a general phenomenon in protein-synthesizing systems. Since, as we have noted, evidence was presented by the Australian workers that the feather keratin messenger RNA concentration was rate-limiting in the synthetic reactions, both quantitative and qualitative control reside at the messenger level. Other areas of potential importance in quantitative control of epidermal and appendageal keratin synthesis such as age (more active synthesis in young animals) remain to be clarified.

Mammalian epidermal keratin messenger RNA has been identified and subsequently purified by Gibbs and Freedberg [76,77] from the skin of young guinea pigs. Bertolino, Gibbs, and Freedberg [78] have done parallel studies with mouse hair root cells while Ward and Kasmarik [79] have reported on the isolation of polysomal RNA from plucked wool roots. This material directs the synthesis of both the high- and low-sulfur wool keratins in a cell-free protein-sythesizing system.

The epidermal and hair root keratin messenger RNAs have polyA tails on their 3' ends and they are capped on their 5' ends [77,78]. The sedimentation value of the active keratin messengers is approximately 18 to 19 S and they direct the synthesis of keratin in heterologous systems such as those derived from wheat germ or reticulocyte lysates. The polypeptides synthesized in these systems have been proved to be keratin by immunologic techniques as well as by biochemical criteria. Parallel studies of epithelial messenger RNAs from mammalian embryonic tooth organs have been published by Zeichner-David and her coworkers [80]. Although not yet definitely identified, the polypeptides synthesized are similar in molecular weight to keratins.

As has been discussed previously, keratins are unique among the intermediate filament components because of their heterogeneity. This heterogeneity has led to a number of questions concerning the control of their synthesis and specifically it has been asked whether any of the keratin polypeptides are related as precursors and products. Studies from laboratories including those of McGuire and Milstone [81], Gibbs and Freedberg [76], Fuchs and Green [82], and Schweizer and Goerttler [83] have shown that each of the keratin polypeptides is encoded separately in the genome and that each has its own messenger. Although the size of the messengers does not correspond directly to the size of their products, all are synthesized de novo. Similar to the situation with feather mRNA, there are variable-sized lengths of nontranslated messenger [82]. In each case, to account for some of the size discrepancy, there is additional modification of the protein molecules following synthesis. The data of Fuchs and Green [84], for example, indicate that there is a reduction in size of some of the keratins during the final stages of epidermal differentiation.

In vivo the translation of the several keratin messenger RNAs occurs at different levels in the epidermis. Green and his associates have shown that the largest keratin polypeptides (MW = ~63,000 to 65,000) are not synthesized primarily in the lower layers of the tissue, but are produced in the more superficial layers, perhaps as direct precursors of stratum corneum proteins [59,84]. This observation is probably related to the findings in the human epidermal cell culture system of Rheinwald and Green [9] that the smaller keratin polypeptides (40,000 to 50,000) are synthesized, while the larger ones are not. As has been discussed

above, the final stages of keratin synthesis do not take place in the culture system.

Since there are multiple genes for the keratins and there is significant processing and posttranslational modification (see below) which takes place during the synthetic reactions, further significant progress will occur only when each of the keratin genes is cloned and appropriate molecular probes are produced. At that time, all of the data detailed above can be applied directly to analysis of normal and pathologic human keratin synthesis. Such cloning studies are close to fruition at this time.

Postsynthetic Modification of Epidermal Constituents

Phosphorylation

A variety of cellular processes are regulated by reversible phosphorylation-dephosphorylation reactions which are controlled in a number of ways. Phosphorylation may be through a specific protein kinase responsive to either cyclic AMP or cyclic GMP or through nonspecific protein kinases independent of such nucleotides [85]. Dephosphorylation, in contrast, depends upon catalysis by phosphoprotein phosphatases. Several of the cytoskeletal constituents from muscle cells, including myosin light chains and α-tropomyosin, were found to be phosphorylated, and it was determined that this phosphorylation was directly related to the biochemical processes involved in muscle contraction [86].

Other components of the cytoskeleton were studied subsequently and it was found that many intermediate filament subunits were phosphorylated both in vitro and in vivo [24]. Desmin and vimentin were shown to exist as both phosphorylated and nonphosphorylated variants [87] and several cyclic AMP–dependent kinases, which can catalyze the phosphorylation reactions, have been identified [88]. The phosphorylation reactions are specific, and in most cases only one or two major peptides serve as the phosphate receptor, with serine usually identified as the phosphorylated amino acid. In several cases the kinases that catalyze the phosphorylation reactions have been identified as being bound to the filamentous structures of the cytoskeleton or nuclear matrix [28, 89], indicating that there may be an important functional role to these reactions. This role remains unknown, however. Among the possibilities are effects upon the polymerization of the filaments themselves, upon their interaction with other intracellular constituents, or upon their role in determining the shape of cells. It is upon this background that we must examine the evidence that phosphorylation of keratin may be of significance in epidermal function.

The importance of cyclic nucleotides in the control of epidermal proliferation has been apparent for a number of years [90,91], but it is only recently that the focus has moved to the substrate for the phosphorylation reactions. Sun and Green [49] showed that some of the charge heterogeneity that exists among the keratins could be related to phosphorylation, and Gilmartin, Culbertson, and Freedberg [92] found that the keratin polypeptides were among the most heavily labled in epidermis following exposure of the tissue either in vivo or in vitro to radiolabeled phosphate. Serine was the phosphate acceptor and many of the major keratin proteins appeared to be phosphorylated simultaneously. Subsequent studies showed that keratin-containing intermediate filaments of esophagus and hair root cells were also phosphorylated [93], indicating that the process was a general one.

No direct data are available concerning the role of this phosphorylation in epidermal function. The possibilities noted above for other intermediate filaments exist but two more specific potential roles must be considered. We have already noted that the precursor of the stratum corneum basic protein is phosphorylated while the final product is not. It is possible, therefore, that phosphorylation of the epidermal intermediate filament proteins plays a role in control of the reactions between keratin and the matrix proteins as the stratum corneum is formed. Finally, it is possible that phosphorylation of the intermediate filament proteins, in general, and keratin polypeptides, specifically, may play a role in transmission of messages from the cell surface to the nucleus. A signal at the cell membrane could activate a protein kinase which subsequently phosphorylates one of several of the keratins. The resulting change in charge could be transmitted along the filament by cyclical phosphorylation-dephosphorylation reactions catalyzed by filament-bound protein kinases. In this way the signal could reach the nuclear membrane. Since intermediate filaments have been seen to insert at nuclear pores and since there are intranuclear matrix proteins which resemble the keratins and which also undergo phosphorylation-dephosphorylation reactions [94], this pathway could be of major biologic significance. For the present, it remains an unproven hypothesis.

Cornified Envelope Formation

The plasma membranes of epidermal stratum corneum cells demonstrate unusual solubility characteristics since they are not dissolved in concentrated alkaline solutions containing reducing agents. This solubility may be of major functional significance and recent studies have shown that it is related to postsynthetic modifications that occur among proteins directly internal to the epidermal cell membranes. Transglutaminase-catalyzed ε-(γ-glutamyl)lysine cross-links are responsible.

The transglutaminase enzyme in epidermis was identified by workers in several laboratories before its substrate became apparent [95,96], although it was believed, even at the beginning, to play a role in terminal differentiation. Rice and Green [97] identified an epidermal ε-(γ-glutamyl)lysine bond which could be produced in vitro and they postulated that epidermal transglutaminase was responsible for its formation. Subsequently, in studies by Buxman and Wuepper, Rice, Green, and their associates [98,99], a soluble substrate precursor of the insoluble material has been identified and calcium has been found to be critical for the polymerization reaction. In cultured cells the envelope forms mainly in the upper, more differentiated cells, and protein synthesis is not required for its formation. The formation of the envelope is directly related to epidermal stratification and differentiation since the precursor envelope proteins are formed only after cells move from the basal layers [59].

Clinical Applications

Although only short periods of time have passed since the several major scientific advances discussed in this chapter have been published, many of them have already been applied to clinical situations. These applications, which are pathophysiologic, diagnostic, and therapeutic, will be described in this section.

Pathophysiology of Epidermal Disease

Soon after the development of methods to separate the several keratin polypeptides, a number of authors [100–104] analyzed the keratin protein pattern from psoriatic scale and the most constant observation has been that the highest-molecular-weight polypeptide (~67,000 to 70,000) is missing or greatly reduced in the involved tissue. Thaler and his coworkers [101,104] have indicated that, in addition, two smaller polypeptides (54,000 to 57,000) are found in psoriatic scale but not in normal tissue. This observation has not been confirmed by Baden [100] or Skerrow [102] and their associates, who have undertaken similar studies. Since the 67,000- to 70,000-dalton keratin is synthesized in the higher layers of the epidermis, as we have already discussed, it is tempting to speculate that it is missing from the psoriatic lesion because the terminal stages of differentiation do not occur in this process. The psoriatic pattern is similar to that of cultured epidermal cells which, as we have noted, also do not undergo terminal differentiation. This possibility is further supported by the fact that the keratin polypeptides revert to normal with reappearance of the larger keratins during therapy [102,105]. LeVine and his coworkers [105] have actually suggested that the keratin polypeptide pattern may be an appropriate way to follow the response to therapy of affected patients.

Levine and McLeod [103] analyzed a number of epidermal disorders using similar techniques and reported that the highest-molecular-weight keratin polypeptide was also missing from the scale of patients with congenital ichthyosiform erythroderma and lamellar ichthyosis. The conclusion of Ogawa and his coworkers [106] was somewhat different, however, since they have reported a patient with bullous congenital ichthyosiform erythroderma (epidermolytic hyperkeratosis) whose stratum corneum lacked only one of the lower-molecular-weight (55,000) keratins. The techniques by which such analyses can be done are now well standardized and further data should soon be available to resolve these discrepencies.

Studies of the keratin patterns obtained from the other types of ichthyosis have not been as rewarding since no consistent polypeptide abnormalities have been noted. Major progress has been made in studies of X-linked ichthyosis, however, since it has been noted that patients with this disease lack a steroid sulfatase [107], the gene for which has been localized to the distal half of the short arm of the X chromosome [108]. As a consequence of the enzyme deficiency, excessive cholesterol sulfate accumulates in the stratum corneum and the material may be related to the abnormal scaling that results [109].

Diagnosis of Epidermal Disorders

Prenatal diagnostic techniques, which rely generally upon the biochemical or cytologic analysis of cultured cells derived from amniotic fluid, have been applied successfully to a number of metabolic diseases with cutaneous changes. More specifically, fetoscopy and prenatal skin biopsy have been used to diagnose epidermolytic hyperkeratosis (bullous congenital ichthyosiform erythroderma) in a fetus being carried by a patient with this severe, dominant trait [110]. Although the procedure is associated with an increased risk of abortion and although it produces scars on the skin of fetuses carried to delivery, fetoscopy and intrauterine biopsy will unquestionably be applied more extensively in the future.

The major applications of the recent scientific advances to clinical diagnosis have been in the immunologic area. Naturally occurring (autoimmune), pathologically generated (graft-versus-host reaction), and specifically raised antibodies to the keratin polypeptides have been used by a number of investigators to diagnose cutaneous and, in some cases, noncutaneous disease. Löning and his coworkers [111] used guinea-pig antiserum to human keratin polypeptides to distinguish the changes that occur in lichen planus and certain squamous cell carcinomas. An antibody to human epidermal callus keratins has been used by Battifora, Sun, and their colleagues [112] to differentiate between thymoma (which contains keratin antigens) and lymphoma (which does not). Koyayashi and Hashimoto [113] have reported that this same antikeratin antibody reacts with amyloid deposits in localized cutaneous amyloidosis. Finally, antibodies to keratin have been shown to decorate the intracellular filaments of the hepatic Mallory bodies in patients with alcoholic cirrhosis as well as filaments in hepatocytes of experimental animals treated with carcinogens or griseofulvin [114,115]. The future will undoubtedly witness an expansion of this new type of immunologic diagnosis which has many forensic as well as clinical applications.

Therapy

As soon as the Rheinwald-Green cell culture system was presented to the biomedical community [4], investigators predicted that it would be applied rapidly for the study of the pathophysiology of a number of epidermal diseases and to the treatment of clinical situations (trauma, burns, ulcers) in which large areas of epidermis are lost. The former prediction has not been completely fulfilled since it has proved difficult to reproduce the pathologic states in vitro, although recent reports [116] indicate that human squamous cell carcinoma lines can be shown to manifest defective differentiation in vitro. Success has been achieved, however, in propagating autologous epidermal cells in vitro and successfully applying them to the skin of burned patients. The first steps were to grow human cells in vitro and prove that they would survive on the skin of an athymic, immunodeficient mouse [117], and to propagate cells from experimental animals and prove that they would be accepted on a wound as an allograft [118]. Subsequently, it has been shown in two patients that skin biopsies can be taken, the epidermis cultured for up to three passages, and that the resulting cells can be placed on a bed of granulation tissue [119]. Extremely large amounts of epithelium can be generated by this technique. After 3 weeks in culture it can be calculated that from a 1-cm^2 biopsy containing 3 million cells, 6000 cm^2 of epithelium may be harvested containing 1.5 billion cells [120]. This technique, or appropriate modifications of it, should be of general importance in a number of clinical situations within the next several years.

References

1. Rheinwald JG, Green H: Formation of a keratinizing epithelium in culture by a cloned cell line derived from a teratoma. *Cell* **6:**317–330, 1975

2. Fischer S et al: Explant methods for epidermal cell culture. *Methods Cell Biol* **21A:**207–227, 1980

3. Price FM et al: A new culture medium for human skin epithelial cells. *In Vitro* **16:**147–158, 1980

4. Rheinwald JG, Green H: Serial cultivation of strains of human epidermal keratinocytes: the formation of keratinizing colonies from single cells. *Cell* **6:**331–344, 1975

5. Fusenig NE, Worst PKM: Mouse epidermal cell cultures. II. Isolation, characterization and cultivation of epidermal cells from perinatal mouse skin. *Exp Cell Res* **93:**443–457, 1975

6. Taichman L et al: In vitro cultivation of human oral keratinocytes. *Arch Oral Biol* **24:**335–341, 1979

7. Stanley MA, Parkinson EK: Growth requirements of human cervical epithelial cells in culture. *Int J Cancer* **24:**407–414, 1979

8. Sun T-T, Green H: Differentiation of the epidermal keratinocyte in cell culture: formation of the cornified envelope. *Cell* **9:**511–521, 1976

9. Rheinwald JG: Serial cultivation of normal human epidermal keratinocytes. *Methods Cell Biol* **21A:**229–254, 1980

10. Marcelo C: Differential effects of cAMP and cGMP on *in vitro* epidermal cell growth. *Exp Cell Res* **120:**201–210, 1979

11. Yuspa SH et al: Epidermal cell culture. *Transplant Proc* **12:**114–122, 1980

12. Rheinwald JG, Green H: Epidermal growth factor and the multiplication of cultured human epidermal keratinocytes. *Nature* **265:**421–424, 1977

13. Keski-Oja J et al: Epidermal growth factor alterations in proliferating mouse epithelial cells. *Exp Cell Res* **128:**279–290, 1980

14. Hennings H et al: Calcium regulation of growth and differentiation of mouse epidermal cells in culture. *Cell* **19:**245–254, 1980

15. Yuspa SH et al: Clonal growth of mouse epidermal cells in medium with reduced calcium concentration. *J Invest Dermatol* **76:**144–146, 1981

16. Yuspa SH: A survey of transformation markers in differentiating epidermal cell lines in culture. *Cancer Res* **40:**4694–4703, 1980

17. Liu S-CC et al: Growth characteristics of human epidermal keratinocytes from newborn foreskin in primary and serial culture. *In Vitro* **15:**813–822, 1979

18. Gilchrest BA et al: Growth of human keratinocytes on fibronectin-coated plates. *Cell Biol Int Rep* **4:**1009–1016, 1980

19. Hawley-Nelson P et al: Optimized conditions for the growth of human epidermal cells in culture. *J Invest Dermatol* **75:**176–182, 1980

20. Peehl DM, Ham RG: Growth and differentiation of human keratinocytes without a feeder layer or conditioned medium. *In Vitro* **16:**516–525, 1980

21. Eisinger M et al: Human epidermal cell cultures: growth and differentiation in the absence of dermal components or medium supplements. *Proc Natl Acad Sci USA* **76:**5340–5344, 1979

22. Peehl DM, Ham RG: Clonal growth of human keratinocytes with small amount of dialyzed serum. *In Vitro* **16:**526–538, 1980

23. Doran TI et al: Intrinsic and extrinsic regulation of the differentiation of skin, corneal and esophageal epithelial cells. *Cell* **22:**17–25, 1980

24. Lazarides E: Intermediate filaments as mechanical integrators of cellular space. *Nature* **283:**249–256, 1980

25. Woodcock CLF: Nucleus-associated intermediate filaments from chicken erythrocytes. *J Cell Biol* **85:**881–889, 1980

26. Fulton AB et al: The spacial distribution of polyribosomes in 3T3 cells and the associated assembly of proteins into the skeletal framework. *Cell* **20:**849–857, 1980

27. Cervera M et al: Messenger RNA is translated when associated with the cytoskeletal framework in normal and VSV-infected HeLa cells. *Cell* **23:**113–120, 1981

28. Eckert BS et al: Association of creatine phosphokinase with the cytoskeleton of cultured mammalian cells. *J Cell Biol* **86:**1–5, 1980

29. Lazarides E: Intermediate filaments—chemical heterogeneity in differentiation. *Cell* **23:**649–650, 1981

30. Sun T-T, Green H: Immunofluorescent staining of keratin fibers in cultured cells. *Cell* **14:**469–476, 1978

31. Sun T-T et al: Keratin cytoskeletons in epithelial cells of internal organs. *Proc Natl Acad Sci USA* **76:**2813–2817, 1979

32. Franke WW et al: Identification and characterization of epithelial cells in mammalian tissues by immunofluorescence microscopy using antibodies to prekeratin. *Differentiation* **15:**7–25, 1979

33. Franke WW et al: HeLa cells contain intermediate-sized filaments of the prekeratin type. *Exp Cell Res* **118:**95–109, 1979

34. Aubin JE et al: Intermediate filaments of the vimentin-type and the cytokeratin-type are distributed differently during mitosis. *Exp Cell Res* **129:**149–165, 1980

35. Schmid E et al: Differential location of different types of intermediate-sized filaments in various tissues of the chicken embryo. *Differentiation* **15:**27–40, 1979

36. Jackson BW et al: Formation of cytoskeletal elements

during mouse embryogenesis. *Differentiation* **17**:161–179, 1980

37. Trotter JA, Kelley RO: A novel technique for high resolution analysis of the cytoskeleton. *Anat Rec* **195**:7–14, 1979

38. Heuser JE, Kirschner MW: Filament organization revealed in platinum replicas of freeze-dried cytoskeletons. *J Cell Biol* **86**:212–234, 1980

39. Steinert PM et al: Subunit structure of the mouse epidermal keratin filament. *Biochim Biophys Acta* **577**:11–21, 1979

40. Huang L-Y et al: Two polypeptide chain constituents of the major protein of the cornified layer of newborn rat epidermis. *Biochemistry* **14**:3573–3580, 1975

41. Inoue N et al: Immunochemical studies of proteins in epidermal cornified cells of human and newborn rat. *Biochim Biophys Acta* **439**:95–106, 1976

42. Culbertson VB, Freedberg IM: Mammalian epidermal keratin. Isolation and characterization of the α-helical proteins from newborn rat. *Biochim Biophys Acta* **490**:178–191, 1977

43. Brysk MM et al: Tonofilament protein from newborn rat epidermis. *J Biol Chem* **252**:2127–2133, 1977

44. Lee LD et al: Intraspecies heterogeneity of epidermal keratins isolated from bovine hoof and snout. *Biochem J* **17**:187–196, 1979

45. Steinert PM et al: Characterization of the keratin filament subunits unique to bovine snout epidermis. *Biochem J* **187**:913–916, 1980

46. Steinert PM et al: Self-assembly of bovine epidermal keratin filaments *in vitro*. *J Mol Biol* **108**:547–567, 1976

47. Baden HP et al: Comparison of stratum corneum and hair fibrous proteins. *J Invest Dermatol* **75**:311–315, 1980

48. Baden HP et al: Modification of polypeptide composition in keratinocyte fibrous protein. *J Invest Dermatol* **75**:383–387, 1980

49. Sun T-T, Green H: Keratin filaments of cultured human epidermal cells. *J Biol Chem* **253**:2053–2060, 1978

50. Fuchs E, Green H: The expression of keratin genes in epidermis and cultured epidermal cells. *Cell* **15**:887–897, 1978

51. Viac J et al: Experimental production of antibodies against stratum corneum keratin polypeptides. *Arch Dermatol Res* **267**:179–188, 1980

52. Woodcock-Mitchell J, Sun T-T: Specific staining of epidermal basal cell layer by a monoclonal antikeratin antibody. *J Invest Dermatol* **76**:312, 1981

53. Bystryn JC: Epidermal antigens. *Int J Dermatol* **16**:645–656, 1977

54. Saurat JH et al: New markers for keratinocyte differentiation. *Front Matrix Biol* **9**:36–56, 1981

55. Steinert PM et al: Intermediate filaments of baby hamster kidney (BHK-21) cells and bovine epidermal keratinocytes have similar ultrastructures and subunit domain structures. *Proc Natl Acad Sci USA* **77**:4534–4538, 1980

56. Milstone LM, McGuire J: Different polypeptides form the intermediate filaments in bovine hoof and esophageal epithelium and in aortic endothelium. *J Cell Biol* **88**:312–316, 1981

57. Rogers GE: Keratins viewed at the nucleic acid level. *TIBS*, 131–133, June 1978

58. Freedberg IM et al: Control of epidermal and hair root protein synthesis, in *Biochemistry of Normal and Abnormal Epidermal Differentiation*. Edited by IA Bernstein, M Seiji. University of Tokyo Press, Tokyo, 1980, pp 295–309

59. Green H: The keratinocyte as differentiated cell type. *Harvey Lect* **74**:101–139, 1979–1980

60. Fukuyama K et al: Differentially localized incorporation of amino acids in relation to epidermal keratinization in the newborn rat. *Anat Rec* **152**:525–535, 1965

61. Fukuyama K, Epstein WL: Sulfur-containing proteins in epidermal keratinization. *J Cell Biol* **40**:830–838, 1969

62. Fukuyama K, Epstein WL: Heterogeneous proteins in keratohyaline granules studied by quantitative radioautography. *J Invest Dermatol* **65**:113–117, 1975

63. Matoltsy AG, Matoltsy MN: The chemical nature of keratohyalin granules of the epidermis. *J Cell Biol* **47**:593–603, 1970

64. Hoober JK, Bernstein IA: Protein synthesis related to epidermal differentiation. *Proc Natl Acad Sci USA* **56**:594–601, 1966

65. Balmain A et al: Protein synthesis during fetal development of mouse epidermis. I. The appearance of "histidine-rich" protein. *Dev Biol* **60**:442–452, 1977

66. Balmain A et al: Protein synthesis during fetal development of mouse epidermis. II. Biosynthesis of histidine-rich and cystine-rich proteins *in vitro* and *in vivo*. *Dev Biol* **73**:338–344, 1979

67. Freinkel RK, Weir KA: Changing patterns of incorporation of [^{14}C]-histidine and [^{3}H]-leucine into epidermal proteins during differentiation of fetal rat skin. *J Invest Dermatol* **65**:482–487, 1975

68. Ball RD et al: Histidine-rich proteins as molecular markers of epidermal differentiation. *J Biol Chem* **253**:5861–5868, 1978

69. Dale BA: Purification and characterization of a basic protein from the stratum corneum of mammalian epidermis. *Biochim Biophys Acta* **491**:193–204, 1977

70. Lonsdale-Eccles JD et al: A phosphorylated keratohyalin-derived precursor of epidermal stratum corneum basic protein. *J Biol Chem* **255**:2235–2238, 1980

71. Dale BA et al: Assembly of stratum corneum basic protein and keratin filaments in macrofibrils. *Nature* **276**:729–731, 1978

72. Dale BA, Ling SY: Evidence of a precursor form of stratum corneum basic protein in rat epidermis. *Biochemistry* **18**:3539–3546, 1979

73. Kemp DJ et al: Translation of pure feather keratin mRNA in a wheat embryo cell-free system. *Mol Biol Rep* **1**:441–446, 1974

74. Powell BC et al: Control of feather keratin synthesis by the availability of keratin mRNA. *Biochem Biophys Res Commun* **68**:1263–1271, 1976

75. Lockett TJ et al: Organization of the unique and repetitive sequences in feather keratin messenger ribonucleic acid. *Biochemistry* **18**:5654–5663, 1979

76. Gibbs PEM, Freedberg IM: Mammalian epidermal messenger RNA: identification and characterization of the keratin messengers. *J Invest Dermatol* **74**:382–388, 1980

77. Gibbs PEM, Freedberg IM: Epidermal keratin messenger RNAs: a heterogeneous family. *Biochim Biophys Acta* **696**:124–133, 1982

78. Bertolino A et al: In vitro biosynthesis of mouse hair keratins under the direction of follicular RNA. *J Invest Dermatol*, in press

79. Ward KA, Kasmarik SE: The isolation of wool keratin messenger RNA from sheep. *J Invest Dermatol* **75**:244–248, 1980

80. Zeichner-David M et al: Isolation and preliminary characterization of epithelial-specific messenger ribonucleic acids and their products during embryonic tooth development. *Biochem J* **185**:489–496, 1980

81. McGuire JS, Milstone LM: A comparison of the abundance of keratin polypeptides in different levels of calf hoof epithelium (abstr). *J Invest Dermatol* **72**:198, 1979

82. Fuchs E, Green H: Multiple keratins of cultured human epidermal cells are translated from different mRNA molecules. *Cell* **17**:573–582, 1979

83. Schweizer J, Goerttler K: Synthesis *in vitro* of keratin polypeptides directed by mRNA isolated from newborn and adult mouse epidermis. *Eur J Biochem* **112**:243–249, 1980

84. Fuchs E, Green H: Changes in keratin gene expression during terminal differentiation of the keratinocyte. *Cell* **19**:1033–1042, 1980

85. Glass DB, Krebs EG: Protein phosphorylation catalyzed by cyclic AMP-dependent and cyclic GMP-dependent protein kinases. *Annu Rev Pharmacol Toxicol* **20**:363–388, 1980

86. Chacko S et al: Effect of phosphorylation of smooth muscle myosin on actin activation and Ca^{++} regulation. *Proc Natl Acad Sci USA* **74**:129–133, 1977

87. O'Conner CM et al: Phosphorylation of subunit proteins of intermediate filaments from chicken muscle and nonmuscle cells. *Proc Natl Acad Sci USA* **76**:819–823, 1979

88. O'Conner CM et al: Phosphorylation of intermediate filament proteins by cAMP-dependent protein kinases. *Cell* **23**:135–143, 1981

89. Browne CL et al: Immunofluorescent localization of cyclic nucleotide-dependent protein kinases on the mitotic apparatus. *J Cell Biol* **87**:336–345, 1980

90. Voorhees JJ et al: Cyclic AMP, cyclic GMP and glucocorticoids as potential metabolic regulators of epidermal proliferation and differentiation. *J Invest Dermatol* **65**:179–190, 1975

91. Green H: Cyclic AMP in relation to proliferation of the epidermal cell: a new view. *Cell* **15**:801–811, 1978

92. Gilmartin ME et al: Phosphorylation of epidermal keratins. *J Invest Dermatol* **75**:211–216, 1980

93. Gilmartin ME et al: Cellular control of keratin phosphorylation. *Clin Res,* in press

94. Berezney R, Coffey DS: The nuclear protein matrix: isolation, structure and functions. *Adv Enzymol Regul* **14**:63–100, 1976

95. Goldsmith LA et al: Vertebral epidermal transamidases. *Biochim Biophys Acta* **351**:113–125, 1974

96. Buxman MM, Wuepper KD: Isolation, purification and characterization of bovine epidermal transglutaminase. *Biochim Biophys Acta* **452**:356–369, 1976

97. Rice RH, Green H: The cornified envelope of terminally differentiated human epidermal keratinocytes consists of cross-linked protein. *Cell* **11**:417–422, 1977

98. Rice RH, Green H: Presence in human epidermal cells of a soluble protein precursor of the cross-linked envelope: activation of the cross-linking by calcium ions. *Cell* **18**:681–694, 1979

99. Buxman MM et al: Epidermal transglutaminase: identification and purification of a soluble substrate and studies of *in vitro* cross-linking. *J Biol Chem* **255**:1200–1203, 1980

100. Baden HP et al: The keratin polypeptides of psoriatic epidermis. *J Invest Dermatol* **70**:294–297, 1978

101. Thaler MP et al: Two tris-urea-mercaptoethanol extractable polypeptides found uniquely in scales of patients with psoriasis. *J Invest Dermatol* **70**:38–41, 1978

102. Skerrow D, Hunter I: Protein modifications during the keratinization of normal and psoriatic human epidermis. *Biochim Biophys Acta* **537**:474–484, 1978

103. Levine M, McLeod A: Fibrous proteins of normal and abnormal human epidermis. *Br J Dermatol* **100**:401–408, 1979

104. Thaler M et al: Comparative studies of keratins isolated from psoriasis and atopic dermatitis. *J Invest Dermatol* **75**:156–158, 1980

105. LeVine MJ et al: Effect of therapy on keratin polypeptide profiles of psoriatic epidermis. *Arch Dermatol* **116**:1028–1030, 1980

106. Ogawa H et al: Abnormal fibrous protein isolated from the stratum corneum of a patient with bullous congenital ichthyosiform erythroderma (BCIE). *Arch Dermatol Res* **266**:109–116, 1979

107. Shapiro LT et al: X-linked ichthyosis due to steroid-sulphatase deficiency. *Lancet* **1**:70–72, 1978

108. Mohandas T et al: Regional assignment of the steroid sulfatase-X-linked ichthyosis locus. Implications for a noninactivated region on the short arm of the human X chromosome. *Proc Natl Acad Sci USA* **76**:5779–5783, 1979

109. Williams ML, Elias PM: X-linked ichthyosis. Elevated cholesterol sulfate in pathologic stratum corneum. *J Invest Dermatol* **76**:312, 1981

110. Golbus MS et al: Prenatal diagnosis of congenital bullous ichthyosiform erythroderma (epidermolytic hyperkeratosis) by fetal skin biopsy. *N Engl J Med* **302**:93–95, 1980

111. Löning T et al: Keratin polypeptide distribution in normal and diseased human epidermis and oral mucosa. *Virchows Arch [Pathol Anat]* **388**:273–288, 1980

112. Battifora H et al: The use of anti-keratin antiserum as a diagnostic tool: thymoma versus lymphoma. *Hum Pathol* **11**:635–641, 1980

113. Koyabashi J, Hashimoto K: Antigenic identity of amyloid in localized cutaneous amyloidosis with keratin. *J Invest Dermatol* **76**:320, 1981

114. Denk J et al: Formation and involvement of Mallory bodies ('alcoholic hyalin') in murine and human liver revealed by immunofluorescence microscopy with antibodies to prekeratin. *Proc Natl Acad Sci USA* **76**:4112–4116, 1979

115. Borenfreund E et al: Intermediate-sized filaments in cultured rat liver tumor cells with Mallory body-like cytoplasm abnormalities. *J Natl Cancer Inst* **64**:323–333, 1980

116. Rheinwald JG, Beckett MD: Defective terminal differentiation in culture as a consistent and selectable character of malignant human keratinocytes. *Cell* **22**:629–632, 1980

117. Banks-Schlegel S, Green H: Formation of epidermis by serially cultivated human epidermal cells transplanted as an epithelium to athymic mice. *Transplantation* **29**:308–313, 1980

118. Eisinger M et al: Wound coverage by a sheet of epidermal cells grown *in vitro* from dispersed single cell preparations. *Surgery* **88**:287–293, 1980

119. O'Conner NE et al: Grafting of burns with cultured epithelium prepared from autologous epidermal cells. *Lancet* **1**:75–78, 1981

120. Green H et al: Growth of cultured human epidermal cells into multiple epithelia suitable for grafting. *Proc Natl Acad Sci USA* **76**:5665–5668, 1979

PYODERMA GANGRENOSUM

Klaus Wolff

Georg Stingl

Definition

Pyoderma gangrenosum (PG) is a rare, destructive, inflammatory skin disease in which a painful nodule or pustule breaks down to form a progressively enlarging ulcer with a raised, tender, undermined border. Lesions may be solitary or multiple and present either as a purely cutaneous disorder or are associated with systemic disease, such as ulcerative colitis, Crohn's disease, polyarthritis, gammopathy, and other conditions.

Etiology and Pathogenesis

When Brunsting, Goeckerman, and O'Leary described PG in 1930 [1], they implicated streptococci and staphylococci as causative agents because of the inflammatory and purulent nature of the condition. Fifty years later the etiology of PG is still unknown, but it is now established that it is neither caused by bacteria nor is infectious in nature. Although a variety of gram-negative and gram-positive microorganisms have been cultured from ulcers, the early lesions are always sterile and the singular observation of virus-like particles in the biopsy material of a patient with PG [2] has not been confirmed.

A key to the etiologic and pathogenic background of this condition might be found in its frequent association with the systemic diseases discussed below, in which autoimmune mechanisms are suspected or are known to occur, but the fact that PG occurs both as a disease sui generis and in association with a systemic disorder calls for a cautious interpretation of the cause-effect relationship of such associations. The phenomenon of pathergy which describes the development of new lesions following trivial trauma, suggests altered, exaggerated, and uncontrolled inflammatory responses to nonspecific stimuli. A circulating dermonecrotic factor has been described in the serum of PG patients [3] which is capable of inducing necrosis in guinea pig skin, but its pathogenic significance in humans is not clear; PG has been considered an example of a Schwartzman phenomenon [4,5], but this idea has been abandoned.

Most authors consider PG a manifestation of altered immunity, but no consistent pattern of immunologic disturbances has emerged so far. Both hyper- and hypogammaglobulinemia occur in PG, but this and its occasional association with gammopathies and myeloma proteins represent insufficient evidence to support the idea that a dysregulation of humoral immune responses is a basic pathogenic event. Autoantibodies against skin and intestinal antigens have been demonstrated [6,7], but there is no evidence that they cause skin lesions.

The evidence implicating a disturbance of cellular immune functions is also equivocal. Cutaneous anergy to recall antigens has been observed by some [8–11], but not by others [12–16], and failure to sensitize PG patients to dinitrochlorobenzene (DNCB) has been reported [8]. Lazarus et al. [8] have observed unresponsiveness to the intradermal injection of purified protein derivative (PPD) of tuberculin, mumps, streptokinase-streptodornase, and *Candida* antigens in four patients, although three of the four exhibited unimpaired antibody production to *Salmonella* and tetanus toxoid antigens. Laboratory studies have revealed that whereas lymphocyte proliferation is readily induced by mitogen and specific antigens in vitro, the production of macrophage inhibitory factor (MIF) is not [8,13]. By contrast, it has also been noted that both antigen-specific and mitogen-induced lymphocyte proliferation are impaired [10,11].

Whereas a defect of monocyte chemotaxis and phagocytosis has been observed in only one patient with PG and chronic active hepatitis [17], abnormalities of neutrophil functions have been more frequently reported [15]; however, consistent patterns have not been observed. Impaired neutrophil chemotaxis was noted in two of seven patients of one series [15] and in one patient with PG and

leukemia [9]; in the latter, neutrophil chemotaxis was defective when studied in vitro in a Boyden chamber, but neutrophil accumulation at a Rebuck skin window was normal and neutrophils did accumulate at sites of pyoderma gangrenosum. A "streaking leukocyte factor" was found in the serum of a patient with PG and juvenile polyarthritis [18], which enhances migration of human leukocytes without altering their chemotactic activity, but others have been unable to confirm the enhancement of leukocyte mobility by homologous and autologous sera [19]. An impairment of microbicidal activity of leukocytes has also been described [15,20].

Thus, while there is evidence that disturbances of immunoregulation and immunologic effector functions occur in some patients with PG, they are not detectable in others and it is not at all clear whether or not they just represent epiphenomena.

Clinical Manifestations

The salient feature of PG is an irregular ulcer with a raised inflammatory border and a boggy, necrotic base [21,22]. It starts as a deep-seated, painful nodule or as a superficial hemorrhagic pustule, either de novo or following minimal trauma (Fig. 1a). The lesions break down and ulcerate, discharging a purulent and hemorrhagic exudate; the irregular, crenated border is elevated and dusky red or purplish (Figs. 1b, c, and d); it is undermined, soggy, and often perforated so that pressure releases pus, both into the ulcer and through these openings.

A halo of bright erythema surrounds the margin of an advancing ulceration (Figs. 1b and d), which may expand rapidly in one direction and more slowly in another, so that a serpiginous configuration of the ulcer results. Peripheral growth results from the burrowing extension of the undermining margin or from new hemorrhagic pustules, which arise on the elevated border (Fig. 1c). The base of such an ulcer is partially covered with necrotic material (Fig. 1c); it is irregular and granulating and studded with small abscesses (Figs. 1b and d). Superficial ulcers may be confined to the dermis, but often they extend into the fat and even down to the fascia.

Lesions are usually solitary or arise in clusters, which then coalesce to form multicentric, irregular ulcerations. Multiple lesions arising simultaneously or consecutively in different parts of the body also occur (Fig. 2). The predilection sites most commonly affected are the lower extremities,

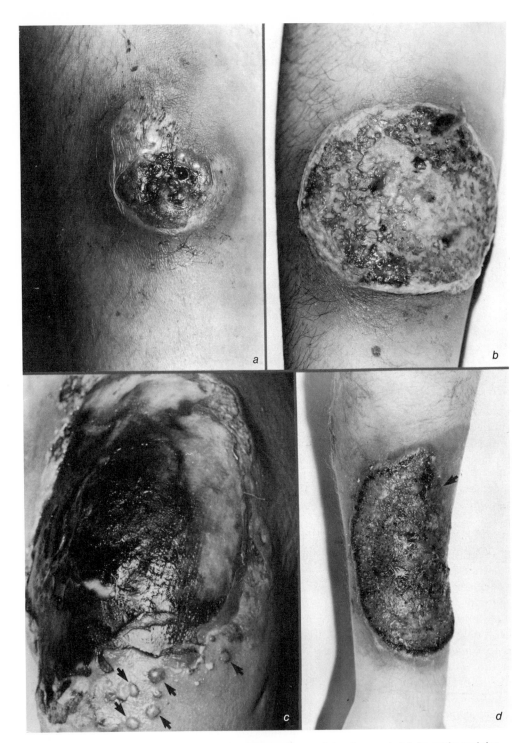

Fig. 1. Pyoderma gangrenosum lesions in various stages of development. (a) An early nodular and partly bullous lesion with small abscesses. (b) A rapidly progressive ulcerative lesion with a soggy, undermined margin, a granulatory necrotic base, and a dusky red inflammatory halo. (c) An acute necrotic ulcer with an elevated purulent border studded with pustules (arrows). (d) A more chronic lesion with an elevated border and a base with small abscesses. While the lesion is expanding on the left, it is spontaneously resolving on the right (arrow). *(Part c from Stingl et al [16], with permission.)*

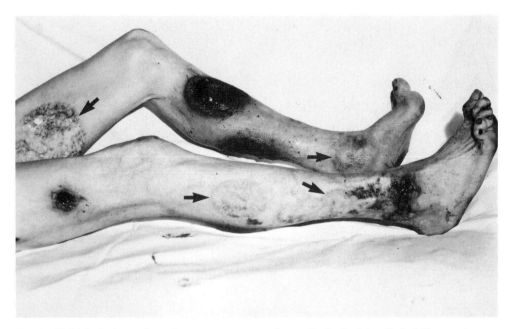

Fig. 2. Multiple lesions of pyoderma gangrenosum in a patient who later died of Wegener's granulomatosis. Note multiple, atrophic scars (arrows), which have resulted from previous flares of PG.

buttocks, abdomen, and face, but any area of the body may be involved. Mucous membranes are usually spared, but aphthous lesions may occur in the oral mucosa; rarely, massive ulcerative involvement of the oral cavity and eyes has been observed.

PG may occur at any age, the course extends over weeks and months, and the growth of the ulcers may be rapid, involving large areas of the body within a few days (Fig. 3), or indolent and slow. Healing usually occurs spontaneously, resulting in a thin, atrophic, usually cribriform scar (Fig. 2). Often an ulcer may heal in the center but progress in the periphery, and as one lesion heals, a new one may arise elsewhere on the body.

Considerable toxicity and fever are usually associated with the acute onset of PG lesions but systemic symptoms may also be absent. Almost invariably, the lesions are painful and cause considerable discomfort.

Exacerbating Factors

The term *pathergy* describes the phenomenon of trivial trauma provoking new lesions or aggravating existing ones. Intradermal skin testing or injections (including even the injection of saline), pricks, insect bites, biopsies, and operations may induce new lesions, and this requires judicious management of these patients. The lesion shown in Fig. 3 arose after laparotomy for a gynecologic prob-

lem. However, pathergy occurs in only 20 percent of the patients [23] and, since even major surgery is tolerated well by some patients, the significance of pathergy is difficult to assess. Pathergy may also be the reason for the rejection of autologous skin grafts [23,24] and the development of new lesions in donor sites, but again skin grafts are not always rejected [16].

Laboratory Findings

There are no laboratory findings that are specific and thus diagnostic. A high erythrocyte sedimentation rate and leukocytosis are invariably present; there may be anemia and low serum iron, and both hyper- and hypoglobulinemia occurs. Specific autoantibodies are not known to be formed in PG, and circulating immune complexes have either not been looked for or have not been detected [11,15,16]. Studies of the complement system in a series of 13 patients, most of whom had arthritis, have revealed depressed total hemolytic complement and C3 levels in only one, but that patient had septicemia [15]. HLA typing has not revealed a consistent pattern [15].

Pathology

The histopathologic features are not diagnostic. They encompass edema, massive neutrophilic

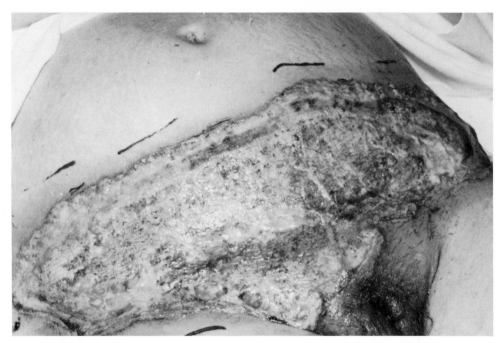

Fig. 3.   Rapidly enlarging pyoderma gangrenosum triggered by laparotomy. The lesion spread to involve the entire lower abdomen within 5 days. *(From Stingl et al [16], with permission.)*

inflammation, engorgement and thrombosis of small- and medium-sized vessels, necrosis, and hemorrhage. The extremely dense infiltrate of polymorphonuclear leukocytes leads to abscess formation and liquefaction necrosis of the collagen with secondary thrombosis of venules. There is disagreement as to the occurrence of necrotizing vasculitis in lesions of PG, as some authors have described fibrinoid necrosis of dermal venules and leukocytoclasia [13,16,25], whereas others have consistently failed to detect features of vasculitis [8,15,19]. In our own series of patients, necrotizing vasculitis indistinguishable from that occurring in immune complex disease (Fig. 4) was seen in 40 percent of the patients. Except for a single report on the deposition of C3 within vessels of a PG lesion [16], intramural deposits of immune complexes or complement components have not been detected by immunofluorescence. Older lesions may show pseudoepitheliomatous hyperplasia in the margins of the ulcer, foreign-body-type granuloma formation, capillary proliferation, and fibrosis.

Associations with Systemic Disease

Pyoderma gangrenosum may present as a disease confined to the skin, but it may also be associated with large and small bowel disease, arthritis, paraproteinemia and myeloma, leukemia, active chronic hepatitis, and Behçet's syndrome. The heterogeneity of these conditions makes it difficult to pinpoint a common denominator responsible for such associations. Data on the prevalence of PG in systemic disease vary greatly because of the screening bias inherent in the referral system by which rheumatologists see PG more often associated with arthritis, gastroenterologists with ulcerative colitis, and dermatologists without associated disease.

Ulcerative Colitis and Crohn's Disease

In its original description PG was associated with ulcerative colitis in four out of five cases [1] and subsequent series have found a prevalence ranging from 30 to 60 percent [21,26,27]. Eleven of 19 cases reported by Perry and Brunsting [21] had ulcerative colitis, as did 31 of 62 patients in a subsequent study from the same center [27]. These figures are probably too high and may represent a sampling bias, for other studies have found a prevalence of only 7 [19] and 15 percent [15]. Also, PG occurs only rarely in ulcerative colitis, the reported prevalence ranging from 0.6 [28] to 5 percent [29]. In most patients symptoms of ulcerative colitis precede PG and exacerbations of the bowel disease frequently correlate with a worsening of the skin lesions, but this is not always the case [30] and PG may persist for long periods

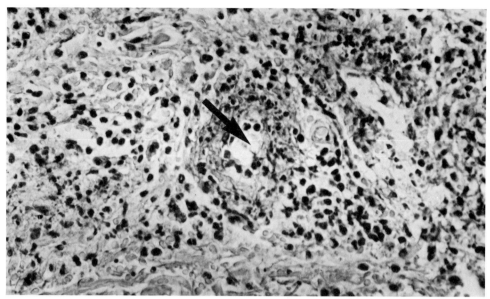

Fig. 4. Dense neutrophilic infiltrate in the dermis of a PG lesion. In the center a venule is shown (arrow) which exhibits fibrinoid necrosis, infiltration by polymorphonuclear leukocytes, and leukocytoclasia. *(From Stingl et al [16], with permission.)*

of time during which bowel disease is quiescent [28]. The fact that PG usually follows the onset of colitis may be taken to suggest that the colitis represents a conditioning factor for the skin disease, but the etiology of ulcerative colitis is as obscure [31] as that of PG. It has been reported that extracts from stools of patients with ulcerative colitis contain epidermolytic proteases [32], but it is difficult to envisage mechanisms by which these enzymes could cause skin lesions; they certainly cannot explain those cases of PG in which ulcerative colitis is not present.

An association of PG is also found with Crohn's disease, but the prevalence is much lower than in ulcerative colitis, ranging from 0.15 [33] to 1.2 percent [29].

Arthritis

Arthritis is frequently associated with PG, which it usually precedes. In one review arthritis was found in 35 of 117 patients collected from the literature [23]. Some patients have classical seropositive rheumatoid arthritis [13,19] and others have the arthritis of ulcerative colitis, which is seronegative, acute, oligoarticular, and nondestructive [34]. The latter form does not occur in PG patients without ulcerative colitis, who instead may present with a seronegative rheumatoid-like arthritic syndrome [8,13,35]. In a recent study of 15 patients with PG [15], inflammatory polyarthritis

was the most frequent associated systemic disease, occurring in 8 patients. Two of the patients with joint disease had classical seropositive rheumatoid arthritis and six an inflammatory polyarthritis, which was seronegative. In four of these patients the polyarthritis was not associated with HLA-B27, psoriasis, or Reiter's syndrome; it was progressive and led to erosive joint destruction and disabling deformities. Depressed levels of total hemolytic complement and cryoprecipitates with anticomplementary activity were present in the synovial effusions, which suggested complement consumption in the inflammatory joints [15].

Hematologic Disease

An increasing number of patients has been reported in whom PG was associated either with myeloma [16,25,35–38] or paraproteinemia without myeloma, mostly of the IgA [23,25,39–41] but also of the IgG [42–44] and IgM [45,46] types. Myeloma usually presents later than PG [37], but one of our own patients had had a micromolecular IgG kappa myeloma for 4 years before her first episode of PG, and the activities of her two diseases were unrelated [16].

PG occurs in acute myeloblastic, myelomonocytic, and chronic myelogenous leukemia [47–54] and has been described in patients with polycythemia vera and osteomyelosclerosis [12,56–58]. In some cases PG preceded the first clinical manifestations of leukemia and thus led to the detection of the hematologic disorder, but usually there is no correlation of the activities of bone marrow and skin. In one patient the lesions of PG bore some resemblance to acute febrile neutrophilic dermatosis [52], which may also be associated with acute leukemia (see article on *Acute Febrile Neutrophilic Dermatosis*).

Other Conditions

PG has been observed in association with active, chronic hepatitis [16,17,59], paroxysmal nocturnal hemoglobinuria [15], SLE [60], and occasionally with gastric and duodenal ulcers, polyps, and diverticulitis [19], but it is questionable whether these associations are not fortuitous. We have seen a patient with PG and features of Behçet's syndrome [16] and others have reported patients with Behçet's syndrome who, in retrospect, may also have had PG [61]. Both diseases share certain features like arthritis, pustulation, aphthous lesions of the mucous membranes, and the phenomenon of pathergy.

PG has been observed with diabetes and vasculitis [62] and in association with Wegener's granulomatosis [63,64]. Figure 2 shows multiple lesions of PG in one of our own patients, who during the course of the disease developed necrotizing urticarial vasculitis and eventually died of Wegener's granulomatosis.

Finally, it should be mentioned that PG has been reported in association with a generalized, grouped, vesiculopustular eruption resembling dermatitis herpetiformis [21,35,65,66], with which it shares its sensitivity to iodides and response to sulfonamides. In some of these cases histologies were not available, and in some histologic features were reported to be not entirely typical for dermatitis herpetiformis; in none were immunofluorescent studies performed. Perry and Brunsting [21], who first drew attention to this association, were troubled by the fact that the distribution of the vesiculopustular lesions did not conform to the lesions of dermatitis herpetiformis, and a clinical photograph of one of the patients bears a striking resemblance to subcorneal pustular dermatosis (Sneddon and Wilkinson's disease). Indeed, we have observed a patient with proven subcorneal pustular dermatosis, IgA paraproteinemia, and PG [24], which may suggest that at least some of the pustular eruptions described in the older literature may have represented Sneddon and Wilkinson's disease. Subcorneal pustular dermatosis can be associated with ulcerative colitis

[67] and IgA myeloma, and it responds to sulfonamides [68], as does PG. The pathogenic significance of these associations is not clear.

Differential Diagnosis

Since there is no specific laboratory test and the histopathology is only suggestive, but not diagnostic, the diagnosis of PG rests entirely on the clinical presentation and course. Postoperative progressive gangrene, ecthyma gangrenosum, atypical mycobacterial and clostridial infection, deep mycoses, amebiasis, and tropical ulcers are excluded by clinical criteria and the demonstration of the causative organisms; bromoderma and North American blastomycosis are more chronic, hyperkeratotic, and present with massive pseudoepitheliomatous hyperplasia; pemphigus vegetans, both of the Hallopeau and Neumann types, can be excluded histologically and by immunofluorescence. Stasis ulcers are easily excluded but artifacts may occasionally cause problems. Wegener's granulomatosis presents with involvement of the upper respiratory tract and is characterized histopathologically by necrotizing and granulomatous vasculitis, but as mentioned above, the two diseases may occur together. The detection of associated systemic disease, such as ulcerative colitis, may help in the establishment of the diagnosis.

Treatment

In patients with underlying disease therapy should not only be directed to PG, but also to control of the systemic disorder. Topical treatment alone is insufficient both in patients with associated systemic disease and in most patients with purely cutaneous PG. While measures directed at cleaning the ulcer and preventing bacterial overgrowth are helpful, more invasive surgical debridement should be discouraged as it may trigger new lesions. This also applies to excision and grafting, unless PG is controlled by systemic treatment.

Corticosteroids

Systemic corticosteroids represent the most effective treatment of PG. They dramatically halt the progression of existing ulceration and prevent the development of new lesions [16,19]. However, high doses may be necessary [69], and these doses are usually higher than those required, for instance, for control of associated ulcerative colitis. Initial doses are 100 to 200 mg/day of prednisone, but sometimes heroic doses are necessary. The patient shown in Fig. 3 required an initial dose of 1000 mg/day for control of PG. Steroid doses are reduced as the inflammatory component of PG disappears and are tapered slowly to be discontinued only after complete resolution has occurred. Very recently pulse therapy with suprapharmacologic doses of methylprednisolone (1 g/day for 5 consecutive days) has been reported to halt progressive PG and side effects were not noted [70a]. Usually, however, corticosteroid side effects occur in up to 50 percent of the patients [15]. Intralesional corticosteroids have been advocated [19,70] but, in our experience, have been disappointing.

Sulfonamides

Dapsone, sulfapyridine, and sulfasalazine (Azulfidine) are beneficial, but not all patients respond equally well [21]. In our experience, sulfasalazine is the most effective of the three, not only in patients with associated ulcerative colitis, but also in some patients with PG who have no systemic disease. Initial daily doses range from 4 to 6 g and, as a response is noted, are gradually reduced to maintenance levels of 0.5 to 1 g. A combination with systemic corticosteroids, particularly in the initial phases of therapy, may be necessary, but we have also seen patients who have failed to respond. An occasional patient can be maintained free of symptoms with either sulfones or sulfapyridine alone, but since PG has an unpredictable course with spontaneous remissions and unpredictable exacerbations, it is not established beyond doubt that such suppression of disease activity is in fact related to treatment.

The mechanism of action of the sulfonamides in PG is unknown but may be related to a stabilizing effect on lysosomes [71] and to their interference with the myeloperoxidase-halide system [72]; it is interesting to note that dapsone is effective in a host of cutaneous disorders, which are all characterized by abnormal accumulation of polymorphonuclear leukocytes, such as erythema elevatum diutinum, dermatitis herpetiformis, Sneddon-Wilkinson disease, and pyoderma gangrenosum.

Immunosuppressive Agents

6-Mercaptopurine [51] and azathioprine [15,60,73,74] have been reported to be beneficial, but have not been universally successful [15]. Azathioprine given in combination with corticosteroids has failed to help a patient with PG and impaired lymphocyte function [11].

Clofazimine

Recent reports have stressed the dramatic efficacy of clofazimine (Lamprene) in PG [75–78]. Doses of 300 mg/day stop progression of lesions within 1 to 2 weeks and lead to complete or partial healing within 2 to 5 months. However, failure of patients to respond to clofazimine is also known [11,15]. Clofazimine enhances intracellular killing of bacteria and increases phagocytosis of neutrophils in vitro and in vivo [79–82]. Since there is some dysregulation of phagocyte function in PG, the effect of clofazimine may be on the phagocyte level; however, just how it works in this disease is unknown. Its side effects are generally less than those of corticosteroids, but splenic infarction has been observed in one patient [83].

Course and Prognosis

The disease behaves in an unpredictable way. PG may have a dramatic onset with pustular and bullous lesions rapidly breaking down to ulcers, which progressively enlarge (Figs. 1a, 1b, 1c, and 3) until arrested by treatment; in these cases there may be toxicity, fever, and considerable pain. More chronic forms show ulcers which extend slowly in a creeping fashion (Fig. 1d), expanding in one direction and healing spontaneously in another or in the center. In both forms, spontaneous healing can occur, but as old lesions resolve, new lesions may arise. The disease may come to a spontaneous halt for no apparent reason, remain quiescent for months and even years, and exacerbate again after minimal trauma, surgery, or without an apparent triggering cause. When associated with ulcerative colitis, the disease activity of PG may parallel that of the bowel disease, but as noted above, it is not always the case. The same is true for patients with associated hematologic disease, where the final prognosis is determined by the underlying condition. All in all the prognosis of PG per se is good, particularly in those patients who readily respond to treatment, but considerable scarring and disfigurement may eventually result.

References

1. Brunsting LA et al: Pyoderma (ecthyma) gangrenosum. Clinical and experimental observations in five cases occurring in adults. *Arch Dermatol* 22:655–680, 1930
2. Gay Prieto J et al: Über die Ätiologie des sogenannten Pyoderma gangraenosum (Phagédénisme géométrique de Brocq). *Hautarzt* 17:26–34, 1966

3. Delescluse J et al: Pyoderma gangrenosum with altered cellular immunity and dermonecrotic factor. *Br J Dermatol* **87**:529–532, 1972

4. Rostenberg A Jr: The Shwartzman phenomenon: a review with a consideration of some possible dermatological manifestations. *Br J Dermatol* **65**:389–405, 1953

5. Goldgraber MB, Kirsner JB: Gangrenous skin lesions associated with chronic ulcerative colitis. *Gastroenterology* **39**:94–103, 1960

6. Brobenger O, Perlmann P: Autoantibodies in human ulcerative colitis. *J Exp Med* **110**:657–674, 1959

7. Samitz MH: Cutaneous vasculitis in association with ulcerative colitis. *Cutis* **2**:383–387, 1966

8. Lazarus GS et al: Pyoderma gangrenosum, altered delayed hypersensitivity, and polyarthritis. *Arch Dermatol* **105**:46–51, 1972

9. Shore RN: Pyoderma gangrenosum, defective neutrophil chemotaxis, and leukemia. *Arch Dermatol* **112**:1792–1793, 1976

10. Deschamps P et al: Déficit immunitaire au cours d'un pyoderma gangrenosum associé à une polyglobulie vraie. *Nouv Presse Med* **6**:2339–2341, 1977

11. Breathnach SM et al: Idiopathic pyoderma gangrenosum and impaired lymphocyte functions: failure of Azathioprine and corticosteroid therapy. *Br J Dermatol* **104**:567–574, 1981

12. Gopinath DK et al: Pyoderma gangrenosum with myelofibrosis. *J Ky Med Assoc* **72**:548–550, 1974

13. Stolman LP et al: Pyoderma gangrenosum and rheumatoid arthritis. *Arch Dermatol* **111**:1020–1023, 1975

14. Callen JP et al: Recurrent pyoderma gangrenosum and agnogenic myeloid metaplasia. *Arch Dermatol* **113**:1585–1586, 1977

15. Holt PJA et al: Pyoderma gangrenosum. Clinical and laboratory findings in 15 patients with special reference to polyarthritis. *Medicine (Baltimore)* **59**:114–133, 1980

16. Stingl G et al: Pyoderma gangränosum. *Hautarzt* **32**:165–172, 1981

17. Norris DA et al: Pyoderma gangrenosum. Abnormal monocyte function corrected in vitro with hydrocortisone. *Arch Dermatol* **114**:906–911, 1978

18. Jacobs JC, Goetzl EJ: "Streaking leukocyte factor," arthritis and pyoderma gangrenosum. *Pediatrics* **56**:570–578, 1975

19. Hickman JG, Lazarus GS: Pyoderma gangrenosum: new concepts in etiology and treatment, in *Dermatology Update. Review for Physicians.* Edited by SL Moschella. Elsevier, New York, 1979, pp 325–342

20. Miller ME, Dooley R: Deficient random mobility, normal chemotaxis and impaired phagocytosis: a new abnormality of neutrophil function. *Pediatr Res* **7**:365–369, 1973

21. Perry HO, Brunsting LA: Pyoderma gangrenosum. A clinical study of nineteen cases. *Arch Dermatol* **75**:380–386, 1957

22. Kresbach H: Ein Beitrag zum Problem der sogenannten Pyodermia ulcerosa. *Arch Klin Exp Dermatol* **208**:128–159, 1959

23. Van der Sluis I: Two cases of pyoderma (ecthyma) gangrenosum associated with the presence of an abnormal serumprotein (beta2A-paraprotein). With a review of the literature. *Dermatologica* **132**:409–424, 1966

24. Long JP, Uesu CT: Pyoderma gangraenosum. *JAMA* **187**:336–339, 1964

25. Thompson DM et al: Studies on a patient with leucocytoclastic vasculitis, "pyoderma gangrenosum" and paraproteinemia. *Br J Dermatol* **88**:117–125, 1973

26. Röckl H: Pyodermia ulcerosa serpiginosa, Pyoderma gangraenosum, Dermatitis ulcerosa, in *Handbuch der Haut- und Geschlechtskrankheiten v. J. Jadassohn*, Erganzungswerk, Bd 1B, Teil 1A. Edited by A Marchionini. Springer-Verlag, Berlin/Göttingen/Heidelberg, 1964, pp 131–147

27. Perry HO: Pyoderma gangrenosum. *South Med J* **62**:899–908, 1969

28. Edwards FC, Truelove SX: The course and prognosis of ulcerative colitis. *Gut* **5**:1–22, 1964

29. Greenstein AJ et al: The extraintestinal complications of Crohn's disease and ulcerative colitis: a study of 700 patients. *Medicine (Baltimore)* **55**:401–412, 1976

30. Johnson ML, Wilson HTH: Skin lesions in ulcerative colitis. *Gut* **10**:255–263, 1969

31. La Mont JTh, Isselbacher KJ: Diseases of the colon and rectum, in *Harrison's Principles of Internal Medicine*, 8th ed. Edited by GW Thorn et al. McGraw-Hill, New York, 1977, pp 1547–1567

32. Stoughton RB: Enzymatic cytolysis of epithelium by filtrates from patients with ulcerative colitis. *J Invest Dermatol* **20**:353–356, 1953

33. Van Pattar WM et al: Regional enteritis. *Gastroenterology* **26**:347–450, 1954

34. Wright V, Watkinson G: The arthritis of ulcerative colitis. *Medicine (Baltimore)* **38**:243–259, 1959

35. Ayers S Jr, Ayers S III: Pyoderma gangrenosum with an unusual syndrome of ulcers, vesicles, and arthritis. *Arch Dermatol* **77**:269–280, 1958

36. Zabel M: Pyoderma gangraenosum mit IgG-Paraproteinämie bei Plasmozytom. *Hautarzt* **27**:603–605, 1976

37. Jablonska S et al: Rapports entre la pyodermite gangreneuse et le myélome. *Ann Dermatol Syphiligr (Paris)* **94**:121–132, 1967

38. Kresbach H: Pyoderma gangraenosum—dermatitis ulcerosa. *Z Haut Geschl Kr* **46**:292–293, 1971

39. Schröpl F: Dermatitis ulcerosa (Pyroderma gangraenosum) mit gamma A-Paraproteinämie. *Arch Klin Exp Dermatol* **228**:430–437, 1967

40. Kövary PM et al: Pyoderma gangraenosum und IgA-Paraproteinämie. *Z Hautkr* **51**:91–96, 1976

41. Wolff K: Subkorneale pustolöse Dermatose (Sneddon-Wilkinson); Pyoderma gangraenosum mit IgA-Paraproteinämie. *Dermatol Monatsschr* **157**:842, 1971

42. Degos R et al: Pyodermite phagédénique avec dysglobulinémie. *Bull Soc Fr Dermatol Syphiligr* **73**:370–373, 1966

43. Imhof JW et al: Monoclonal gammopathy (IgG) and chronic ulcerative dermatitis (phagedenic pyoderma). *Acta Med Scand* **186**:289–292, 1969

44. Zabel M, Brändle I: Pyoderma gangränosum mit IgG-Paraproteinämie. *Med Klin* **74**:358–360, 1979

45. Cream JJ: Pyoderma gangrenosum with a monoclonal IgM red cell agglomerating factor. *Br J Dermatol* **84**:223–226, 1971

46. Badanoiu A et al: Bemerkungen über einen Fall von Dermatitis ulcerosa mit gamma M-Paraproteinämie (beta 2 M-Makroglobulinämie). *Hautarzt* **21**:324–328, 1970

47. Bazex A et al: Pyoderma gangrenosum et leucémie aigue myéloblastique. *Bull Soc Fr Dermatol Syphiligr* **80**:440–447, 1973

48. Fayolle J et al: Pyoderma gangrenosum et leucose aigue myéloblastique. Cas personnel et revue de la litterature. *Bull Soc Fr Dermatol Syphiligr* **81**:334–336, 1974

49. Perry HO, Winkelmann RK: Bullous pyoderma gangrenosum and leukemia. *Arch Dermatol* **106**:901–905, 1972

50. Pye RJ et al: Bullous pyoderma as a presentation of acute leukemia. *Clin Exp Dermatol* **2**:33–38, 1977

51. Maldonado N et al: Pyoderma gangrenosum treated with 6-mercaptopurine and followed by acute leukemia. *J Pediatr* **72:**409–414, 1968

52. Burton JL: Bullous pyoderma of leukaemia. *Br J Dermatol* **95:**209–210, 1976

53. Goldin D, Wilkinson DS: Pyoderma gangrenosum with chronic myeloid leukemia. *Proc R Soc Med* **67:**1239–1240, 1974

54. Cramers M: Bullous pyoderma gangrenosum in association with myeloid leukaemia. *Acta Derm Venereol (Stockh)* **56:**311–312, 1976

55. Barrière H et al: Pyoderma gangrenosum et hémopathie. A propos de 3 observations. *Ann Dermatol Venereol (Paris)* **106:**427–435, 1979

56. Basset A et al: Pyodermite phagédénique (pyoderma gangrenosum) associée à une leucopénie. *Bull Soc Fr Dermatol Syphiligr* **78:**159–160, 1971

57. Duverne J et al: Pyodermites en placards extensifs et sphacéliques au cours d'une maladie de Vaquez stabilisée par le P 32. *Bull Soc Fr Dermatol Syphiligr* **76:**86–89, 1969

58. Feuerman E, Potruch-Eisenkraft S: Pyoderma gangrenosum. Un cas de polycythémie vraie. *Bull Soc Fr Dermatol Syphiligr* **78:**260–261, 1971

59. Byrne JPH et al: Pyoderma gangrenosum associated with active chronic hepatitis. *Arch Dermatol* **112:**1297–1301, 1976

60. Olson K: Pyoderma gangrenosum with systemic lupus erythematosus. *Acta Derm Venereol (Stockh)* **51:**233–234, 1971

61. Fromer JL: Behcet's syndrome. *Arch Dermatol* **102:**116–117, 1970

62. Philpott JA et al: Pyoderma gangrenosum, rheumatoid arthritis, and diabetes mellitus. *Arch Dermatol* **94:**732–738, 1966

63. Reed WB et al: The cutaneous manifestations in Wegener's granulomatosus. *Acta Derm Venereol (Stockh)* **43:**250–264, 1963

64. Ryan TJ, Wilkinson DS: Cutaneous vasculitis: "angiitis," in *Textbook of Dermatology,* 3d ed. Edited by A Rook et al. Blackwell, Oxford, 1979, pp 993–1058

65. Lorincz AL, Pearson RW: Sulfapyridine and sulfone type drugs in dermatology. *Arch Dermatol* **85:**2–14, 1962

66. Potter B, Malkinson FD: Atypical dermatitis herpetiformis with arthritis and pyoderma gangrenosum successfully treated with sulphamethoxypyridazine. *Arch Dermatol* **80:**354–355, 1959

67. Wilkinson DS: Subcorneal pustular dermatosis (Dermatose pustuleuse souscornée). *Bull Soc Fr Dermatol Syphiligr* **69:**674–679, 1962

68. Hönigsmann H, Wolff K: Subcorneal pustular dermatosis (Sneddon–Wilkinson disease), in *Dermatology in General Medicine.* Edited by TB Fitzpatrick et al. McGraw-Hill, New York, 1979, pp 347–349

69. Mehregan AH: Pyoderma gangrenosum. *Arch Dermatol* **109:**269, 1974

70. Moschella SL: Pyoderma gangrenosum. A patient successfully treated with intralesional injections of steroid. *Arch Dermatol* **95:**121–123, 1967

70a. Johnson RB, Lazarus GS: Pulse therapy. Therapeutic efficacy in the treatment of pyoderma gangrenosum. *Arch Dermatol* **118:**76–84, 1982

71. Barranco VP: Inhibition of lysosomal enzymes by dapsone. *Arch Dermatol* **110:**563–566, 1974

72. Stendahl O et al: The inhibition of polymorphonuclear leukocyte cytotoxicity by dapsone. *J Clin Invest* **62:**214–220, 1978

73. August PJ, Wells GC: Pyoderma gangrenosum treated with Azathioprine and prednisolone. *Br J Dermatol* **91:(suppl 10):**80–82, 1974

74. Schöpf E et al: Azathioprin-Behandlung der Dermatitis ulcerosa (Pyoderma gangraenosum). *Hautarzt* **20:**558–563, 1969

75. Michaelsson G et al: Clofazimine. A new agent for the treatment of pyoderma gangrenosum. *Arch Dermatol* **112:**344–349, 1976

76. Beurey J et al: Pyoderma gangrenosum: thérapeutique par clofazimine. *Ann Dermatol Venereol (Paris)* **104:**631–634, 1977

77. Thomsen K, Rothenborg HW: Clofazimine in the treatment of pyoderma gangrenosum. *Arch Dermatol* **115:**851–852, 1979

78. Kark EC et al: Pyoderma gangrenosum treated with clofazimine. *J Am Acad Dermatol* **4:**152–159, 1981

79. Brandt L: Enhancing effect of clofazimine on the phagocytosis of neutrophil leucocytes in vitro. *Scand J Haematol* **8:**265–269, 1971

80. Cline MJ: Drug potentiation of macrophage function. *Infect Immun* **2:**601–605, 1970

81. Michaelsson G: Decreased phagocytic capacity of the neutrophil leucocytes in patients with atopic dermatitis. *Acta Derm Venereol (Stockh)* **53:**279–282, 1973

82. Molin L: Clofazimine-enhanced phagocytosis in pustulosis palmaris et plantaris. *Acta Derm Venereol (Stockh)* **55:**151–153, 1975

83. McDougall AC et al: Splenic infarction and crystallization associated with the use of clofazimine (Lamprene-B 663) in the treatment of pyoderma gangrenosum. *Br J Dermatol* **102:**227–230, 1980

VARIEGATE PORPHYRIA
A Potentially Fatal Porphyric Syndrome That Mimics Porphyria Cutanea Tarda

Jan E. Muhlbauer

Madhu A. Pathak

Variegate porphyria (VP) is an hereditary disorder of heme metabolism expressed in adults as either fragility and blistering of sun-exposed skin, acute attacks of abdominal and neuropsychiatric symptoms, or both [1–4]. Biochemical analysis of feces of adults with either manifest or latent VP shows increased excretion of porphyrins, including coproporphyrin (COPRO) and especially protoporphyrin (PROTO) [5,6]. Early literature was confused by use of terminology such as protocoproporphyria, porphyria cutanea tarda hereditaria, mixed porphyria, and South African genetic porphyria. In 1959, Dean and Barnes [7] proposed the name *porphyria variegata* to describe this type of porphyria, seen commonly in South African white Afrikaners; porphyria variegata could be manifest as an acute form similar to acute intermittent porphyria (AIP) and/or a cutaneous form similar to porphyria cutanea tarda (PCT). This confusion in nomenclature has been resolved and the disease is now commonly referred to as variegate porphyria. The differentiation of VP from PCT is critical, since patients with VP are vulnerable to life-threatening paralytic attacks, often provoked by drugs; in contrast, patients with PCT do not have acute attacks.

VP has been recognized in many nations, but always with much less frequency than reported from South Africa. About 80 cases have been reported from the United States [2,8,9]. Recently, we have identified five additional families with VP from New England (*JAMA* 1982, in press. [9a]), so that the disease may be more common in the United States than previously recognized. VP may be misdiagnosed as PCT or AIP, depending on whether the presenting symptoms are cutaneous or visceral, respectively.

Epidemiology

In 1971, Dean [1] estimated 12,000 people in South Africa to be affected with VP; he suggested a prevalence of 3 per 1000 in the white population. Dean [1] and Eales et al. [10] showed that almost all individuals with VP from South Africa are descendants of a fertile Dutch couple who married in Cape Town in 1688. The disease is seen not only in Afrikaners but also in English-speaking and so-called Cape Coloured of South Africa as a result of intermarriage. Outside of South Africa, VP has been found most frequently in Finland, where the prevalence is at least 1.3 per 100,000 in the adult population [11]. VP has been reported also from Britain, Ireland, France, Italy, Sweden, Holland, Denmark, Belgium, Germany, Spain, Yugoslavia, Japan, Egypt, India, and Taiwan, as well as the United States [2,12]. For the most part, these families do not share common ancestry with the large South African family. VP has not been reported in blacks of entirely African descent.

Family studies of VP in South Africa and elsewhere have uniformly showed an autosomal dominant pattern of inheritance [1,8,10–15]. Penetrance is high and not altered by the presence or absence of symptoms in the parent who transmits the trait. Family studies suggest that the expressivity of the VP gene is less than 50 percent [8,11,13,14]. It is impossible to predict whether skin disease, visceral attacks, both, or neither will occur in the lifetime of a specific genetic carrier. It is not known whether the homozygous form of VP is compatible with life. Cartwright et al. [16] predicted that 10 to 12 marriages between two carriers of VP exist at the present time in South Africa; however, to date, the offspring of such a union have not been studied intensively.

Dean pointed out that the so-called Cape Coloured of South Africa, who are descendants of white European immigrants who intermarried with the native black population, may have VP and PCT in different members of the same family [1]. Watson et al. [17] reported fecal porphyrin excretion patterns consistent with VP and PCT in different members of one family of German-American ancestry.

In South Africa, both VP and PCT are quite common, and the coexistence of both types of porphyria in the same individual has been suggested by biochemical studies [18].

Etiology

The specific cause of VP has not been established. The search for a specific enzyme defect in VP has existed since 1965, when Tschudy et al. [19] found that the activity of hepatic δ-aminolevulinic acid synthase (ALA-S), the rate-limiting enzyme in heme biosynthesis, was markedly increased in the acute phase of AIP. Before 1973, VP was also believed to be an overproduction disease of ALA-S [20]. However, it was reported that activity of ALA-S was increased in hereditary coproporphyria (HC) as well, and this finding is now thought to be a secondary phenomenon in all forms of acute hepatic porphyria [21]. Diminished activity of uroporphyrinogen-1-synthase (URO-S) and coproporphyrinogen oxidase (COPRO-O) are currently held to be the primary enzymatic defects in AIP and HC, respectively [22,23] (Fig. 1).

Data relating to the specific enzymatic defect in VP is conflicting. Initially, ferrochelatase activity was reported to be normal in skeletal muscle of patients with VP [24]. Becker et al. [25] reported decreased activity of ferrochelatase in both intact and lysed normoblasts from patients with VP, but reduced activity of ferrochelatase only in lysed normoblasts of patients with erythropoietic protoporphyria (EPP). Skin fibroblasts from patients with VP also had reduced activity of this enzyme when compared to normal fibroblasts [26]. These authors hypothesized that patients with VP have a structural gene mutation coding for a stable but less active form of the enzyme, whereas patients with EPP have an unstable variant of the enzyme. However, Smith et al. [27], based on indirect evidence, proposed that protoporphyrinogen oxidase (PROTO-O), the enzyme that catalyzes the oxidation of protoporphyrinogen to PROTO, may be deficient in patients with VP (Fig. 1). Recently, Brenner and Bloomer [28] performed assays for ferrochelatase in intact and sonicated skin fibroblasts; in this system ferrochelatase activity was reduced in patients with EPP but not in patients with VP. Instead, PROTO-O was reduced to 43 percent of normal in sonicated skin fibroblasts from patients with VP. Thus, their data indicate normal ferrochelatase activity and a marked reduction in PROTO-O activity in patients with VP. Certainly, further investigation will be needed to clarify the enzymatic defects in VP.

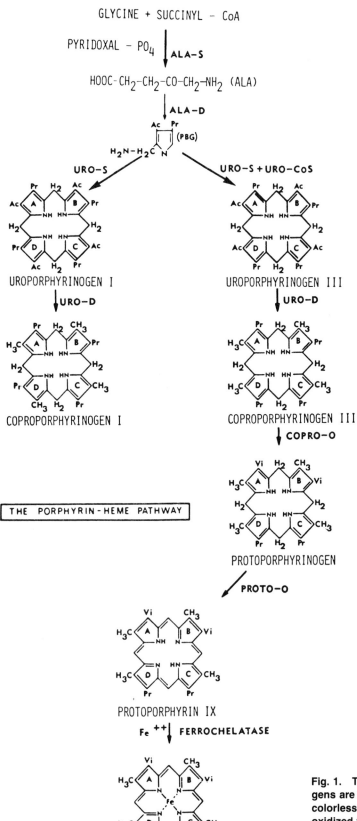

THE PORPHYRIN-HEME PATHWAY

Fig. 1.   The porphyrin-heme pathway. The porphyrinogens are the reduced form of the porphyrins. They are colorless nonfluorescing compounds which are readily oxidized to the corresponding porphyrins. ALA-S is the rate-limiting step in heme synthesis, except during an acute attack of porphyria, in which later enzymatic steps may become rate-limiting. Ac = acetic acid, Pr = propionic acid, Vi = vinyl.

A reduction in hepatocyte ferrochelatase activity in patients with VP could account for the excess PROTO in feces (Fig. 1). A defect in PROTO-O could also explain this porphyrin excretion pattern if protoporphyrinogen is released by the liver and oxidized to protoporphyrin in the bile or feces. However, Day et al. [29] have found low levels of COPRO and PROTO in hepatocytes of patients with VP. They hypothesize that the excess fecal porphyrins originate in the mucosa of the small intestine and colon. Direct evidence to support this theory is not available.

A reduction in activity of ferrochelatase or PROTO-O cannot explain the enhanced excretion of COPRO in the urine of patients with VP. Day and Eales [30] have assembled data from patients with chronic renal failure and from rats with experimental porphyria that suggest the kidney may be the source of excess COPRO excretion.

The acute attack of VP may be preceded by the following biochemical events [31,32]. A partial enzyme deficiency of either PROTO-O or ferrochelatase reduces free heme production and thereby causes derepression of ALA-S activity. Lipophilic chemicals such as allyl-containing barbiturates or ethynyl-substituted steroids are converted by the liver cytochrome P_{450} system, thus further depleting the free pool of heme and enhancing ALA-S activity. The consequence is a massive production of the porphyrin precursors, δ-aminolevulinic acid (ALA), and porphobilinogen (PBG). These porphyrin precursors may be directly neurotoxic to the nervous system [3,33]. Alternatively, defective heme metabolism within nerve tissue may produce dysfunction of the nervous system [34]. In either case, damage to the peripheral, autonomic, and bulbar nervous system is held to be responsible for almost all the clinical manifestations of acute porphyric attacks in VP.

Clinical Features

The age of onset of symptoms of VP ranges from 12 to 77 years, with most patients presenting during the third or fourth decades of life [4,35,36] (Table 1). Over 50 percent of South African patients have been shown to have cutaneous symptoms as their initial complaint [4]. Review of several large series of patients with symptomatic VP indicates that 80 percent demonstrate skin disease at some point in life [4,8,11,13,14]. The cutaneous manifestations occur equally in males and females [4]. The most common cutaneous symptom is fragility of the backs of the hands or face; minimal trauma induces separation of the epidermis from the dermis with formation of blisters and erosions (Fig. 2). Lesions heal with mild scars and milia formation. Secondarily infected lesions may produce more significant scarring. Hyperpigmentation and hypopigmentation may appear on the hands and face. Hirsutism in a periorbital distribution and scleroderma-like thickening of sun-exposed skin have been reported in patients from South Africa [37]. It is important to note that the cutaneous manifestations in patients with VP are indistinguishable from those that occur in patients with PCT.

Sunlight may exacerbate cutaneous manifestations in some patients with VP. Immediate photosensitivity, defined by the acute onset of pruritus, erythema, and edema after specific exposure to sunlight, is rare, but not unheard of, in patients with VP [2,37,38]. None of 53 Finnish patients reported by Mustajoki [11] had evidence of direct photosensitivity. In our experience from New England, immediate photosensitivity was not observed in eight patients with cutaneous features of VP (unpublished observation). In a large series from South Africa, Eales [37] recorded photosensitivity in 20 percent of patients with cutaneous symptoms of VP, but he did not specify whether such sensitivity was immediate or delayed.

Seasonal exacerbation of skin disease in sun-exposed sites is not uncommon in patients with VP. Eight of 17 patients with cutaneous VP had more severe skin fragility in the summer as compared to the winter [11]. In our experience, six of eight patients with cutaneous VP had exacerbation of skin symptoms in the summer (unpublished observation). Seasonal flaring of skin fragility and blistering may be due to delayed photosensitivity; alternatively, increased physical activity in the summer could be associated with more mechanical trauma to the skin leading to enhanced blistering.

Women with VP given estrogens may develop a drug-induced cholestatic hepatitis associated with an acute flare of blistering in sun-exposed skin [38–40]. In these individuals, porphyrin excretion is probably diverted from the bile to the blood and urine.

A relationship between the severity of skin disease and the likelihood or severity of acute attacks has not been found. Although skin manifestations most commonly precede an acute attack, they may occur at the same time as, or follow, the acute attack. Skin fragility or blistering was present in 77 percent of South Africans during the acute attack [41]. In contrast, Mustajoki [11] observed that Finnish patients with VP displayed

Table 1 Précis of variegate porphyria (VP)

Patients with VP have a heritable metabolic disease with cutaneous manifestations indistinguishable from those that occur in patients with porphyria cutanea tarda (PCT). However, acute attacks of visceral and neurologic symptoms related to autonomic, sensory, and motor neuropathy may occur in VP, but not in PCT. These acute episodes are often precipitated by drugs such as barbiturates or sulfonamides, with serious consequences, including fatality.

Epidemiology and Etiology

Age	Twenty to 50, not before puberty
Sex	Skin manifestations occur equally in males and females. Acute attacks predominate in females.
Heredity	Autosomal dominant with high penetrance and variable expressivity
Factors that Provoke acute attacks	Drugs, particularly barbiturates; hydantoin; griseofulvin, sulfonamides; hormone preparations containing estrogens and progestins; ethanol; infection; acute illness; and starvation
Induce skin disease	Rarely, estrogens, in the context of cholestasis resulting from this hormone

History

Skin symptoms	The period of onset and symptoms in the skin are identical to those that occur in PCT.
Systems review	A history of acute episodes of abdominal pain, nausea, vomiting, constipation, behavioral disturbances, paralysis, and seizures (similar to acute intermittent porphyria) may or may not be elicited. Adverse reactions to drugs and anesthetics may also be recalled.

Physical Examination

Skin lesions Type and distribution	Same as PCT
Abdomen (acute attack only)	Diffuse tenderness to palpation without peritoneal signs

Differential Diagnosis

	Patients who present only with skin manifestations are indistinguishable from PCT. Acute attacks in VP are similar to those that occur in acute intermittent porphyria, but skin findings are always absent in the latter disease.

Laboratory Examinations

Porphyrin studies	In feces: Increased coproporphyrin but especially protoporphyrin. These fecal porphyrins are elevated in almost all adults with the VP trait, in the presence or absence of any symptoms.
	In urine: Positive Watson-Schwartz test and increased porphobilinogen during systemic attacks with normal or slightly elevated values between attacks; coproporphyrin and uroporphyrin are elevated during the acute attack; coproporphyrin excretion may be increased and usually exceeds uroporphyrin excretion when skin manifestations are present without acute symptoms (in direct contrast to PCT, in which urinary uroporphyrin excretion exceeds coproporphyrin excretion).

Management

Acute attacks	Stop provoking drugs, give high carbohydrate diet, treat infections; supportive care for electrolyte and neurologic abnormalities, propranolol, hematin infusions

Table 1   Précis of variegate porphyria (VP) (*continued*)

Skin disease	No specific therapy is available. Protection from sun by use of clothes or opaque sunscreens may be helpful, as well as avoidance of mechanical trauma. Oral β-carotene (120–240 mg/day) may diminish the cutaneous responses to trauma (skin fragility of the sun-exposed skin).
Preventive measures	Affected individuals should be cautioned to avoid porphyrinogenic drugs as well as ethanol and low-carbohydrate diets. All adult family members should be screened for latent VP by testing the feces for protoporphyrin and coproporphyrin.

minimal skin manifestations. Fragility and blistering were infrequent, both during attacks and in remission. This difference may be due to less intense sunlight in Finland as compared to South Africa, but genetic differences cannot be excluded. The clinical significance is that patients from northern latitudes may be at greater risk of being misdiagnosed as having AIP, in which skin manifestations are totally absent. As a result, family members would not be screened appropriately with fecal porphyrin analysis and thus patients with latent VP would not be alerted to their diagnosis and the possible danger of porphyrinogenic drugs.

Review of the reported cases indicates that 16 percent of patients with VP present in an acute attack without cutaneous disease; about one-half of patients with symptomatic VP develop an acute attack in the course of their disease [4,11,41]. South African and Finnish investigators tabulated the most frequent symptoms and signs of the acute attack of VP [4,11,41]. These symptoms and signs are similar to those that occur in acute attacks of AIP and HC. The chief complaint is abdominal pain, present in almost all acute attacks. It is associated with extremity and back pain in 50 and 25 percent of cases, respectively. Nausea, vomiting, and constipation are observed in 60 to 80 percent of cases with acute attacks. A behavioral disturbance or confusional state occurs in a majority of cases. Seizures, stupor, and coma are present in a minority of patients. Eales et al. observed that limb pains may be precipitated by administration of certain drugs, leading to motor neuropathy and sometimes to generalized life-threatening quadriplegia and bulbar paralysis [4].

The signs and their frequency during an acute attack in patients with VP include tachycardia (85 percent), nonlocalized abdominal tenderness without rigidity (80 percent), dark urine (80 percent), hypertension (60 percent), motor neuropathy (63 to 80 percent), and bulbar paralysis (18 to 40 percent). Chemical abnormalities in the blood include hyponatremia, hypochloremia, hypokalemia, azotemia, and leukocytosis. Hyponatremia may be related to sodium losses from vomiting, but overzealous intravenous infusions of glucose in water, primary renal tubular sodium loss, and inappropriate secretion of antidiuretic hormone may also be responsible [4]. Radiographic examination of the abdomen often reveals dilated loops of bowel. The acute attack of VP must be differentiated from the acute hepatotoxic reaction that may occur in patients with PCT who are given large doses of antimalarial drugs [42].

Acute attacks may be precipitated by the ingestion of certain drugs, especially barbiturates [32,43–49] (Table 2). Patients with VP as well as those with AIP and HC may be vulnerable to these medications. Attacks tend to be most severe when multiple porphyrinogenic drugs have been administered over a short period of time [35]. Hormonal factors may be important as acute attacks do not occur before puberty and most attacks occur in women of childbearing age. The female/male ratio for acute attacks is 3:1 [4]. Acute attacks may be precipitated by the menstrual cycle or by pregnancy; however, this is more common in patients with AIP than with patients with VP [50,51]. Other provoking factors include infection, emotional stress, alcohol abuse, and low carbohydrate diets; at least 10 percent of acute attacks occur without a recognized precipitant, however [35]. Attacks do not always occur with exposure to a potentially dangerous drug; likewise, a history of tolerance to a particular drug does not preclude an acute attack on readministration [35,43,52]. Mustajoki and Heinonen [52] found that the risk of inducing an attack of VP was low when patients were given barbiturates during remission. The majority of patients had an acute worsening of their symptoms, however, if barbiturates were given during an acute attack [52].

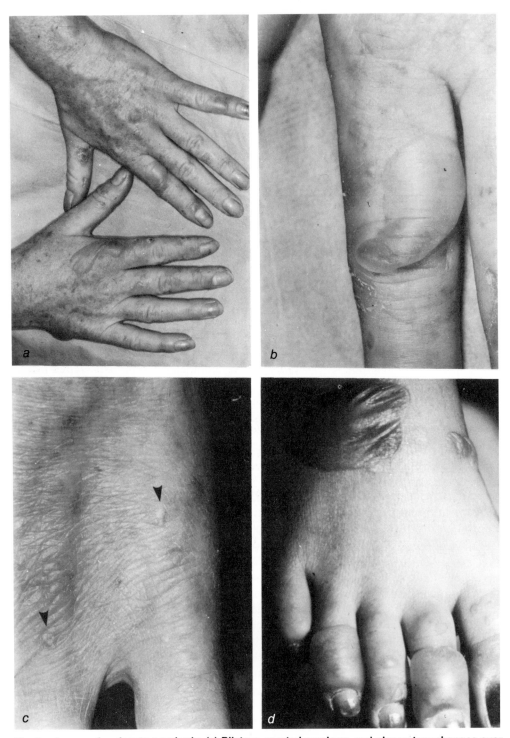

Fig. 2. A case of variegate porphyria. (*a*) Blisters, crusted erosions, and pigmentary changes over the dorsa of the hands and fingers. (*b*) Close-up view of index finger shows an intact blister with milia and pigmentary changes. (*c*) Healing phase shows milia (arrows) and pigmentary changes. (*d*) Large bullae of dorsum of foot and toes. *Note:* Patients with porphyria cutanea tarda have indistinguishable cutaneous findings.

The prognosis of the acute attack has been improved dramatically in the last 20 years. Virtually all deaths from VP were recorded before 1960, when the mortality rate from an acute attack exceeded 20 percent [11,41]. Although acute attacks continue to occur, there were no deaths in 53 patients who were followed by Mustajoki for an average of 6 years [11]. Similarly, Eales et al. have observed no deaths in a large group of patients with VP followed for an average of 9 years [4].

Table 2   Drugs potentially hazardous in patients with acute porphyrias*

Amphetamines
Analgesics
    Aminopyrine, antipyrine, amidopyrine, dichloralphenazone,
    diclophenac, phenylbutazone, fentanyl
Anesthetics
    Althesine, barbiturates (Pentothal), enflurane, halothane,
    methoxyflurane
Anticonvulsants
    Carbamazepine, diphenylhydantoin, ethosuximide,
    mephenytoin, methsuximide, phensuximide, primidone,
    trimethadione, valproate
Antihypertensives
    Clonidine, hydralazine, methyldopa, pargyline,
    phenoxybenzamine, spironolactone
Antimicrobial agents
    Chloramphenicol, griseofulvin, pyrazinamide, novobiocin,
    sulfonamides
Barbiturates
Chloroquine
Dapsone
Diethylpropion
Dramamine
Ergot preparations
Ethchlorvynol
Ethyl alcohol
Furosemide
Hormones
    Estrogens, progesterones
Hyoscine-*N*-butylbromide
Imipramine
Nikethamide
Nonbarbiturate hypnotics
    Chlormezanone, glutethimide, meprobamate, methyprylon,
    sulphonal, trional
Pentazocine
Pyrazinamide
Sedormid
Sulfonylureas
    Tolbutamide, chlorpropamide
Theophylline
Tranquilizers
    Chlordiazepoxide, clonazepam, diazepam, oxazepam,
    flurazepam

* This list includes drugs known to precipitate attacks of acute porphyria
in humans [43–45] as well as drugs shown to induce porphyrin
production or ALA-S activity in cell cultures or whole animals [46–49].

Increased awareness of the entity as well as advanced methods of supportive care for treatment of the acute attack may be responsible for these encouraging findings.

Various authors have reported patients with VP who complain of neuropsychiatric or abdominal symptoms in the absence of an acute attack [8,9,14,15,37]. These symptoms include headaches, depression, paresthesias, personality disorders, constipation, and abdominal pain. Relevant to these clinical observations is the finding of abnormal nerve conduction velocities in asymptomatic patients with acute hepatic porphyria [53].

However, the nonspecificity and high frequency of these symptoms in a normal population would appear to lessen their significance to the VP gene.

Barnes and Boshoff [54] performed ocular examinations on 38 South Africans of European ancestry with porphyria; many of these patients had VP, although biochemical data were not included in the study. They found eyelid scarring, blepharochalasis, symblepharon, conjunctival thickening, acute conjunctivitis, scleral ulcerations, and corneal scars in some of these patients. During the acute attack, patients had lesions of the fundus of two types: edematous cotton-wool patches and thin flat edematous films. Thirty years later, this ophthalmologic study still awaits confirmation.

Laboratory Diagnosis

Urine and fecal porphyrin analyses are important in separating VP from PCT, AIP, and HC (Tables 3 and 4). Qualitative analysis of the urine for PBG, such as the Watson-Schwartz test, is consistently positive during the acute attack of VP, AIP, or HC. False-negative results may be obtained, however, if the urine is allowed to stand too long. A positive test should always be followed up by quantitative urine examination for ALA and PBG [55–57]. Eales and Linder observed that the total porphyrin precursor excretion (ALA and PBG) correlated reasonably well with the severity of the acute attack of VP and diminished rapidly as an acute attack subsided [41,58]. During the quiescent phase of VP, the Watson-Schwartz test is usually negative and the urinary excretion of porphyrin precursors is normal or slightly elevated [11]. During the quiescent phase of AIP, however, the Watson-Schwartz test is positive and the urinary excretion of porphyrin precursors is significantly increased in most cases. The finding of increased PBG in the urine in patients with abdominal pain and a history of skin fragility often indicates VP. Conversely, the presence of an acute attack of abdominal symptoms with a negative Watson-Schwartz test suggests the absence of acute porphyria.

Quantitative analysis for uroporphyrin (URO) and COPRO fractions in the urine are helpful in the diagnosis of VP [55,57]. During an acute attack, both fractions are usually markedly elevated; the apparent increase in URO excretion is believed to be secondary to nonenzymatic conversion from PBG [4,5,11,41]. During remission, the COPRO fraction may be elevated, but the URO fraction is

Table 3   Distinguishing biochemical features of the hepatic porphyrias

Type of porphyria	Fecal porphyrins		Urine				Other features
			Precursors		Porphyrins		
	COPRO	PROTO	ALA	PBG	URO	COPRO	
AIP							
Latent	N to +	N to +	+	+	N	N to +	↓ URO-S
Acute	N to +	N to +	2+ to 3+	2+ to 4+	3+	2+	
VP							
Latent	2+	3+	N to +	N to +	N	N to 2+	↓ Ferrochelatase or PROTO-O;
Acute	3+	4+	2+ to 3+	2+ to 3+	3+	3+	↑ fecal X-porphyrin; ↑ plasma PU
PCT	1+ to 2+	N to +	N	N	4+	2+	↓ URO-D; ↑ ISOCOPRO in urine and feces; ↑ urine URO (I > III); ↑ 7-carboxyporphyrin (III > I)
HC							
Latent	3+ to 4+	N to +	N to +	N to +	N	N	↓ COPRO-O
Acute	3+ to 4+	N to +	2+ to 4+	2+ to 4+	2+	4+	

Note: N = Normal, + = above normal, 2+ = moderately increased, 3+ and 4+ = greatly increased; URO = uroporphyrin, COPRO = coproporphyrin, PROTO = protoporphyrin; AIP = acute intermittent porphyria, VP = variegate porphyria, PCT = porphyria cutanea tarda, HC = hereditary coproporphyria; ISOCOPRO = isocoproporphyrin, URO-S = uroporphyrinogen-1-synthase, URO-D = uroporphyrinogen decarboxylase, PROTO-O = protoporphyrinogen oxidase, COPRO-O = coproporphyrinogen oxidase.

usually normal; the URO/COPRO ratio is almost always less than 1. Asymptomatic patients with previous symptoms of VP and latent carriers may have entirely normal urine porphyrin analysis as measured by solvent extraction methods. In contrast, patients with active PCT excrete large amounts of URO in the urine with lesser amounts of COPRO; the URO/COPRO ratio is generally greater than 1. Wood's light (emitting 320 to 400 nm) examination of acidified fresh urine may reveal pink-red fluorescence in patients with either PCT or VP, but false-negative results are too common for one to rely exclusively on this screening test.

Fecal porphyrin tests should be performed in all patients suspected of having VP. Abnormal levels of fecal porphyrins may be qualitatively confirmed by examination of a stool specimen (nickel size) with a mixture of equal parts of amyl alcohol, glacial acetic acid, and ether. The solvent layer, upon Wood's light examination, shows marked orange-red fluorescence, indicative of abnormal levels of COPRO and PROTO. Qualitative stool tests are sensitive, but a false-positive result may occur in patients with PCT or gastrointestinal disorders [1,3,6]. Whenever possible, and certainly in the presence of a positive qualitative test, quantitative analysis of fecal COPRO and PROTO should be performed [57,59]. Stool specimens should be kept frozen until analysis can be performed. Adults with manifest VP tested either during an acute attack or during remission will have markedly increased fecal porphyrin excretion. Both the COPRO and PROTO fractions are increased, usually with a COPRO/PROTO ratio that is less than 1; the total of two fractions usually exceeds 200 μg/g dry weight of feces and is frequently in excess of 500 μg/g dry weight [4,6,11,36]. Patients with PCT have fecal porphyrin excretion of COPRO and PROTO that rarely exceeds 200 μg/g dry weight, and the COPRO/PROTO ratio is greater than 1 [6,60]. In addition, patients with PCT have enhanced excretion of fecal isocoproporphyrin, whereas patients with VP do not [61].

The diagnosis of latent VP in family members of patients with VP is made by demonstration of elevated fecal porphyrins. The lowest level of fecal porphyrin excretion necessary for a diagnosis of latent VP has not been determined [62]. Fecal porphyrin excretion may vary considerably from one collection to another in the same individual; patients suspected of having latent VP may require

Table 4   Procedures for evaluation of patients with variegate porphyria

Detailed family history
Skin biopsy of intact vesicle/bulla
Quantitative urine analysis for uroporphyrin and coproporphyrin (24-hr specimen, keep refrigerated)
Quantitative stool analysis for coproporphyrin and protoporphyrin (spot specimen, keep frozen until analysis)
Quantitative urine ALA and PBG (24-hr specimen)
Research methods
  Thin-layer chromatography
  High-pressure liquid chromatography
  Red blood cell ferrochelatase activity
  Skin fibroblast protoporphyrinogen oxidase activity

multiple stool examinations to demonstrate increased fecal porphyrins [62].

Urine and fecal porphyrin studies are almost always normal in children from families with VP. Subsequent testing of some of these individuals as adults will often demonstrate biochemical evidence of VP [11]. In addition, several investigators have reported normal biochemical studies in adult obligate genetic carriers [8,11,14,63]. Nevertheless, the fraction of adults with latent VP undetectable by solvent extraction methods is probably small.

Rimington et al. [64] found large amounts of a hydrophilic porphyrin-peptide complex they termed *porphyrin-X* in the feces of patients with VP. Elder et al. [65] demonstrated that porphyrin-X is also increased in the feces of patients with PCT; thus, the qualitative presence of porphyrin-X in stools cannot be used as a diagnostic test for VP. Chromatographic techniques subsequently showed that the porphyrin moiety in porphyrin-X is mostly hematoporphyrin in VP, and a mixture of uroporphyrin, 7-carboxyporphyrin, and isocoproporphyrin in PCT [4,65].

Several investigators have achieved excellent separation of porphyrins in samples of urine, plasma, feces, bile, and other tissues from patients with VP by first converting the porphyrins to their methyl esters and then using thin-layer chromatography [5,63,66–68]. In the urine and fecal specimens tested, a characteristic "fingerprint" pattern was obtained that distinguished VP from other forms of porphyria and confirmed the data previously obtained by extraction methods. Day et al. [68] combined thin-layer chromatography with enhancement of porphyrin fluorescence with a dodecane-hexadecane solvent to show that the plasma of patients with VP had a characteristic lipid-coproporphyrin complex called *PU*. It is present in the plasma of patients with latent VP as well as in those with manifest VP (personal communication, L. Eales).

Observations by Poh-Fitzpatrick and Lamola [69,70] showed that saline-diluted plasma specimens from patients with VP have characteristic fluorescence emission maxima that distinguish these patients from those with other forms of acute hepatic porphyria, PCT, erythropoietic protoporphyria, and lead poisoning. The method appears simple and may prove useful in the rapid diagnosis of VP; however, confirmation of this finding is needed.

Lastly, high-pressure liquid chromatography has allowed excellent separation of porphyrins from tissues of patients with VP [71]; the method is rapid but expensive.

Histopathology

The histopathology of skin lesions from patients with VP is indistinguishable from that observed in patients with PCT [72]. Examination of biopsy specimens shows subepidermal bullae with intact dermal papillae (Fig. 3). Elastosis and homogeneous thickening of vessels of the upper portion of the dermis are observed. Thickening of vessels is highlighted by PAS-positive diastase-resistant staining, which also may occur at the epidermal basement membrane zone. Direct immunofluorescence studies of skin from patients with PCT and VP show IgG, less commonly IgM or complement, around vessels and to a lesser extent at the epidermal basement membrane zone [72]. Deposition of these immunoreactants is most likely due to previous vessel damage rather than to a specific immune process. Electron microscopic examination of one case of VP showed reduplication of the basal lamina of vessels and the epidermal basement membrane zone, deposition of a fine fibrillar material in the upper dermis, and evidence of elastosis. The regeneration of basal lamina material is evidence for injury to endothelial and basal cells [72].

Differential Diagnosis

PCT must be differentiated from VP, since patients with PCT are not subject to life-threatening paralytic attacks, often provoked by drugs, as are patients with VP. The cutaneous and biochemical abnormalities in PCT respond to treatment with phlebotomy or low-dose chloroquine whereas such therapies are ineffective in VP [8,60]. Since the cutaneous and histopathologic features of PCT and VP are indistinguishable, reliable separation depends on accurate quantitative analysis of porphyrins in the urine and feces. Eales et al. have shown that almost all patients with VP and PCT from South Africa may be delineated by taking into consideration the results of both urine and fecal tests [36]. Thin-layer chromatography, high-pressure liquid chromatography, and emission fluorescence spectrophotometry are research techniques at the present time; they may prove useful in resolving diagnostic difficulties or in the diagnosis of latent VP. It cannot be overemphasized that the omission of fecal porphyrin analysis may result in the misdiagnosis of VP as PCT, with potentially fatal consequences for the undiagnosed VP patient who is given a porphyrinogenic drug.

VP must be differentiated also from AIP and

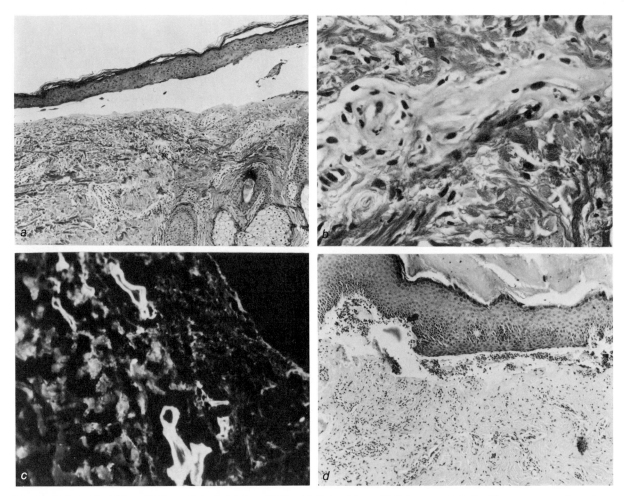

Fig. 3. Cutaneous histopathology of variegate porphyria. (*a*) Subepidermal blister associated with sparse lymphocytic dermal infiltrate in an early lesion. X 60. (*b*) Higher magnification of same biopsy specimen shows hyalinized thickening of superficial dermal vessels. X 400. (*c*) Direct immunofluorescence of same biopsy specimen shows deposition of IgG in vessel walls with a glassy or homogeneous pattern. X 250. (*d*) Subepidermal cleft with marked dermal sclerosis in a chronically sun-exposed site. Hemorrhage in the blister cavity and chronic inflammatory cells in the dermis are present. X 100. *Note:* Patients with porphyria cutanea tarda have indistinguishable cutaneous histopathologic and immunopathologic findings.

HC. Patients with AIP do not develop skin lesions; the cutaneous manifestations of HC are generally restricted to acute attacks. Reliable differentiation can be made by quantitative fecal porphyrin analysis or by enzyme assays for URO-S in red blood cells and COPRO-O in leukocytes [22,23].

Treatment

Prevention of acute attacks is of prime importance. Patients and their physicians should be given lists of potentially hazardous drugs (Table 2). Avoidance of barbiturates at the time of surgical procedures is especially important. Starvation-type diets and alcohol abuse should be discouraged. Patients should be observed for early signs of an acute attack during periods of illness, infection, fever, emotional stress, and pregnancy. Identifi-

cation bracelets are useful. Adult family members of a patient with VP should be screened by qualitative, or, if available, quantitative porphyrin analysis of the feces. Patients with latent VP should follow the same precautions advised for those with manifest disease.

Treatment of the acute attack includes early hospitalization and withdrawal of any provoking drugs [4,31,43,73]. Supportive care includes rehydration when nausea and vomiting are severe and appropriate restriction of free water in the presence of hyponatremia. Intubation should be performed at the first sign of respiratory failure. Patients often respond to intravenous and oral loading with carbohydrates; this so-called glucose effect may be due to suppression of ALA-S activity in the liver [4,74]. Beta blockers such as propranolol ameliorate symptoms of tachycardia and hypertension [3,75,76]. Infusions of hematin have shown therapeutic promise in the United States in patients with acute attacks of AIP and VP [77]. The drug is taken up by hepatocytes and appears to replenish the free heme pool, resulting in reduced ALA-S activity. A common side effect of hematin infusions is phlebothrombosis.

Drugs considered safe to give patients with an acute attack of VP include morphine and meperidine for pain; phenothiazines for nausea or behavioral disturbances; ether and nitrous oxide for anesthesia; bromides for seizures; and penicillins for infection. Extensive lists of drugs for specific use in patients with acute attacks of porphyria are available [45].

Specific treatment for cutaneous manifestations of VP has not been discovered. In an uncontrolled study we have observed a striking amelioration of blistering of sun-exposed skin in two patients with VP who were given β-carotene (Solatene) in divided doses of 180 to 210 mg/day. Both of these patients had previously observed summer exacerbation of their skin fragility and blistering. In contrast, South African physicians have had mixed results with β-carotene and a related drug, canthaxanthin [78]; Eales does not believe these drugs to be efficacious. Chloroquine has not helped in two patients with VP [8,79]. At the present time, therapy of skin disease is directed toward avoidance of skin trauma, protection from sunlight by use of opaque clothing or sunscreens, and oral β-carotene.

References

1. Dean G: *The Porphyrias: A Story of Inheritance and Environment,* 2nd ed. Lippincott, Philadelphia, 1971
2. Mustajoki P: Variegate porphyria. *Ann Intern Med* **89**:238–244, 1978
3. Kramer S: Porphyria variegata. *Clin Haematol* **9**:303–322, 1980
4. Eales L et al: The clinical and biochemical features of variegate porphyria: an analysis of 300 cases studied at Groote Schuur Hospital, Cape Town. *Int J Biochem* **12**:837–853, 1980
5. Elder GH: The porphyrias: clinical chemistry, diagnosis, methodology. *Clin Haematol* **9**:371–398, 1980
6. Eales L et al: The place of screening tests and quantitative investigations in the diagnosis of the porphyrias, with particular reference to variegate and symptomatic porphyria. *S Afr Med J* **40**:63–71, 1966
7. Dean GD, Barnes HD: Porphyria in Sweden and South Africa. *S Afr Med J* **33**:246–253, 1959
8. Fromke VL et al: Porphyria variegata: study of a large kindred in the United States. *Am J Med* **65**:80–88, 1978
9. Corey TJ et al: Variegate porphyria: clinical and laboratory features. *J Am Acad Dermatol* **2**:36–43, 1980
9a. Observations of New England families with VP will appear in *JAMA* 1982 (in press)
10. Eales L et al: The clinical biochemistry of the human

11. Mustajoki P: Variegate porphyria: twelve years' experience in Finland. *Q J Med* **49**:191–203, 1980
12. Eales L: The common cutaneous porphyrias of South Africa: studies of symptomatic and variegate porphyria considered against the background of African and world experience, in *Essays on Tropical Dermatology,* vol II. Edited by J Marshall. Excerpta Medica, Amsterdam, 1971, pp 129–153
13. Husquinet H et al: Porphyria variegata. A study of a large family. *J Genet Hum* **26**:367–383, 1978
14. Hamnström B et al: Three Swedish families with porphyria variegata. *Br Med J* **4**:449–453, 1967
15. Tu J et al: Clinical and biochemical studies of hereditary hepatic porphyria in Chinese subjects in Taiwan. *Metabolism* **20**:629–641, 1971
16. Cartwright JD et al: Porphyria variegata—studies of an affected couple and their children. *S Afr Med J* **53**:669–671, 1978
17. Watson CJ et al: Porphyria variegata and porphyria cutanea tarda in siblings: chemical and genetic aspects. *Proc Natl Acad Sci USA* **72**:5126–5129, 1975
18. Day RS et al: Co-existent variegata and symptomatic porphyria in South African families. *South African Medical Research Council News* **10**:1–2, 1978
19. Tschudy DP et al: Acute intermittent porphyria: the first "overproduction disease" localized to a specific enzyme. *Proc Natl Acad Sci USA* **53**:841–847, 1965
20. Dowdle EB et al: δ-Aminolaevulinic acid synthetase activity in normal and porphyric human livers. *S Afr Med J* **41**:1093–1096, 1967
21. McIntyre N et al: Hepatic δ-aminolaevulinic acid synthetase in an attack of hereditary coproporphyria and during remission. *Lancet* **1**:560–564, 1971
22. Magnussen CR et al: A red cell enzyme method for the diagnosis of acute intermittent porphyria. *Blood* **44**:857–868, 1974
23. Brodie MJ et al: Hereditary coproporphyria: demonstration of the abnormalities in haem biosynthesis in peripheral blood. *Q J Med* **46**:229–241, 1977
24. Pimstone N et al: Enzymatic defects in hepatic porphyria: preliminary observations in patients with porphyria cutanea tarda and variegate porphyria. *Enzyme* **16**:354–366, 1973
25. Becker DM et al: Reduced ferrochelatase activity: a defect common to porphyria variegata and protoporphyria. *Br J Haematol* **36**:171–179, 1977
26. Viljoen DJ et al: Reduced ferrochelatase activity in fibroblasts from patients with porphyria variegata. *Am J Hematol* **6**:185–190, 1979
27. Smith SG et al: Incubation of double labelled coproporphyrinogen with chicken red cell haemolysates, chemical and TLC fractionation of extracts. *Ann Clin Res* **8(Suppl 17)**:53–55, 1976
28. Brenner DA, Bloomer JR: The enzymatic defect in variegate porphyria: studies with human cultured skin fibroblasts. *N Engl J Med* **302**:765–769, 1980
29. Day RS et al: Hepatic porphyrins in variegate porphyria. *N Engl J Med* **303**:1368, 1980
30. Day RS, Eales L: Porphyrins in chronic renal failure. *Nephron* **26**:90–95, 1980
31. Brodie MJ, Goldberg A: Acute hepatic porphyrias. *Clin Haematol* **9**:253–272, 1980
32. Smith AG, De Matteis F: Drugs and the hepatic porphyrias. *Clin Haematol* **9**:399–425, 1980
33. Becker DM, Kramer S: The neurological manifestations

of porphyria: a review. *Medicine (Baltimore)* 56:411–423, 1977

34. Shanley BC et al: Pathogenesis of neural manifestations in acute porphyria. *S Afr Med J* 51:458–460, 1977

35. Eales L: Acute porphyria: the precipitating and aggravating factors. *S Afr J Lab Clin Med, Special Issue,* 17:120–125, 1971

36. Eales L et al: The diagnostic importance of faecal porphyrins in the differentiation of the porphyrias: values in the cutaneous porphyrias. *S Afr J Lab Clin Med* 9:126–136, 1963

37. Eales L: Cutaneous porphyria: observations on 111 cases in three racial groups. *S Afr J Lab Clin Med* 6:63–94, 1960

38. McKenzie AWP, Acharya U: The oral contraceptive and variegate porphyria. *Br J Dermatol* 86:453–457, 1972

39. Dean G: Oral contraceptives in porphyria variegata. *S Afr Med J* 39:278–280, 1965

40. Fowler CJ, Ward JM: Porphyria variegata provoked by contraceptive pill. *Br Med J* 1:663–664, 1975

41. Eales L: Porphyria as seen in Cape Town. A survey of 250 patients and some recent studies. *S Afr J Lab Clin Med* 9:151–162, 1963

42. Felsher BF, Bedeker AG: Effects of chloroquine on hepatic uroporphyrin metabolism in patients with porphyria cutanea tarda. *Medicine (Baltimore)* 45:575–583, 1966

43. Eales L: Porphyria and the dangerous life-threatening drugs. *S Afr Med J* 56:914–917, 1979

44. Wetterberg L: Report on an international survey of safe and unsafe drugs in acute intermittent porphyria, in *Supplement to the Proceedings of the First International Porphyrin Meeting "Porphyrins in Human Disease."* Edited by M Doss, P Nawrocki. Karger, Basel, 1976, pp 191–202

45. Moore MR: International review of drugs in acute porphyria—1980. *Int J Biochem* 12:1089–1097, 1980

46. Blekkenhorst GH et al: Screening of certain anaesthetic agents for their ability to elicit acute porphyric phases in susceptible patients. *Br J Anaesth* 52:759–762, 1980

47. Blekkenhorst GH et al: Drug safety in porphyria. *Lancet* 1:1367, 1980

48. Anderson KE: Effects of antihypertensive drugs on hepatic heme biosynthesis, and evaluation of ferrochelatase inhibitors to simplify testing of drugs for heme pathway induction. *Biochim Biophys Acta* 543:313–327, 1978

49. Marks GS: The effect of chemicals on hepatic heme biosynthesis. Differences in response to porphyrin-inducing chemicals between chick embryo liver cells, the 17-day-old chick embryo and other species, in *Heme and Hemoproteins: Handbook of Experimental Pharmacology,* vol 44. Edited by F De Matteis, WN Aldridge. Springer-Verlag, Berlin, 1978, pp 201–237

50. Brodie MJ et al: Pregnancy and the acute porphyrias. *Br J Obstet Gynaecol* 84:726–731, 1977

51. Tschudy DP et al: Acute intermittent porphyria: clinical and selected research aspects. *Ann Intern Med* 83:851–864, 1975

52. Mustajoki P, Heinonen J: General anesthesia in "inducible" porphyrias. *Anesthesiology* 53:15–20, 1980

53. Mustajoki P, Seppäläinen AM: Neuropathy in latent hereditary hepatic porphyria. *Br Med J* 2:310–312, 1975

54. Barnes HD, Boshoff PH: Ocular lesions in patients with porphyria. *Arch Ophthalmol* 48:567–580, 1952

55. Rimington C: Quantitative determination of porphobilinogen and porphyrins in urine and porphyrins in faeces and erythrocytes. *Association of Clinical Pathologists,* broadsheet 70 (revised broadsheet 36), August 1971

56. Mauzerall D, Granick S: The occurrence and determination of δ-aminolaevulinic acid and porphobilinogen in urine. *J Biol Chem* 219:435–446, 1956

57. Schwartz S et al: Determinations of porphyrins in biological materials, in *Methods of Biochemical Analysis,* vol 8. Edited by D Glick. Interscience, New York, 1960, pp 221–293

58. Eales L, Linder GC: Porphyria—the acute attack. An analysis of 80 cases. *S Afr Med J* 36:284–292, 1962

59. Holti G et al: An investigation of "porphyria cutanea tarda." *Q J Med* 27:1–17, 1958

60. Muhlbauer JE, Pathak MA: Porphyria cutanea tarda. *Int J Dermatol* 18:767–780, 1979

61. Elder GH: Differentiation of porphyria cutanea tarda symptomatica from other types of porphyria by measurement of isocoproporphyrin in faeces. *J Clin Pathol* 28:601–607, 1975

62. Cochrane AL, Goldberg A: A study of faecal porphyrin levels in a large family. *Ann Hum Genet* 32:195–208, 1968

63. Perrot H et al: Faecal porphyrin excretion in various types of porphyria. Thin layer chromatographic study. *Arch Dermatol Res* 263:67–73, 1978

64. Rimington C et al: The excretion of porphyrin-peptide conjugates in porphyria variegata. *Clin Sci* 35:211–247, 1968

65. Elder GH et al: Faecal "X porphyrin" in the hepatic porphyrias. *Enzyme* 17:29–38, 1974

66. Day RS et al: Quantitation of red cell porphyrins by fluorescence scanning after thin-layer chromatography. *Clin Chim Acta* 89:25–33, 1978

67. Grosser Y, Eales L: Patterns of faecal porphyrin excretion in the hepatocutaneous porphyrias. *S Afr Med J* 47:2162–2168, 1973

68. Day RS et al: The diagnostic value of blood plasma porphyrin methyl ester profiles produced by quantitative TLC. *Int J Biochem* 9:897–904, 1978

69. Poh-Fitzpatrick MB, Lamola AA: Direct spectrofluorometry of diluted erythrocytes and plasma: a rapid diagnostic method in primary and secondary porphyrinemias. *J Lab Clin Med* 87:362–370, 1976

70. Poh-Fitzpatrick MB: A plasma porphyrin fluorescence marker for variegate porphyria. *Arch Dermatol* 116:543–547, 1980

71. Gray CH et al: The differentiation of the porphyrias by means of high pressure liquid chromatography. *Clin Chim Acta* 77:167–178, 1977

72. Epstein JH et al: Cutaneous changes in the porphyrias. *Arch Dermatol* 107:689–698, 1973

73. Sergay SM: Management of neurologic exacerbations of hepatic porphyria. *Med Clin North Am* 63:453–463, 1979

74. Perlroth MG et al: The effect of diet in variegate (South African genetic) porphyria. *Metabolism* 17:571–581, 1968

75. Atsmon A et al: Treatment of an acute attack of porphyria variegata with propranolol. *S Afr Med J* 46:311–314, 1972

76. Blum I, Atsmon A: Reduction of porphyrin excretion in porphyria variegata by propranolol. *S Afr Med J* 50:898–899, 1976

77. Watson CJ et al: Use of hematin in the acute attack of the "inducible" hepatic porphyrias. *Adv Intern Med* 23:265–286, 1978

78. Eales L: The effects of canthaxanthin on the photocutaneous manifestations of porphyria. *S Afr Med J* 54:1050–1052, 1978

79. Cramers M, Jepsen LV: Porphyria variegata: failure of chloroquin treatment. *Acta Derm Venereol (Stockh)* 60:89–91, 1980

MASTOCYTOSIS
Chemical Mediators
and Therapeutic
Interventions

Robert A. Lewis

K. Frank Austen

The similarity in normal pulmonary mast cells and cutaneous mastocytosis cells of histamine and heparin content and capacity to generate prostaglandin D_2 (PGD_2) suggests that much of the recent information concerning human pulmonary mast cells may be relevant to understanding the full complex of symptoms and signs in mastocytosis. In addition, it is possible to offer a rationale for and clinical experience with new therapeutic interventions in mastocytosis, namely cromolyn, cimetidine, and nonsteroidal anti-inflammatory drugs.

Definition

Mastocytosis is an uncommon disease of mast cell proliferation, which occurs in both cutaneous and systemic forms. Since the mast cell is a connective tissue cell, the systemic disease has been reported to directly involve virtually all organs except the central nervous system. The most common locations for excess mast cells are skin, bone, gastrointestinal tract, liver, spleen, and lymph nodes. Mast cells in lesional sites are generally identifiable by their metachromatic granules when histologic sections are stained with basic thionine dyes.

Incidence and Prevalence

Fewer than 1000 cases of mastocytosis have been reported in the literature. As the hallmark of this disease is based on cutaneous manifestations, over 95 percent of mastocytosis patients are said to have skin lesions [1]. However, the actual percentage of patients with visceral mastocytosis and lacking the dermatologic stigmata may be underestimated, based upon the recent description of patients with cardiovascular manifestations and no fixed cutaneous lesions [2]. The first occurrence of cutaneous lesions is more prevalent in early childhood than after maturity and is not sex-linked for any age of onset [3]. Visceral disease is not commonly associated with skin lesions arising in infancy or early childhood. However, approximately one-quarter of individuals with adult-onset cutaneous lesions have visceral involvement [1].

Clinical Manifestations

Mastocytosis lesions of the skin are designated urticaria pigmentosa. The lesions may be isolated mastocytomas or generalized and multiple (Fig. 1), and they are generally reddish brown and plaquelike or nodular. Much less common are the telangiectatic and the doughy-feeling erythrodermic forms. When a cutaneous lesion is stroked firmly, it often becomes pruritic and raised with surrounding erythema (Darier's sign). Stroked cutaneous lesions of very young children with the disease may vesiculate. In up to 50 percent of patients, stroking of macroscopically uninvolved skin produces a wheal of dermographia due to microscopic dermal mastocytosis. However, gen-

eralized pruritus and flushing may occur with or without cutaneous lesions.

Systemic symptoms of an acute nature (Table 1) reflect a sudden and greatly elevated level of released mast cell mediators. An acute symptomatic systemic episode may focus on the vasculature and present with headache, flushing, dizziness, tachycardia, hypotension, syncope and even frank shock, rarely irreversible and fatal, and/or on the gastrointestinal tract, causing anorexia, nausea, vomiting, and diarrhea. Occasionally rhinorrhea and, rarely, audible wheezing occur, reminiscent of the signs of rhinitis and asthma, respectively.

More chronic problems include ill-defined neuropsychiatric symptoms, ranging from malaise to decreased attention span and irritability, and such gastrointestinal manifestations as malabsorption [4] or even a possible predilection for peptic ulceration [1]. Malabsorption with or without steatorrhea may be due to the chronic release of mediators from mast cells infiltrating small bowel mucosa and lamina propria. Hepatomegaly or hepatosplenomegaly occurs in about 5 to 10 percent of patients and is directly related to infiltrative disease of those organs [5]. Biopsy specimens in patients with hepatomegaly may reveal periportal proliferation of mast cells, eosinophil infiltration, and fibrosis [6], and these findings may account for the rare manifestations of portal hypertension and gastroesophageal varices. More than 10 percent of all mastocytosis patients, and a greater proportion of those with systemic disease, are estimated to have osseous lesions [7], most commonly in the pelvis, ribs, vertebrae, skull, and proximal long bones. Bone pain may occur with or without pathologic fractures. Anemia, leukopenia, thrombocytopenia, and even mast cell leu-

Fig. 1. Skin lesions of mastocytosis.

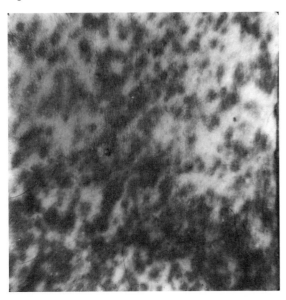

Table 1   Clinical manifestations of mastocytosis

Cutaneous	Reddish-brown papules
	Flush
Cardiovascular	Tachycardia, hypotension, and syncope (rarely fatal)
Gastrointestinal	Nausea, vomiting, diarrhea (exacerbated by alcohol)
	Malabsorption (rare)
	Portal hypertension (rare)
Bone	Pain
Neurologic	Neuropsychiatric symptoms (malaise, irritability)
Respiratory	Rhinorrhea, wheezing (rare)
Hematologic	Anemia, leukopenia, thrombocytopenia (rare)
	Eosinophilia
	Coagulopathies
	Leukemia (rare)

kemia have been rarely reported in association with severe bone marrow infiltration by mast cells.

Pathobiology

When mast cells degranulate, they both release their preformed granule-associated mediators [8] and generate PGD_2 [9,10] (Table 2). These cells are abnormal in number in mastocytosis, but not in the types or concentrations of mediators contained or generated per mast cell [11]. The apparent ease with which the cells degranulate in response to physical stimuli, such as gentle stroking (Darier's sign) and moderate heat or cold, and to chemical stimuli known to be histamine releasers, such as codeine and radiopaque dyes, is most likely due to the quantities of products released by the increased mast cell numbers rather than some unusual fragility or responsiveness. Once a skin lesion urticates, it requires up to 3 days to regenerate adequate granule histamine to form a second wheal at that site.

The heparin released from concentrations of mastocytoma cells has been implicated in the prolonged local bleeding time at the sites of excised lesions, the occasional purpura underlying cutaneous mastocytomas, and the rare incidence of significant gastrointestinal bleeds related to local mast cell infiltration. The moderate eosinophilia noted in 10 to 20 percent of mastocytosis patients does not have a mechanistic explanation at present, while the prominent association of tissue eosinophilia with mastocytosis lesions in bone and in periportal spaces most likely reflects the action of eosinophilotactic granule peptides [12,13] and the generation from arachidonate of monohydroxyeicosatetraenoic acids (HETEs) [14,15] and leukotriene B_4 [16,17]. The development of osseous lesions which are porotic and sclerotic [18] may relate to the action of mast cell tryptase [19,20] and acid hydrolases [20,21] on extracellular proteoglycans. Hepatic periportal fibrosis may also be a result of the action of these enzymes.

Table 2 Pathobiologic factors in mastocytosis

Histamine	Urticaria
	Gastrointestinal symptoms
PGD_2	Flush
	Cardiovascular symptoms
	Gastrointestinal symptoms
Heparin	Bleeding at biopsy site
	Purpura and hemorrhage (rare)
Neutral protease and acid hydrolases	Patchy hepatic fibrosis
	Bone lesions

Prior to the recognition of the lipid mediators, the majority of the manifestations of mastocytosis were ascribed to effects of released histamine. The primacy of histamine in causing local cutaneous whealing and pruritus as well as rhinitis, when it occurs, remains likely. However, the causative mediators of vasodilation and of the spectrum of gastrointestinal symptoms in this disease are likely multiple. Because the combined use of antihistamines of both the classical H-1 antagonist group, such as chlorpheniramine maleate, and the more recently described H-2 antagonists, exemplified by cimetidine, has failed to control either the gastrointestinal symptoms or the hypotension in some mastocytosis patients, the identification of a vasodilating prostaglandin (PGD_2) may be relevant to both pathophysiology and therapy.

Arachidonic acid, a 20-carbon fatty acid with four olefinic bonds, is released from perturbated mast cell plasma membrane phospholipid stores by the actions of one or more acyl hydrolases, as exemplified by phospholipase A_2 [22]. The free fatty acid is then metabolized via the cyclooxygenase pathway in rat peritoneal mast cells to PGD_2 and prostacyclin (PGI_2) (Fig. 2), with the former being the predominant product by almost an order of magnitude [9]. In human mast cells dispersed from lung parenchyma, only PGD_2 is generated via the cyclooxygenase pathway after immunologic activation with anti-IgE antibody [10]. Further, elevated levels of PGD_2 metabolites have been detected in urines obtained from mastocytosis patients with flushing, hypotension, and even shock in the absence of cutaneous lesions [2]. An initial report described measurement by gas chromatography–mass spectrometry (GC–MS) of one urinary metabolite, 9α-hydroxy-11,15-dioxo-2,3,4,5-tetranorprostane-1,20-dioic acid (PGD-M₁) (Fig. 2), from two such patients, as contrasted to the undetectable levels of this metabolite in urines of over 200 normal individuals [23]. Elevated urinary excretion of a second metabolite, 9α-hydroxy-11,15-dioxo-2,3,18,19-tetranorprost-5-ene-1,20-dioic acid (PGD-M₂) (Fig. 2), also described in the first two patients, was quantitated from an additional eight mastocytosis patients with attacks of flushing and dizziness [2]. Since PGD_2 has been shown to be potent as both a vasodilator and a bronchoconstrictor in the dog [24], the release of the compound from lesional mast cells may be causatively related to the flushing and hypotension and the less-common wheezing described in patients with this disease. Since these same patients also excreted increased amounts of histamine, the relative clinical effects of histamine and PGD_2 can

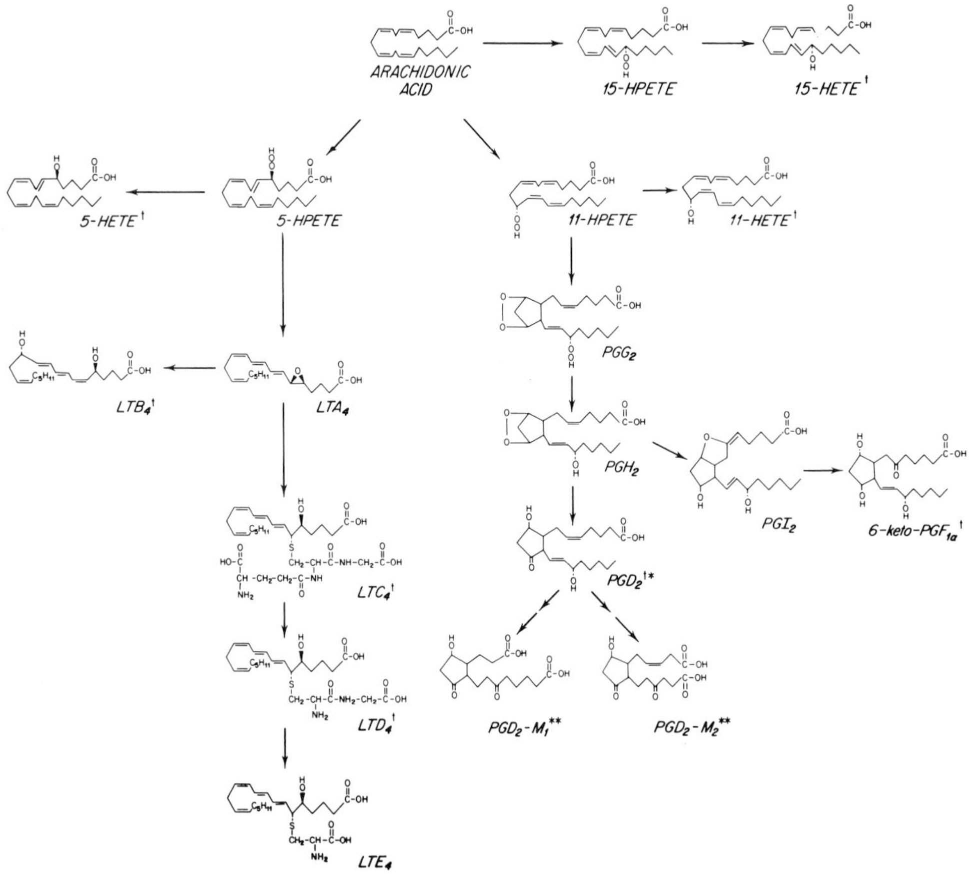

Fig. 2. Mast cell pathways of oxidative metabolism of arachidonic acid. Products identified from rat mast cells (†), human mast cells (*), and mastocytosis patient urines (**).

only be surmised from data on therapeutic intervention noted below. Further, the importance of quantities of histamine and PGD$_2$ released in the tissue locations of mastocytosis are not known and do not necessarily correlate with those levels of each compound measured in the urine.

In addition to PGD$_2$, a number of other biologically active oxidative metabolites of arachidonic acid have been appreciated in extracts and release supernatants of rat serosal mast cells incubated with the calcium ionophore A23187. Among these compounds are included several products of the 5-lipoxygenase pathway: the granulocyte-chemotactic lipid 5(S)-hydroxy-6,8,11,14-eicosatetraenoic acid (5-HETE) and the slow-reacting substance leukotrienes (LTs) 5(S)-hydroxy-6(R)-S-glutathionyl-7, 9-trans-11,14-cis-eicosatetraenoic acid (LTC$_4$), and 5(S)-hydroxy-6(R)-S-cysteinylglycyl-7, 9-trans-11,14-cis-eicosatetraenoic acid (LTD$_4$) [25,26] (Fig. 2). LTC$_4$ and LTD$_4$ have been generated in mast cell–containing human lung fragments by IgE-dependent activation for histamine release [27]. Both LTC$_4$ and LTD$_4$ evoke peripheral airway bronchospasm in guinea pigs and humans [28,29] and also increase vasopermeability in both species [28,30]. The 15-lipoxygenase product 15-HETE and 11-HETE, which is a cyclooxygenase metabolite and possibly a product of a specific lipoxygenase, are both modest granulocyte chemotactic factors and are produced by ionophore-stimulated rat mast cells [31]. None of these compounds or their known metabolites has been measured in biologic fluids from patients with mastocytosis. It is nonetheless possible that administration of nonsteroidal anti-inflammatory drugs to these patients may not only decrease PGD$_2$ generation by inhibiting the cyclooxygenase, but also increase the biosynthesis of lipoxygenase products by redirecting available arachidonic acid as substrate for the latter pathways.

Diagnosis

While the cutaneous lesions in conjunction with Darier's sign are pathognomonic, especially with biopsy confirmation of mastocytosis (Fig. 3), additional criteria are helpful in establishing the

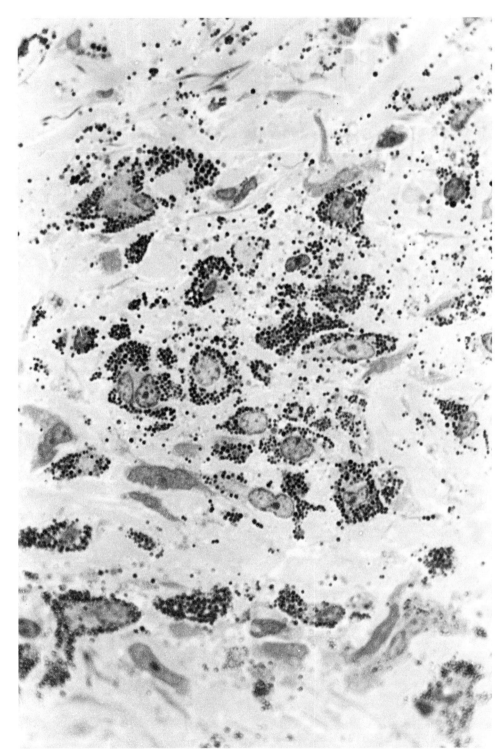

Fig. 3.   A 1-μm epon-embedded, Giemsa-stained lesional skin biopsy specimen, showing mast cell proliferation in the dermis. X 520. *(Photomicrography by John P. Caulfield, M.D.)*

diagnosis, especially in the absence of skin lesions (Table 3). Osseous infiltration by mast cells may be suspected from radiologic lesions with adjacent areas of osteoporosis and mottled osteosclerosis and proved by bone marrow biopsy, demonstrating areas of abnormally high mast cell numbers, along with rarefaction of the spongiosa or, alternatively, myelofibrosis and sclerosis. In the absence of radiologic abnormalities, ^{99}Tc bone scans may define areas of increased radionuclide uptake [32].

Table 3 Diagnosis of mastocytosis

Darier's sign
Tissue biopsy enriched for mast cells
Skin
Bone marrow
24-Hr urine collection
Histamine
Increased to > 50 μg/24 hr
9α-Hydroxy-11,15-dioxo-2,3,18,19-tetranorprost-5-ene-1,20-dioic acid
Increased to > 350 ng/24 hr
5-Hydroxyindoleacetic acid
Generally normal

Bone marrow aspiration or biopsy may be positive for increased numbers of mast cells even without localizing laboratory findings. Histaminuria of 2 to 3 times normal 24-hr levels (36 ± 15 μg) [33] is common among patients with extensive cutaneous involvement with or without acute symptoms of visceral disease, although both episodic normal values and striking elevations of over 1000 μg per 24 hr occur. Twenty-four-hour urinary excretions of 9α-hydroxy-11,15-dioxo-2,3,18,19-tetranorprost-5-ene-1,20-dioic acid, even during asymptomatic periods, may range from 1.5- to 120-fold above normal levels of 286 ± 75 ng [2].

For the patient with flushing, intermittent hypotension, diarrhea, tachycardia, and possibly hepatomegaly and peptic ulceration, the main differential diagnosis is with the carcinoid syndrome. The most direct criterion is a biopsy demonstrating mast cell proliferation, as opposed to argentaffin cell infiltration in an involved organ. Failing this, the measurement of grossly elevated levels of histamine and its metabolites in the urine favors mastocytosis, while elevated urinary levels of 5-hydroxyindoleacetic acid (5-HIAA) are noted in carcinoid syndrome. However, it should be recalled that gastric carcinoids lead to increased urinary excretion of both histamine and 5-HIAA [34] and that elevated urinary 5-HIAA have been reported in mastocytosis, although rarely [35].

Treatment

Treatment of patients with asymptomatic cutaneous lesions may be unnecessary or limited to H-1 antihistamines if pruritus and whealing are bothersome and can be controlled by such an agent. The addition of an H-2 blocker, cimetidine, has been reported to be helpful [36], but the efficacy of a combination of H-1 and H-2 blockers has not been established by any controlled studies or objective measurements.

Drugs known to cause mast cell degranulation,

such as alcohol, morphine, and codeine, are to be prohibited. The former is well described to exacerbate diarrhea, occasionally to the extent of a malabsorption syndrome, in patients with intestinal mastocytosis. It is particularly for the gastrointestinal symptoms that oral therapy with disodium cromoglycate (cromolyn), given at 100 mg 4 times daily has been effective in a double-blind controlled trial [33]. While the mode of cromolyn action is incompletely defined, it is thought to prevent mast cell degranulation by interfering with cellular calcium flux [37]. As less than 2 percent of the drug is known to be absorbed, a local action on the gastrointestinal mast cell proliferative infiltrate seems likely. It is less convenient to explain the therapeutic effects of this agent in decreasing cutaneous symptoms of pruritus, whealing, and flushing, as well as normalization of some of the neuropsychiatric complaints [33]. Cromolyn may prove useful in combination with antihistamines and aspirin, but this is unproved and the introduction of a nonsteroidal agent requires the precautions noted below.

Since aspirin and other nonsteroidal anti-inflammatory drugs (NSAIDs) inhibit prostaglandin synthesis, it is reasonable to relax judiciously the previous prohibition of aspirin use in these patients, with careful monitoring and pretreatment with H-1 and H-2 blockers. The occasional reports of hypotensive episodes induced by administration of aspirin and other NSAIDs seem valid on the basis of a repetitive episode with a second administration [38,39]. Thus, because of the theoretical possibilities of effecting increases in both lipoxygenase product synthesis by diversion of arachidonate and mast cell histamine release by augmentation of secretion with NSAIDs, it is advisable to administer therapeutic doses of both H-1 and H-2 antihistamines prior to the use of aspirin and then to employ very small initial doses of the latter agent. In a recently employed protocol for use in adult mastocytosis patients, therapy was initiated with 8 mg chlorpheniramine maleate and 300 mg cimetidine 4 times daily. After 2 days, aspirin therapy was added at initial doses of 16 mg (0.25 gr) 4 times daily, and the dose doubled on each subsequent day until either symptomatic relief was achieved or the side effect of tinnitus required maintenance at that dose [2,23]. In these patients, the minimum therapeutic aspirin dose, in combination with the antihistamines, is then maintained chronically. Of eight patients treated on this protocol for 1 to 15 months, none has reported severe flushing or hypotensive episodes while on therapy [2].

Isolated cutaneous mastocytomas of infancy commonly involute spontaneously; when this does not occur, the single lesions may be excised surgically. None of the recently recognized medical therapies [23,33] effects involution of either cutaneous or visceral lesions. In a preliminary report, the use of oral 8-methoxypsoralen and long-wave ultraviolet irradiation (PUVA) has been purported to effect a partial involution of cutaneous lesions [40].

Malignant mastocytosis is a very rare disorder with high mortality within 2 years of diagnosis. It may occur either as a cutaneous or a systemic disease and reportedly may appear by malignant transformation of a benign neoplasm, especially of the systemic variety. Histopathologic analysis utilizing special staining procedures, such as the naphthol-AS-chloracetate esterase technique, may be necessary to detect the immature granules of malignant cells [41,42]. No particular cytotoxic drug protocol has been established or recommended. Leukemias associated with mastocytosis may be monocytic, mastocytic, or myeloid, in approximately equal frequencies, of which the sum appears in few of all mastocytosis patients. The relationship of mastocytosis to such leukemias has been unclear but possibly may relate to the recent evidence that mast cells, at least in some portion, are derived from bone marrow stem cells [43–46].

References

1. Sagher F, Even-Paz Z: *Mastocytosis and the Mast Cell.* Year Book Medical Publishers, Chicago, 1967
2. Roberts LJ II et al: Shock syndrome associated with mastocytosis: pharmacologic reversal of the acute episode and therapeutic prevention of recurrent attacks, in *Advances in Shock Research.* Liss Publishers, New York, in press
3. Shaw JM: Genetic aspects of urticaria pigmentosa. *Arch Dermatol* **97**:137–138, 1968
4. Scott BB et al: Involvement of the small intestine in systemic mast cell disease. *Gut* **16**:918–924, 1975
5. Cryer PE, Kissane JM: Clinicopathologic conference: systemic mastocytosis. *Am J Med* **61**:671–680, 1976
6. Capron JP et al: Portal hypertension in systemic mastocytosis. *Gastroenterology* **74**:595–597, 1978
7. Lucaya J et al: Mastocytosis with skeletal and gastrointestinal involvement in infancy. *Pediatr Radiol* **131**:363–366, 1979
8. Austen KF: Biologic implications of the structural and functional characteristics of the chemical mediators of immediate hypersensitivity. *Harvey Lectures* **73**:93–161, 1979
9. Roberts LJ II et al: Prostaglandin, thromboxane and 12-hydroxy-5,8,10,14-eicosatetraenoic acid production by ionophore-stimulated rat serosal mast cells. *Biochim Biophys Acta* **575**:185–192, 1979
10. Lewis RA et al: Preferential generation of prostaglandin

11. Metcalfe DD et al: Identification of sulfated mucopolysaccharides, including heparin, in the lesional skin of a patient with mastocytosis. *J Invest Dermatol* **74**:210–215, 1980
12. Goetzl EJ, Austen KF: Purification and synthesis of eosinophilotactic tetrapeptides of human lung tissue: identification as eosinophil chemotactic factor of anaphylaxis. *Proc Natl Acad Sci USA* **72**:4123–4127, 1975
13. Boswell RN et al: Intermediate molecular weight eosinophil chemotactic factors in rat peritoneal mast cells: immunologic release, granule association, and demonstration of structural heterogeneity. *J Immunol* **120**:15–20, 1978
14. Goetzl EJ et al: The regulation of human eosinophil function by endogenous monohydroxyeicosatetraenoic acids (HETEs). *J Immunol* **124**:926–933, 1980
15. Goetzl EJ et al: Modulation of human neutrophil function by monohydroxyeicosatetraenoic acids. *Immunology* **39**:491–501, 1980
16. Borgeat P, Samuelsson B: Metabolism of arachidonic acid in polymorphonuclear leukocytes. Structural analysis of novel hydroxylated compounds. *J Biol Chem* **254**:7865–7869, 1979
17. Goetzl EJ, Pickett WC: The human PMN leukocyte chemotactic activity of complex hydroxyeicosatetraenoic acids (HETEs). *J Immunol* **125**:1789–1794, 1980
18. Gagnon JH et al: Mastocytosis: unusual manifestations; clinical and radiologic changes. *Can Med Assoc J* **112**:1329–1332, 1975
19. Montagna W: Histology and cytochemistry of human skin. XI. The distribution of β-glucuronidase. *J Biophys Biochem Cytol* **3**:343–347, 1957
20. Schwartz LB et al: Acid hydrolases and tryptase from secretory granules of dispersed human lung mast cells. *J Immunol* **126**:1290–1294, 1981
21. Glenner GG, Cohen LA: Histochemical demonstration of a species-specific trypsin-like enzyme in mast cells. *Nature* **185**:846–847, 1960
22. Hirata F et al: Concanavalin A stimulates phospholipid methylation and phosphatidyl serine decarboxylation in rat mast cells. *Proc Natl Acad Sci USA* **76**:4813–4816, 1979
23. Roberts LJ II et al: Increased production of prostaglandin D_2 in patients with systemic mastocytosis. *N Engl J Med* **303**:1400–1404, 1980
24. Wasserman MA et al: Bronchopulmonary and cardiovascular effects of prostaglandin D_2 in the dog. *Prostaglandins* **13**:255–269, 1977
25. Yecies LD et al: Slow reacting substance (SRS) from ionophore A23187-stimulated peritoneal mast cells of the normal rat. *J Immunol* **122**:2083–2089, 1979
26. Falkenhein SF et al: Effect of the 5-hydroperoxide of eicosatetraenoic acid and inhibitors of the lipoxygenase pathway on the formation of slow reacting substance by rat basophilic leukemia cells: direct evidence that slow reacting substance is a product of the lipoxygenase pathway. *J Immunol* **125**:163–168, 1980
27. Lewis RA et al: Slow reacting substances of anaphylaxis: identification of leukotrienes C-1 and D from human and rat sources. *Proc Natl Acad Sci USA* **77**:3710–3714, 1980
28. Drazen JM et al: Comparative airway and vascular activities of leukotrienes C-1 and D *in vivo* and *in vitro*. *Proc Natl Acad Sci USA* **77**:4354–4358, 1980
29. Weiss JW et al: Bronchoconstrictor effects of leukotriene C in human subjects. *Science* **216**:196–197, 1982

D_2 by rat and human mast cells, in *Biochemistry of the Acute Allergic Reactions, 4th International Symposium.* Edited by EL Becker et al. Alan R Liss, New York, 1981, pp 239–254

30. Lewis RA et al: Local effects of synthetic leukotrienes on monkey and human skin (abstr). *Clin Res* **29**:492A, 1981

31. Lewis RA et al: Generation of oxidative metabolites of arachidonic acid from rat serosal mast cells (abstr). *J Allergy Clin Immunol* **63**:220, 1979

32. Sostre S, Handler HL: Bony lesions in systemic mastocytosis: scintigraphic evaluation. *Arch Dermatol* **113**:1245–1247, 1977

33. Soter NA et al: Oral disodium cromoglycate in the treatment of systemic mastocytosis. *N Engl J Med* **301**:465–469, 1979

34. Oates JA, Sjoerdsma A: The unique syndrome associated with secretion of 5-hydroxytryptophan by metastatic gastric carcinoids. *Am J Med* **32**:333–342, 1962

35. Demis DJ: The mastocytosis syndrome: clinical and biological studies. *Ann Intern Med* **59**:194–206, 1963

36. Gerrard DM, Ko C: Urticaria pigmentosa: treatment with cimetidine and chlorpheniramine. *J Pediatr* **94**:843–844, 1979

37. Foreman JC, Garland LG: Cromoglycate and other antiallergic drugs: a possible mechanism of action. *Br Med J* **1**:820–821, 1976

38. Brogren H et al: Urticaria pigmentosa (mastocytosis). *Acta Med Scand* **163**:223–233, 1959

39. Hamrin B: Release of histamine in urticaria pigmentosa. *Lancet* **1**:867–868, 1957

40. Christopher E et al: PUVA-treatment of urticaria pigmentosa. *Br J Dermatol* **98**:701–702, 1978

41. Leder LD: Subtle clues to diagnosis by histochemistry in mast cell disease. *Am J Dermatopathol* **1**:261–266, 1979

42. Lennert K, Parwaresch MR: Mast cells and mast cell neoplasia: a review. *Histopathology* **3**:349–365, 1979

43. Razin E et al: Growth of a pure population of mouse mast cells *in vitro* with conditioned medium derived from concanavalin A-stimulated splenocytes. *Proc Natl Acad Sci USA* **78**:2559–2561, 1981

44. Schrader JW et al: The persisting (P) cell: histamine content, regulation by a T cell-derived factor, origin from a bone marrow precursor, and relationship to mast cells. *Proc Natl Acad Sci USA* **78**:323–327, 1981

45. Tertian G et al: Long term *in vitro* culture of murine mast cells. I. Description of a growth factor-dependent culture technique. *J Immunol* **127**:788–794, 1981

46. Nabel G et al: Another inducer T cell function: synthesis of a factor that stimulates proliferation of cloned mast cells. *Nature*, in press

VITILIGO
Etiology, Pathogenesis,
Diagnosis, and Treatment

David B. Mosher

Madhu A. Pathak

Thomas B. Fitzpatrick

Vitiligo is a pigmentary problem of prime concern to hundreds of thousands of darkly pigmented peoples of all races throughout the world. Unfortunately, only a few investigators are concentrating on the etiology and pathogenesis of this common disfiguring disorder that can often be a medical catastrophe, far more important than is generally perceived. Much more research effort is needed, but the enigma of vitiligo is no easier to unravel than many other unsolved diseases with multifactorial etiologies. The pathogenesis of vitiligo is still incompletely understood.

Despite the lack of definitive knowledge of the etiology, two effective treatments are available and both of these were discovered by serendipity: (1) oral PUVA photochemotherapy for repigmentation of vitiligo macules, and (2) topical application monobenzylether of hydroquinone cream to bleach the normal skin of a vitiligo patient to achieve permanent depigmentation.

This chapter summarizes the present knowledge of the pathogenesis of vitiligo and the results of a controlled, double-blind treatment of a large series of vitiligo patients using oral PUVA photochemotherapy. The good to excellent results obtained in this study should encourage physicians to elect to treat those patients with vitiligo who have severe disfigurement, now that sophisticated high-intensity UVA lighting systems are commercially available throughout the world; these lighting units make it possible to treat patients throughout the year, and repigmentation can be achieved more rapidly and more completely than when sunlight is used as the source of UVA.

Definition

Vitiligo is an idiopathic, acquired, circumscribed amelanoderma characterized by evolving chalk-white macules resulting from gradual destruction of melanocytes, pigment-producing cells (Fig. 1). The amelanosis of the skin results from an acquired often inherited loss of functional melanocytes of skin and hair. A positive family history is reported in at least 30 percent of cases. This disorder affects 1 to 2 percent of the population worldwide, with males and females probably equally affected [1,2]. Incidence figures from 0.14 to 8.8 percent have been reported from various populations. It appears that the incidence of vitiligo is rising, especially in countries like India, Pakistan, and the Far Eastern countries. Based on outpatient attendance in clinics and the cosmetic concerns of females, there is an apparent preponderance of females with vitiligo. However, this is considered to be a bias of reporting; vitiligo likely affects men and women equally. Vitiligo can appear at any age. We have seen it appear in babies within 3 months after birth and in adults after age 50. In half of cases it develops before the age of 21.

Classification

There are two general types of vitiligo and a mixed type. Several subtypes exist within each group:

I. Localized or patterned
   A. Focal—one or several isolated macules in one general anatomic area
   B. Segmental—one to many macules in a dermatomal or quasidermatomal array (Fig. 2)
II. Generalized
   A. Widespread (vulgaris)—scattered macules with no special pattern of distribution, though often symmetrical (Fig. 3)
      1. Small macular type [many small (0.5- to 2.0-cm macules)]
      2. Large macular type (large macules widely distributed)
      3. Lip-tip macular type (primarily confined to distal digits, lips, and oral mucosa)
   B. Universal
III. Mixed (widespread and segmental)

Of all types, focal vitiligo is the most difficult to characterize for in most cases it represents the initial stage of a developing disease that may

Fig. 2. Segmental vitiligo is an uncommon type of localized vitiligo; it involves one to several quasidermatomal areas of skin. It is unusual for additional new macules to develop outside of this general area.

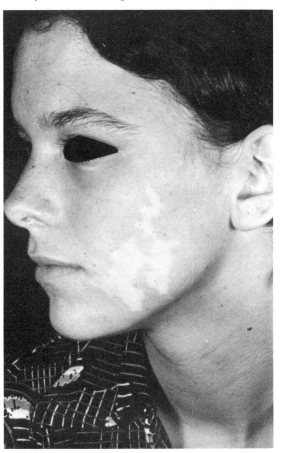

Fig. 1. Typical macule of vitiligo with amelanosis and concave borders.

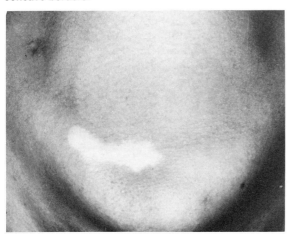

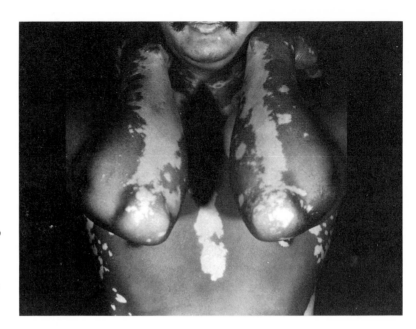

Fig. 3. Generalized symmetrical vitiligo is the most common form of vitiligo. Involvement of bony prominences such as elbows, knees, and interphalangeal joints is common; distal digits are commonly depigmented. Gradual progression is the rule.

eventually become widespread. In about 5 percent of cases the disease is limited to such a single macule, which is generally less than 3 cm in diameter and is usually readily treatable.

Segmental vitiligo may be slow to respond to psoralen plus UVA therapy (PUVA). Once manifested, it does not appear to spread beyond the presenting region of depigmentation.

Vitiligo in the majority of patients is of the generalized type—the large macular type being much more common than the small macular variety. The latter is particularly responsive to psoralen photochemotherapy. The lip-tip variant, with depigmentation of distal digits (tips of fingers and toes) and lips alone or including the gums, is quite common and generally unresponsive to PUVA. Large macular vitiligo is usually quite responsive to PUVA. Universal vitiligo may at times also be quite responsive, though such individuals usually have involvement of lips and fingertips and toes also—areas that are all unlikely to be repigmented. Universal vitiligo can be associated with multiple endocrinopathies, alopecia areata, and chronic mucocutaneous candidiasis.

While vitiligo has traditionally been considered a cutaneous disorder, findings of ocular depigmentation (5 percent of our patients, higher in patients of other investigators [3]) and high frequency of vitiligo-associated diseases (up to 50 percent in our patients) suggest that vitiligo is a cutaneous expression of a systemic disorder. Over 40 percent of vitiligo patients are at risk for thyroid disease [4]. Among our patients the frequency increases with age and is often insidious. Of 18 patients over 40 years of age, 6 of the 7 found to have abnormal thyroid-stimulating hormone (TSH) determinations and thyrotropin-releasing hormone (TRH) stimulation tests reported no symptoms and felt well (though one patient developed symptomatic hyperthyroidism during the course of study). The group of patients at highest risk appears to be women over the age of 40, with a positive family history of vitiligo, diabetes mellitus and/or thyroid disease, and with generalized though not necessarily extensive vitiligo. Diabetes mellitus may occur in about 8 percent, pernicious anemia in about 1 percent, and Addison's disease uncommonly (and then most often with other endocrinopathies and/or alopecia areata and mucocutaneous candidiasis) [5,6].

Up to 50 percent [7] of vitiligo patients have also been found to have elevated titers of antithyroid cell, antithyroglobulin, antiparietal cell, and antiadrenal cell antibodies; the frequency of the latter far exceeds the frequency of associated pernicious anemia or Addison's disease. While there are no hematologic or clinical markers that can segregate those vitiligo patients at risk for systemic disease, associated diseases are so common (up to 50 percent of our older patients) that vitiligo must alert the physician to look for associated general medical diseases. Although the mechanism for a common pathogenesis is unknown, vitiligo and vitiligo-associated disease probably represent separate expressions of a single defect.

Pathogenesis

The pathophysiology of vitiligo is poorly understood because of the lack of cohesive findings to unify most of the significant clinical, genetic, and laboratory observations. There remain three classical hypotheses of vitiligo: self-destruction of melanocytes, a neurogenic or neurochemical mediator destroying melanocytes, and immunologic disturbance. The following discussion summarizes the evidence supportive of each hypothesis.

The self-destruction hypothesis suggests that vitiligo results from overproduction of toxic intermediates that are generated in the biosynthesis of melanin. Lerner [8] has proposed that normal melanocytes are protected from toxic intermediates generated when tyrosine is converted to melanin. Tyrosine and dopa at high concentrations are toxic to melanocytes; intermediates dopachrome and 5,6-dihydroxyindole are more toxic to melanoma cells than either tyrosine or dopa. The identification of phenolic derivatives, which cause depigmentation in animals and humans, is cited as supportive evidence. Chemical leukoderma, whether due to monobenzylether of hydroquinone, p-tert-butyl phenol, 4-isopropylcatechol, or other agents, is often (though not always) clinically indistinguishable from vitiligo [9]. Such occupational leukoderma shares many of the histologic and ultrastructural features commonly seen in vitiligo. The mechanism is less likely direct tyrosinase inhibition than the uncontrolled generation of damaging melanin free radicals and melanin destabilization. Cutaneous depigmentation in vitiligo most probably results from the formation of diffusible free radicals (OH^-) and/or singlet oxygen ($^1O_2$) and superoxide anions (O_2^-) generated within melanocytes, which in turn initiate cell membrane damage and lipid peroxidation in melanocytes and thus their eventual destruction [9,10]. These cytotoxic products can arise from tyrosinase-mediated oxidation of the depigmenting agent, as well as the chemical and physical interactions of the depigmenting agent with pigment melanin. Some observations suggest that stimulation of melanin synthesis increases the risk for leukoderma; vitiligo may develop or spread following intense UV exposure, and normally hyperpigmented areas—axillae, nipples, genitalia—are particularly at risk as are habitually sun-exposed cutaneous surfaces. Destruction of melanocytes in the embryonic stage of development of the White Leghorn chicken is a model for spontaneous genetically programmed pigment cell death [11]. Further, there are several reported series of industrial occupational leukoderma associated with goiter or elevated TSH levels [12,13].

The neurogenic hypothesis purports defective neurotransmitter function or other defect at the peripheral nerve ending that results in melanocyte destruction. A neurochemical mediator (e.g., acetylcholine, epinephrine, or norepinephrine) liberated by the peripheral nerve endings is postulated to destroy melanocytes. Melanocytes are of neural crest origin and both melanin and catecholamines have tyrosine as a precursor substrate. Disruption of the neural end plate in the vicinity of melanocytes displaying cytotoxic changes has been observed in vitiligo macules and suggests that peripheral nerve changes could precede melanocytic autophagy [14]. Certain animal model systems clearly have a neural control mechanism. In fish, electrical stimulation of cutaneous nerves causes blanching, and sectioning the nerve causes darkening. Pigment cells of fish, amphibians, and reptiles have α- and/or β-adrenergic receptors. In amphibians, dispersion of chromatophores (pigment lightening) follows β-adrenergic stimulation, and aggregation (pigment darkening) follows α-adrenergic stimulation or nerve section [15]. Melatonin, released by light exposure, inhibits melanocyte-stimulating hormone (MSH) and lightens dermal melanocytes of the frog but has no effect on the melanocytes in humans. Both Fabian [16] and Voulot [17] have demonstrated that denervation in guinea pigs slows the rate of pigment spread. In the frog, acetylcholine causes lightening, though darkening results in some fish. In humans, four cases of eserine-induced depigmentation have been observed; eserine potentiates acetylcholine [18]. However, acetylcholine has not been shown to be cytotoxic to melanocytes in vivo or in vitro. Decreased cholinesterase levels have been observed in vitiligo macules with leukotrichia [19]. Many other studies of neuromediated functions affecting melanocytes have been reported in vitiligo macules but the results have been disappointingly inconclusive [20–23]. The compelling clinical observation is the occurrence of segmental vitiligo in a quasidermatomal pattern. Development of vitiligo selectively in neurologically compromised cutaneous regions, following psychologic trauma and following cutaneous injury (with disruption of normal cutaneous peripheral nerves), is best explained by the neurogenic hypothesis.

The immunologic hypothesis is currently the most championed. Antithyroid cell, antithyroglobulin, antiadrenal, and antiparietal cell antibodies have been found in up to 50 percent of vitiligo patients [5–7]. Demonstration of antimelanin antibodies has been reported by Langhof et al. [24] and positive indirect immunofluorescence has been reported by several investigators [25,26] and also observed by us in one case of inflammatory vitiligo. Attempts to reproduce the work of Langhof et al. have been unsuccessful however [27]. Certain patients with vitiligo exhibit an inflammatory phase in evolution where lymphocytes are present in the dermis and Langerhans cells are increased in the epidermis [28]. Electron microscopy has revealed the presence of lymphocytes in close proximity to melanocytes. The melanocytes show varying degrees of destructive changes, including autophagic vacuoles. Changes in halo nevi are more dramatic and provide an example of the capacity of lymphocytes to destroy melanocytes. Destruction of melanocytes is apparent in the areas of active regression; antigenically active lymphocytes have been found to infiltrate nevus cells in halo nevus [29].

In vitro cytotoxicity of antimelanoma antibodies to cutaneous melanoma has been demonstrated [30,31]. A cytotoxic factor to normal melanocytes in culture has been described in the serum of several patients with multiple halo nevi [32], and lymphocytes of patients with halo nevi (without melanoma) have been found cytotoxic to melanoma cell lines (W. H. Clark, Jr., unpublished data). T-cell and B-cell levels have been reported to be normal [33], though decreased T-cell levels were reported in one study [34]. Abnormally high blastoid formation against premelanosomal antigens has also been reported in a series of cases of generalized vitiligo [35], though not in segmental or focal types. Occurrence of leukoderma in halo nevi with characteristic lymphocytic infiltrate and remote from the halo nevus in up to 50 percent of patients and in the otherwise normal skin of some patients with melanoma suggests melanocytes are antigenic; antimelanoma cell antibodies have been described in these patients with or without vitiligo but not in those with vitiligo alone [36]. A Vogt-Koyanagi-Harada-like syndrome has been observed both spontaneously and following bacillus Calmette-Guérin (BCG) therapy, in melanoma patients. Association of vitiligo with immunologically mediated disorders such as thyroiditis, alopecia areata, halo nevi, pernicious anemia, and Addison's disease (of nontuberculous origin) suggests a common immunologic pathogenesis. Animal models—Lippizaner horses [37] and Sinclair swine [38]—develop leukoderma associated with melanotic tumors. Certain Arabian, Lippizaner, Percheron, and Camargue horses are born dark and spontaneously become white by age 9, and at the same time the horses frequently develop melanoma. The Rhode Island Red chicken develops alopecia and lightening of the feathers [39]. There is, however, no clear animal model for isolated macular leukoderma. Patients with vitiligo have discrete pigmentary lesions of the fundus, and patients with uveitis may have a high incidence of vitiligo [40]. Several unpublished findings of our laboratory describing light and electron microscopic observations of vitiligo biopsies indicate in vitiligo macules (a) a cellular infiltrate consisting of lymphocytes, (b) lymphocytes in close contact with melanocytes, and (c) a varying degree of destructive changes in melanocytes, including autophagic vacuoles. These observations support the hypothesis that vitiligo is a systemic disease in which pigment cells in any part of the body may be destroyed by immunologic mechanism.

Many of the observations supportive of these hypotheses are incontrovertible truths. Accepting this, one must assume either all hypotheses are at least partially incorrect or that there is an hypothesis that must encompass them all. These can be interrelated if vitiligo is considered in precipitating and sustaining steps. The self-destruction of melanocytes or neurogenic hypotheses explain induction; the resultant sustained depigmentation is immunologically mediated. Either disruption of the normal melanocyte–peripheral nerve axis or melanocyte injury by mechanical or chemical injury exposes antigenic melanocyte receptors or other antigens. An unidentified chemotactic factor is liberated so that Langerhans cells migrate into the involved epidermis. Langerhans cells represent the afferent limb of the immunologic mechanism and the final step in the induction. Lymphocytes represent the effector limb that perpetuates sustained melanocyte destruction. The distribution of vitiligo macules for both the evolving generalized vitiligo and for the relatively localized quasidermatomal disease deserves explanation. Segmental vitiligo may be best explained by an abnormal clone of melanocytes that migrates from the neural crest in embryonic life or by a localized defect in the neuron-melanocyte axis; only these localized areas are at risk. In generalized vitiligo all melanocytes are at risk and either the defect is universal or a melanin precursor or its metabolite has rendered all melanocytes potentially vulnerable.

Diagnosis

The diagnosis of vitiligo is usually straightforward and is based on the presence of amelanotic macules that are chalk-white. Almost all vitiligo is invariably acquired and dynamic. Usually, as time lapses, established macules enlarge and new discrete macules appear. The shape of the lesions is round to oval, although irregular lesions or patterned ones may correspond to recent or remote injury that has Koebnerized. The distribution of lesions in generalized vitiligo is often, though not universally, symmetrical and is most likely to involve distal digits (beginning distally and progressing proximally), extensor joints, axillae, periorificial regions, and lower back. Segmental vitiligo is most common on the face and neck and least so on the legs. The color of the lesions is alabaster or chalk-white, reflecting the absence of melanocytes. When examined under Wood's light (UVA of 320–400 nm), the lesions appear white; they are amelanotic and only rarely hypopigmented. Most lesions are surrounded by a narrow rim of trichrome (an intermediate hypomelanotic color—tan), but, occasionally, large macular margins of trichrome will be apparent; rarely an entire macule will be trichrome. A familial or an acquired amelanoderma, which is characterized by evolving white macules in a segmental or symmetrically patterned distribution, is invariably vitiligo (if chemical leukoderma is excluded).

When the history is vague and the individual is fair-skinned, with a few or segmental lesions, confusion with tuberous sclerosis or nevus depigmentosus is possible. *Tuberous sclerosis* may be characterized by segmental and/or small discrete macules, but these are congenital and fixed; with Wood's light the lesions clearly are off-white as a reflection of the presence of normal melanocyte numbers with decreased capacity to synthesize melanin [41]. *Nevus depigmentosus* is a cutaneous disorder and is not readily confused as it is congenital, not amelanotic but hypomelanotic or "off-white," and nonevolutionary. Further, nevus depigmentosus usually appears more "nevoid" than does segmental vitiligo.

Perhaps the most difficult to diagnose are those cases in which the amelanoderma is of abrupt onset after an identifiable event. We have seen depigmentation follow chemical burns, allergic reactions, surgical procedures, dermabrasion, and medication usage; in such cases the awareness of the amelanoderma is sudden and the relationship to the "culpable" event usually within 2 to 3 weeks (although up to 6 months has been described and we have seen a patient depigment an area of plastic surgery some 8 years after the procedure). Diagnosis in such cases may be readily apparent—Koebnerization—in an individual with a family or personal history of vitiligo, diabetes mellitus, or thyroid disease in particular. Careful examination with a Wood's light in a well-darkened room to examine for other macules of leukoderma is always indicated. Diagnosis is most difficult when family history is negative and there are no other macules of leukoderma. Biopsy to identify dopa-positive melanocytes after incubating the sodium bromide–split epidermis in dopa solution may be helpful—if no melanocytes are present, vitiligo (presenting as a Koebner phenomenon) is the likely diagnosis; if some melanocytes are present, postinflammatory hypomelanosis may be the diagnosis (the latter being unassociated with endocrinopathies, having no general medical implications, and being totally self-limited). Nevertheless the diagnosis may remain uncertain until the disease course reveals itself.

Piebaldism [42], Woolf's syndrome [43], Waardenburg's syndrome [44], and the Ziprkowski-Margolis syndrome [45] all share the color of vitiligo except for the absence of trichrome but are readily segregated by their congenital and nonprogressive character. Piebaldism is congenital, stable, has characteristic frontal macule with white forelock, and spares the dorsal spine; islands of hyperpigmented or normally pigmented macules are present in the white patches. Waardenburg's and Woolf's syndromes manifest hearing defects and, in the former, other distinct features that are absent in vitiligo.

The Vogt-Koyanagi-Harada syndrome is characterized by meningeal, ocular, and cutaneous phases, the latter marked by vitiligo-like depigmentation with autophagocytosis. Nordlund et al. [46] have rightly stated that the Vogt-Koyanagi-Harada syndrome and vitiligo may represent varied limits of expression of a disease process. Those presenting with acquired poliosis of the eyebrows and lashes, with or without alopecia areata, tinnitus, deafness, or a history of meningeal symptoms should be carefully screened as possible cases with Vogt-Koyanagi-Harada syndrome for uveitis, which may lead to residual and permanent blindness. Careful ophthalmologic examinations in over 200 cases of vitiligo have failed to reveal any signs of uveitis in otherwise normal patients with vitiligo (personal observations).

Because vitiligo is a marker for other diseases and thereby an important medical diagnosis, these common cutaneous disorders with which vitiligo may be confused should be noted. *Pityriasis alba* involves indiscrete hypomelanotic macules of the face, less so the arms and legs, particularly in deeply pigmented peoples; the lesions always have a powdery scale. *Tinea versicolor* is characterized by erythematous, tan or hypomelanotic, round lesions, which, if abundant, coalesce, particularly on the upper back and chest. Examination by Wood's light shows hypomelanotic lesions in contrast to amelanotic lesions of vitiligo, chartreuse (greenish-yellow) flourescence, and a KOH scraping that is positive for hyphae and yeast forms. Resolved tinea versicolor may be difficult to distinguish from vitiligo if there has been inadequate UV exposure to induce melanogenesis following effective antimycotic therapy. *Idiopathic guttate hypomelanosis* (IGH) gives very sharply circumscribed, porcelain-white macules less than 5 mm in diameter on the legs, particularly anteriorly and occasionally elsewhere, and is common in deeply pigmented peoples. IGH is unrelated to vitiligo and probably represents a functional degenerative process of melanocytes.

Treatment

No affected individual should be turned away without at least some consideration to the five possible approaches to the patient with vitiligo: (1) Reassurance about the lack of medical seriousness of vitiligo itself, with awareness of the risk for associated diseases. (2) Photoprotection with sunscreens to decrease acute and chronic effects of UVB and to reduce the contrast between the normal skin and vitiliginous areas. (3) The camouflaging or disguising of the socially interactive areas (exposed regions of face, neck, and hands) with cosmetically acceptable makeup products that approximate the normal color of the skin. (4) Repigmentation, which usually means photochemotherapy with oral psoralens (either 8-methoxypsoralen or trimethylpsoralen) plus sunlight or oral psoralens plus UVA from high-intensity PUVA therapy units emitting long-wave UV radiation in the 320- to 400-nm range (see below). (5) Depigmentation with monobenzylether of hydroquinone applied to the remaining normally melanized skin of older patients with 40 percent or more vitiligo. All patients deserve an awareness of these options with their attendant risks and benefits. The bias of the dermatologist and his experience will help determine which of these the patient opts to select.

The purpose of the following sections is to emphasize the role of, success with, and limitations of each approach. That treatment of vitiligo is available is hardly widely known to many practicing physicians. Too often patients are summarily

dismissed with "that's vitiligo and there is nothing you can do about it."

The only reasonable objective of the treatment of vitiligo is to satisfy the cosmetic needs of the patient, who may desire "normal-looking skin," especially of socially interactive areas such as the face, neck, chest, and hands. Among many very fair-skinned whites (Skin Types I and II), treatment may be unnecessary because the white amelanotic macules are hardly noticeable unless the skin is exposed to the sun, which will increase the contrast between the normal and the vitiliginous skin. Such patients can camouflage the disfigurement with certain cosmetic makeup preparations and, as long as they avoid the sun, learn to accept the pigmentary abnormalities without treatment. But vitiligo in brown or black skin is a serious disfigurement that often leads to personal unhappiness, social discrimination at work or school, career advancement limitations, marital discord, and other severe psychosocial disasters. For these millions of vitiligo patients throughout the world, particularly in Asia, Africa, and South America, and the blacks of the United States, vitiligo carries a dire social stigma; nearly all these patients desperately wish to be treated. The search for an effective treatment for achieving uniform repigmentation or "cure" among these vitiligo patients is intense, constant, endless, and even frantic.

Reassurance

Most patients experience considerable confusion about their vitiligo. Some are fearful of skin cancer, others of some dreaded contagious disease. Historically, dating from thousands of years B.C., vitiligo has been confused with leprosy. Much of biblical leprosy as noted in Leviticus XIII was surely vitiligo. Even to the present day in some areas of the world, such as India, Pakistan, and Asiatic countries, social stigma accompanies vitiligo. It is not unusual for Indians to make a pilgrimage for the cure of vitiligo—in hopes that this dreaded blight be removed, that they may advance in their jobs and social position, and perhaps more importantly that marriages for their affected daughters can be arranged. In perhaps no lesser sense, many afflicted with vitiligo plot a pilgrimage to nondermatologists renowned for a "secret formula" for repigmentation, which is invariably acquired from folk remedies or through the local ancient art of medical practice. The patient, with the hope of achieving instantaneous results, goes from one curer to the other. Although some of these ancient remedies are effective in restoring normal color to some of the amelanotic macules, the mystical and often unscientific approach more often perpetuates anecdotes and blind faith. Having been disappointed, a few of these patients eventually return to the dermatologist (or internist) in a never-ending search for understanding their disease, reassurance of favorable prognosis, and guarantee of ready cure.

In the discussion of their vitiligo with patients we elaborate on the potential medical significance of the disorder and then on what can be done about the appearance and the presence of vitiligo. While some are satisfied to learn of the benign nature of vitiligo, few are reassured only by exclusion of associated disease. However, even in those who insist they feel well, laboratory testing for at least thyroid function and diabetes mellitus must be performed. The authors have identified three cases of thyroid disease in the past 2 months just by the insistence on such screening procedures. Most patients are seeking some successful modality of therapy; to dismiss vitiligo with "Don't worry about it" or "It doesn't look bad to me" is to be insensitive to the patient's plea for assistance.

Patients with vitiligo are often concerned about the inheritance of disease. In about 30 percent of vitiligo patients, there is a history of vitiligo in another family member. And often only one other family member is affected with the disease. Vitiligo appears to be an autosomal dominant disorder with variable expression and incomplete penetrance [47]. Direct transmittance of the disease is by no means proved or guaranteed. Children of patients with a personal and family history of vitiligo, diabetes, and thyroid disease are most at risk. Genetic transfer is least likely if the family history for vitiligo is not well established.

Sunscreen Protection

Most patients have observed their exposed vitiligo macules to be particularly susceptible to the acute (sunburn) and chronic (actinic elastosis) effects of UV radiation. Use of broad-spectrum sunscreens with a sun protection factor (SPF) of 15 or greater will usually provide maximum protection without the cosmetic liabilities of opaque formulations. Daily use is mandatory, and reapplication during prolonged exposure in tropical zones or on the beach in temperate zones in the summer is often essential. Routine usage not only prevents acute sunburn reaction, but also may retard the rate of actinic degeneration and the degree of delayed melanogenesis of the normal skin so that the contrast between the vitiliginous skin and the normally pigmented skin is minimized. Daily, year-round use of such sunscreens is indicated for those in whom reduction of contrast is a desired goal. Sunscreens containing 5% p-aminobenzoic acid (PreSun, Pabanol) or combination sunscreens containing benzophenones and cinnamates (Piz Buin-8 cream, milk, or lotion) or benzophenones and PABA esters (Super Shade 15, Total Eclipse) appear to be helpful.

Camouflage

Cosmetic coverup with lotions containing dihydroxyacetone and certain aniline dyes (e.g., Vita-Dye of Paul B. Elder Co., Bryan, Ohio, or Dy-O-Derm of Owens Laboratories, Dallas, Texas) or with makeup creams containing zinc oxide and various shades of pigments, etc. (e.g., Covermark, Lydia O'Leary, New York, or Reflecta, Texas Pharmaceuticals) may be acceptable to some patients (Fig. 4). Because these are eluted by water washing, daily reapplication is usually required. Artificial suntan formulations containing 5% dihydroxyacetone are satisfactory to an occasional patient with light skin. If these formulations are freshly compounded, they often give satisfactory skin color, but because they are unstable, they often impart an unnatural greenish hue to the skin if used after 6 to 9 months. The opaque formulations (Covermark, Reflecta) are often acceptable to women, and some patients can indeed learn to normalize the appearance of their skin color. However, these formulations can be messy to use and often discolor clothing.

Use of oral β-carotene (60 to 120 mg daily of Solatene, Hoffmann-LaRoche) may be recommended to certain patients with generalized vitiligo (universalis). For a few patients, mild carotoderma is preferable to the alabaster or chalk-white skin of vitiligo. Use of β-carotene is most successful in patients with extensive depigmentation. The accompanying yellow-orange discoloration of the palms is distressing to some and the color match may be only fair. Topical dyes or makeup may be used conjointly.

Repigmentation

Return of normal melanin pigmentation in vitiliginous areas is the goal and the burning desire of most patients. There are probably as many folk remedies as there are cultures. Some of these

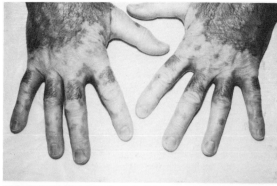

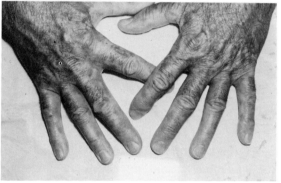

Fig. 4. Camouflage with topical dihydroxyacetone solution containing a dye. Top: Macules without cosmetic cover-up. Bottom: Same macules are much less apparent after one application of the dye solution. Reapplication after a washing with soap and water is generally necessary. Unwashed skin tends to retain the color for two to three days.

remedies are the foundations of present-day therapy with use of powder or suspensions of *Ammi majus* Linn (Umbelliferae) or *Psoralea corylifolia* (Leguminosae) seeds. There have been brief periods of enthusiasm for PABA, vitamin B, dopa, clofazimine, and others, but few modalities of therapy have survived the tests of predictability, reproducibility, efficacy, and safety. Topical steroids may produce repigmentation in some limited cases. In fact, for children under 12 with vitiligo, we suggest the use of 2.5% hydrocortisone cream twice daily. Monthly monitoring for the possible development of telangiectasia is necessary, particularly if hydrocortisone is to be used on periorbital skin. Several months of application may be required before perifollicular macules appear. On nonfacial, nonaxillary, nonintertriginous skin, more potent topical corticosteroid creams may occasionally be used, but never without regular patient monitoring. We have seen striae develop on the anterior legs of individuals applying fluorinated corticosteroid creams for as short a period of time as 4 months. In our view, and despite reports of some success [48], there is no role for the use of oral corticosteroids or adrenocorticotropic hormone (ACTH) in the treatment of vitiligo.

Routine sun exposure may possibly augment the effects of topical steroids. Topical steroids may suppress T cells to create a favorable environment for melanocyte mitosis and migration to occur in response to solar radiation.

PUVA (Psoralens + UVA—Oral Photochemotherapy). Photochemotherapy has been found to be an effective therapeutic modality for vitiligo. Based on the observation that oral 8-methoxypsoralen and sunlight stimulate melanin pigmentation of normal skin, the goal of photochemotherapy of vitiligo is to restore the normal color of the skin by use of UV radiation (UVA—320 to 400 nm) and a photosensitizing agent such as 8-methoxypsoralen, 4,5′,8-trimethylpsoralen, or psoralen. Historically, photochemotherapy of vitiligo can be traced back as far as 2000 to 1500 B.C. in India and Egypt. Folk medicine in several cultures treated vitiligo with topical extracts of plants (e.g., Bavachee or *Psoralea corylifolia* or *Ammi majus* Linn), which are known to contain photosensitizing and pigment-stimulating furocoumarins such as psoralen, 8-methoxypsoralen, 5-methoxypsoralen, etc. [49]. In Western countries, early results of vitiligo therapy with exposure to sunlight or UV irradiation were reported in the early 1900s. Kuske [50] reviewed the nature of skin pigmentation stimulated by several plant extracts (figs, limes, lemons, etc.) that are now known to contain furocoumarins. The Finsen lamp, carbon-arc lamp, and Kromayer lamp were generally used to stimulate melanogenesis [51,52]. Encouraging results with the topical and oral psoralens were initially reported by Uhlmann [53,54], El Mofty [55], and Lerner et al. [56].

The most frequently recommended treatment of vitiligo involves the ingestion of either 8-methoxypsoralen (8-MOP, methoxsalen) or 4,5′,8-trimethylpsoralen (TMP, trioxsalen) followed by exposure to solar radiation or to long-wave UV radiation from artificial light sources (UVA or 320 to 400 nm). At the present time, administration of oral psoralens (either 8-MOP or TMP) and exposure to UV radiation remains the only effective method which offers a hope of achieving repigmentation of vitiliginous macules.

The following are criteria for patient selection for PUVA repigmentation of vitiligo: (1) age 12 or over, (2) ability to follow protocol and be available for 12 to 24 months of continuous therapy, (3) ophthalmologic examination, and (4) vitiligo other than lip-tip variant (q.v.). Those criteria used for

Table 1 Percent of patients with over 75 percent repigmentation

Site	Lo-8-MOP + Me-TMP Years		Me-TMP Years		Hi-TMP Years		VH-TMP Years		Lo-8-MOP Years		Me-8-MOP Years		Me-Ps Years		Hi-Ps Years		Placebo Years	
	1	2	1	2	1	2	1	2	1	2	1	2	1	2	1	2	1	2
Face	33	64	10	25	22	42	40	—	35	60	52	27	14	23	46	40	0	—
Neck	16	56	28	18	18	24	25	—	17	67	50	26	100	25	11	50	25	—
Chest	27	48	14	25	13	35	33	—	25	69	42	39	25	30	29	20	9	—
Arms	21	43	9	25	18	23	10	—	40	32	39	35	14	6	45	33	10	—
Legs	16	43	28	29	14	24	12	—	10	22	35	39	0	10	14	0	20	—
Hands	14	15	0	0	3	4	0	—	0	0	6	15	0	0	0	0	0	—
Total	24	38	19	17	11	14	9	—	19	31	23	25	7	3	9	29	0	—

selection of psoriasis patients for PUVA in general do apply. Pregnant and lactating women should not be treated. The following sections summarize our recent experience with PUVA (oral psoralens plus UVA) and PUVASOL (oral psoralens plus sunlight) in the treatment of vitiligo.

Light Source. For repigmentation of vitiligo, irradiation with UVA (320 to 400 nm) is necessary. The biologic action spectrum for psoralen-induced stimulation of melanin pigmentation is in the 320- to 360-nm UVA range.

Excellent results with oral 8-MOP or TMP can be achieved with sunlight, but for many, particularly in temperate zones, regular sun exposures may be problematic. Daily and seasonal variations in solar UV intensity make the sun an unreliable light source and the weather is often unpredictable. Furthermore, adolescents requiring therapy must remain in school during the obligatory sun-exposure period of 10:00 a.m. to 2:00 p.m., and working adults may not be able to use their lunch hours for sunlight exposure. These factors make sunlight a capricious light source for therapy.

The development of a high-intensity UVA-emitting light system [57], which does not have these problems, has made successful photochemotherapy of vitiligo realistic. Total-body light exposures can be taken any time of the day, throughout the year, and under well-defined controlled exposure conditions with proper dosimetry and careful follow-up. Necessary equipment involves a standard walk-in PUVA phototherapy unit equipped with 36 to 60 fluorescent tubes, control devices for measuring UVA dosimetry, and standard electrical safety features. A properly trained and careful phototherapist to monitor UV exposures is equally essential. The success of PUVA is often a function of the commitment of the patient, the dermatologist, and the phototherapy technician; of paramount importance is the presence of a concerned and observant phototherapist whose thoughtful interaction with the patient seems essential for compliance and good results.

Sunlight and high-intensity fluorescent tubes emitting UVA (320 to 400 nm) with peak emission at 360 nm (FR40-T12HO PUVA lamps) appear to be equally effective [58]. 4,5′,8-Trimethylpsoralen (trioxsalen 0.6 to 0.9 mg/kg) or 8-methoxypsoralen (methoxsalen 0.3 to 0.6 mg/kg) is ingested 2 hr before exposure to the light source. Exposures should begin with 1 to 2 J/cm^2 or 5 to 10 min of summer sun and be increased by 0.5 to 1.0 J/cm^2 or 5 min of sun until a maximum treatment exposure of 8 to 12 J/cm^2 or 45 min of sun is reached. These values are for stationary standing (PUVA) or supine (PUVASOL) exposures. The objective of the UV dosimetry is to expose the skin to minimal phototoxic doses of UVA so that mild ($\pm$ to 1+) and persistent erythema is apparent 36 to 48 hr after exposure. Suberythemal UV exposures may induce repigmentation, so that even minimal phototoxicity is not necessarily required in many cases. If mild erythema is observed, subsequent increases in the UVA dosages must be carefully monitored to minimize cutaneous phototoxicity which could, otherwise, precipitate a Koebner reaction. If no erythema develops, the dose of UVA or sun exposure may be increased. Overexposure must be avoided. Repigmentation develops as small, brown, perifollicular macules that enlarge and coalesce or may also begin from the margins and spread centripetally (Fig. 5). Evidence of repigmentation is usually first seen within 15 to 25 treatments. Complete repigmentation usually requires 100 to 300 treatments.

The question of which psoralen is most effective must be addressed. Although 8-methoxypsoralen and 4,5′,8-trimethylpsoralen were introduced between 1947 and 1960 for the treatment of vitiligo,

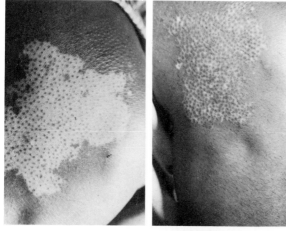

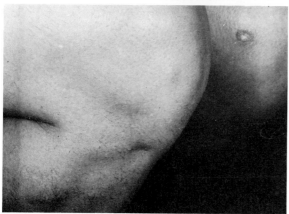

Fig. 5. Topical therapy with 0.1% 8-MOP solution and sunlight. Upper left: Macule has begun to repigment after a month of thrice weekly sun exposures 2 hours after topical applications of 0.1% 8-MOP. Upper right: Over 60 percent of the macule shows repigmentation after four months of therapy. Bottom: Complete repigmentation after 6 months of therapy. The perifollicular pigmentation resembles that repigmentation stimulated by oral 8-MOP + UVA radiation therapy.

they had never before been evaluated in a controlled randomized, double-blind comparative manner. A large double-blind controlled study of vitiligo involving 365 East Indian patients with vitiligo was recently reported [59]. This study was designed to examine the relative effectiveness of three psoralens in various dosages that are used in the treatment of vitiligo throughout the world. These patients were treated for over 2 years with one of several doses of either 8-methoxypsoralen (8-MOP), 4,5′,8-trimethylpsoralen (TMP), or psoralen (Ps), and sunlight. The patient population was selected from outpatients of the Bangalore Baptist Hospital, Bangalore, India[1]; most had generalized

[1] The investigators wish to acknowledge the tireless help and cooperation of Russell Rowland, M.D., Rebecca Naylor, M.D., John Wickman, M.D., and their staff.

vitiligo with 1 to 70 percent skin involvement of 1 to 50 years' duration. Males and females were equally represented. Patients from ages 8 to 70 were randomly assigned to eight treatment groups. They were instructed to ingest their psoralen tablets 2 hr before midday sun exposure of 30 to 45 min 3 times weekly, not 2 days in a row. The various dosage schedules were as follows:

Group	Code	Drug dose
Combination low-dose Oxsoralen + medium-dose Trisoralen	Lo-8-MOP + Me-TMP	0.3 mg/kg 8-MOP + 0.6 mg/kg TMP
Low-dose Oxsoralen	Lo-8 MOP	0.3 mg/kg 8-MOP
Medium-dose Oxsoralen	Me-8-MOP	0.6 mg/kg 8-MOP
Medium-dose Trisoralen	Me-TMP	0.8 mg/kg TMP
High-dose Trisoralen	Hi-TMP	1.8 mg/kg TMP
Very-high-dose Trisoralen	VH-TMP*	3.6 mg/kg TMP
Medium-dose psoralen	Me-Ps	0.6 mg/kg psoralen
High-dose psoralen	Hi-Ps	1.2 mg/kg psoralen

* *Note:* One-year treatment only; this group received placebo for the first year of the study.

In addition, for the first year of the study there was a control group that received placebo (no oral psoralens) and sunlight. Patients were seen bimonthly and evaluated extensively on a yearly basis. Assessment of repigmentation was based on comparison of the patient to previous photographs taken at the commencement of the study, as judged by at least two evaluator-physicians.

Of those treated for 2 years or more, 45 percent of the patients treated with combination Lo-8-MOP + Me-TMP and Lo-8-MOP fully repigmented their faces and nearly 60 percent achieved over 75 percent repigmentation of the head and neck (Figs. 6 to 8). The neck, abdomen, and back repigmented nearly as well and better than the arms and legs (see Table 1). Seventy-five percent or more repigmentation of all vitiligo macules occurred in 38 percent of patients on Lo-8-MOP + Me-TMP, 31 percent of patients on Lo-8-MOP, 29 percent of patients on Hi-Ps (though the number of patients was small), and less than 19 percent of patients with all TMP groups. Patients receiving Hi-TMP and Hi-Ps had a better repigmentation response than those on lower dosage schedules but were not so successful as with 8-MOP schedules. Results of 2 years of treatment with VH-TMP were not available. After 2 years of therapy, patients receiving Lo-8-MOP had done better than

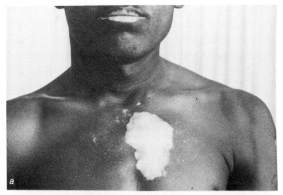

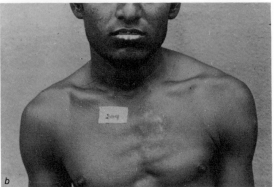

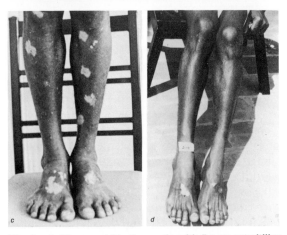

Fig. 6. A 20-year-old Indian male with 5 percent vitiligo of over 3 years' duration treated with 40 mg 8-MOP thrice weekly for 24 months. (*a*) Chest before therapy. (*b*) After 2 years of therapy the large macule on the chest is nearly fully repigmented. Even partial repigmentation of the lips is apparent. (*c*) Legs and feet before therapy. (*d*) After 2 years of therapy legs are fully repigmented, but dorsal feet only about 50 percent repigmented. The patient was very satisfied with his response.

those receiving Me-8-MOP (see later). The lips, hands, feet, palms, and soles repigmented poorly in all groups.

Several specific observations could be made. Initially, higher doses of 8-MOP (Me-8-MOP) gave a quicker response than lower doses (Lo-8-MOP), yet after 2 years the latter was associated with a much better response rate (60 to 69 percent on the

face, neck, and chest after 15 months). High-dosage TMP (Hi-TMP) gave a favorable response in the first year (except for arms and legs, though this may not be significant). After 2 years of therapy, the combination therapy (Lo-8-MOP + Me-TMP) gave repigmentation rates that exceeded those with Me-TMP or Hi-TMP. Lo-8-MOP results, except for arms and legs, were as good as the combination. Curiously, the combination did much better than Me-8-MOP, particularly in 2 years of treatment of the head and neck. Hi-Ps also did better than Me-Ps, but the results on the legs were disappointing. Only the combination and Me-8-MOP gave any degree of repigmentation of the hands (15 percent). The overall 2-year 75 percent repigmentation response appeared to be best with Lo-8-MOP + Me-TMP (38 percent) followed by Lo-8-MOP (31 percent).

Several useful conclusions about PUVASOL may be drawn in general from our outdoor experience in India. First, some areas of the skin respond better than others regardless of the psoralen used. The face and neck tend to do best, but the chest, arms, and legs in some cases respond almost as well. The back and abdomen are comparable. The hands (also feet, lips, palms, soles, and nipples) respond poorly. Second, longer duration of therapy is correlated with more extensive repigmentation unless severe phototoxicity persists; this may cause melanocyte destruction and Koebnerization. Third, the figures for total repigmentary response may be poor standards for comparison as they may reflect undue weight placed upon areas unresponsive to any modality of phototherapy. Face, neck, trunk, upper arms and legs are the best criteria for comparison.

The PUVA treatment of vitiligo was virtually without adverse reactions; there were no abnormal laboratory results of CBC, liver function tests, or urinalysis in serial determinations over the 2 years of study (and also after an additional 2-year follow-up).

Subjective complaints—particularly nausea, gastrointestinal distress, pruritus, lightheadedness, and headache—were recorded with all groups. These were most common with Me-8-MOP (especially nausea and giddiness). In all groups the occurrence was dose-related. Nausea was least likely with TMP, even VH-TMP, but gastrointestinal distress occurred with average frequency. Pruritus was also less common with TMP than with 8-MOP or Ps. Headaches were infrequent but when they occurred probably were related to the heat of solar radiation rather than to the psoralens themselves.

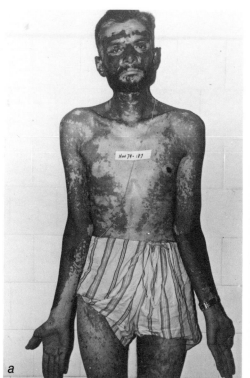
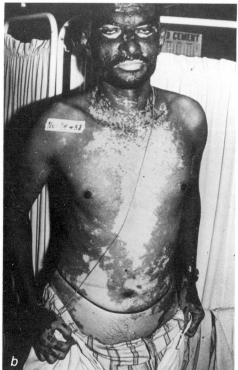
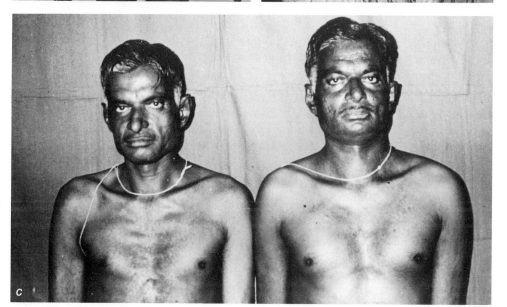

Fig. 7. Forty-three-year-old twin brothers with hyperthyroidism of 6 years' and vitiligo of 13 years' duration. (*a*) and (*b*) Prior to therapy some repigmentation had been apparent in normally sun-exposed areas. (*c*) After a year of therapy with thrice-weekly 40 mg 8-MOP and sunlight (approximately 1 hour), complete repigmentation of the face, chest, and upper arms (as well as lower arms, abdomen, back, and legs) was observed. Distal digits and knuckles, however, did not respond even after 2 years of therapy.

Acute and chronic phototoxicity occurred with all dosage schedules for all psoralens. These were most common with Me-8-MOP and least so with Me-TMP and Me-Ps. That they appeared less frequently with Me-8-MOP than with Lo-8-MOP or Lo-8-MOP + Me-TMP in this study suggests

an aberration of the data; severe phototoxicity may have selected against continuation of some Me-8-MOP patients.

Although photosensitivity reactions were noted, severe disabling photosensitivity reactions (erythema, edema, blistering, etc.) were absent. No

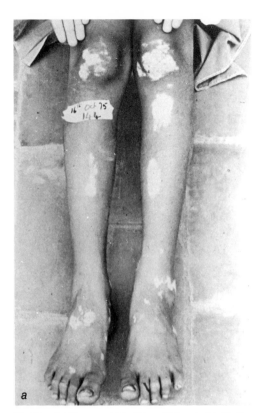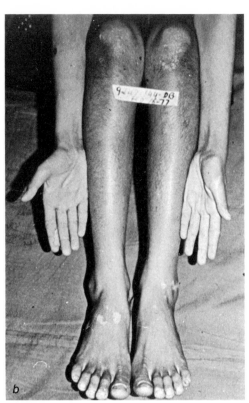

Fig. 8. A 10-year-old Indian girl treated initially with placebo and sunlight for a year, with gradual worsening of her vitiligo. (*a*) After a year she was switched to 3.6 mg/kg TMP. (*b*) A year later her knees are nearly fully repigmented as are her legs. The dorsal feet repigmented nearly 75 percent.

keratoses were noted at 26 months of treatment; however, when 220 patients were seen at 4 years, 13 percent (29/220), most of whom had been treating for over 48 months, had developed at least one keratosis in the vitiliginous macules located mostly on the lower legs. Fifteen patients had more than one lesion, and five had multiple lesions of several types. Clinically, the lesions were (1) keratotic papules, (2) actinic keratosis-like macules, (3) nonscaling dome-shaped papules, and (4) lichenoid porokeratotic-like papules. No morphologic-type lesion could be associated with any one of the three psoralen derivatives except that dome-shaped papules were found only with VH-TMP, and this group had the highest percentage (32 percent) of patients with lesions. Histologically, the lesions showed benign papillary epidermal hyperplasia with hyperkeratosis, papillary actinic keratoses, and atrophic actinic keratoses. Only seven lesions were actinic keratoses; atypia was mild. Apoptotic bodies (colloid bodies) were occasionally numerous. None of these lesions had been noted at 1- or 2-year examinations of the patients. It is not certain whether these lesions were related to the psoralens plus sunlight exposure or to the prolonged exposure of these amelanotic areas to sunlight over several years. Many patients had also had prior therapy involving topical remedies very difficult to identify. No squamous cell carcinomas, basal cell carcinomas, or melanomas were observed [60].

Despite some chronic phototoxicity and occasional complaints of nausea and pruritus and gastrointestinal distress, patients were generally pleased with their results. In this study, 8-MOP was the most effective single drug, and use of 0.3 mg/kg gave optimal results. Combination therapy with 8-MOP + TMP seemed to improve results, particularly on the arms and legs. It is possible that VH-TMP (continued for similar periods of time) may do as well and better than 0.6 to 0.9 mg/kg TMP in this study. Ps (0.6 mg/kg) was not an effective therapy, but higher dosage (1.2 mg/kg) appeared to be better than medium-dose Ps, as judged on a limited number of patients.

Despite the Indian study results, we have been impressed with repigmentation induced with TMP (0.6 to 0.9 mg/kg) and sunlight or artificial UVA (Fig. 9). Because orally administered TMP is less phototoxic than 8-MOP and thereby can be used out of doors for Skin Types III and IV, over the past 2 years we have treated 42 patients with 0.6

to 0.9 mg/kg of TMP. All patients were treated in a conventional stand-up commercial UVA unit composed of 44 vertically mounted FR40-T12HO PUVA bulbs (Psoralite, Paul B. Elder Co., Bryan, Ohio). Patients were treated twice weekly, not 2 days in a row. All were treated with suberythemal to trace-erythemal UVA dosages ranging from 4 to 20 J/cm² per treatment (average, 6 to 12 J/cm²). The overall results correlating number of treatments with percent of patients achieving 80 percent or more repigmentation response were as follows:

	No. of patients	No. of treatments	No. (%) with repigmentation > 80%	
	11	< 50	2	(18%)
	25	50–200	7	(28%)
	6	> 200	5	(83%)
Total	42		14	(33%)

Of these 42 patients who treated regularly, 28 (69 percent) had involvement of the face and neck. The best assessment of responsiveness is data involving such normally responsive areas as follows:

No. of treat-ments	No. of patients	Face and neck response		
		< 25% repig-mented	26%–80% repig-mented	> 80% repig-mented
< 50	6	67%	17%	17%
50–200	16	38%	12%	50%
> 200	6	0	17%	83%

Response clearly correlates with duration of continuous therapy.

The most limiting factor in therapy is the slow rate of response. Other problems do occur, though they infrequently limit therapy. Pruritus occurs in about 25 percent, but in only one case has it been intractable. Marked phototoxicity occurs in 5 to 10 percent of patients. Development of polymorphous light eruption (PMLE)–like small erythematous papules within vitiliginous macules occurs in about 15 percent; these develop either at the energy level of the minimum phototoxic dose (MPD) or, in a few cases, significantly below that. In the latter, gradually increasing increments of UVA will usually result in clearing. Topical corticosteroids may be used as a temporary adjuvant.

For indoor PUVA therapy, patients are preferably treated with oral 4,5′,8-trimethylpsoralen (TMP), Trisoralen, or trioxsalen. Patients initially receive 0.6 mg/kg of TMP. The schedules of treatments for patients with Skin Types II or III (fair-skinned people who burn easily or burn moderately and tan minimally or moderately) require twice-weekly UVA exposures 2 hours after psoralen ingestion. Thrice-weekly treatments on every alternate day may be prescribed to patients with pigmented skin (Skin Types IV, V, or VI). Treatments are not given on two consecutive days. Preliminary experience suggests that weekly treatments are inadequate and more than thrice-weekly treatments may be unnecessary. Ideally, an MPD

Fig. 9. A 50-year-old woman with vitiligo of the extensor knees. (a) After initiating therapy with 40 mg TMP (0.6 mg/kg) and artificial high-intensity UVA twice weekly. (b) After 18 months of therapy complete repigmentation is apparent.

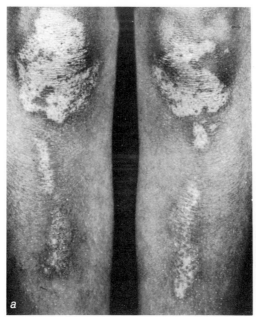
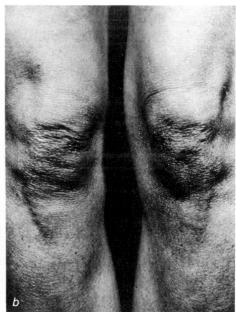

determination precedes therapy. The initial UVA exposure dose for repigmentation therapy is approximately 60 to 70 percent of that MPD, the UVA dose which initially produced a 1+ erythematous reaction. Otherwise, for fair-skinned people, UVA exposure dose should begin with 1.0 J/cm² and be increased at each subsequent therapy session by 0.5 to 1.0 J/cm² until a faint (±) or 1+ erythema results in vitiligo macules. Patients with Skin Types V or VI may receive 2 to 3 J/cm² of UVA in the first treatment and an increment of 1 to 1.5 J/cm² at subsequent treatments until a faint erythematous reaction is observed. In our experience, erythema is not essential for stimulating repigmentation and the minimum melanogenic dose (MMD) is less than MPD; therefore, photochemotherapy can be successfully performed at suberythemal exposure doses. Some incremental increase or decrease in exposure doses may be required periodically to limit the skin exposure at MPD levels. Severe phototoxicity must be avoided since this may retard or even inhibit melanogenesis or even result in Koebnerization and appearance of new areas of depigmentation.

With any treatment regimen (outdoor PUVA-SOL or indoor PUVA), between 15 and 25 treatments are required before perifollicular macules of repigmentation are observed. The appearance of myriads of small perifollicular dots of repigmentation is a good prognostic sign and should encourage continuation of the course of therapy. Generally, all macules in any given area (face, neck, trunk, etc.) tend to respond equally well unless UVA exposure is not uniform. As treatments continue, the small perifollicular macules enlarge and coalesce until an amelanotic macule is completely repigmented.

Topical Therapy. Topical psoralens are recommended only for small localized lesions (Fig. 5). Commercially available Oxsoralen lotion containing 1% 8-MOP should be diluted to 0.1% concentration with a 1:1 mixture of ethanol and propylene glycol. (Nine parts of this alcoholic propylene glycol solution are mixed with one part of 1.0% Oxsoralen solution to obtain a 0.1% 8-MOP solution. The vitiliginous macules are painted uniformly once with this 0.1% 8-MOP solution.) A carefully applied application will deliver about 0.25 mL to a macule of about 50 cm²; this provides approximately 250 μg of 8-MOP per 50 cm² of skin (5 μg/cm²). Application of 8-MOP solution should be restricted to the lesional skin only, with minimal application of the lotion to the surrounding normal skin. Thirty to 45 min after application, the skin is exposed to UVA or to solar radiation. Initial UVA exposures must be minimal, beginning at 0.25 J/cm². Likewise, sun-exposure doses are kept low (1 to 2 min for the first treatment), and sunlight exposures should be carried out preferably between 11:00 a.m. and 2:00 p.m. Subsequent treatments are no more frequent than every other day; with each exposure, the dose of UVA is increased by 0.25 J/cm² up to a total dose of 2 to 3 J/cm². Sunlight exposures should be increased cautiously to a maximum of approximately 10 min (± 5 min). The goal of the UV dosimetry is to irradiate the skin with a minimal phototoxic dose of UVA so as to achieve barely perceptible erythematous reaction 36 to 48 hr after exposure. Occasionally patients overexpose and develop blistering phototoxic reactions with accompanying edema and/or marked pruritus. Treatments are then discontinued until the acute phototoxicity has abated and the skin has returned to "normal" appearance. Subsequently, treatments are resumed with caution and UVA doses are carefully regulated. Evidence of repigmentation is usually apparent after 10 to 20 treatments. Continuation of therapy should be encouraged until the small lesion is uniformly repigmented. After each treatment, patients must wash the treated areas with soap and water and apply a broad-spectrum sunscreen containing cinnamate and benzophenone (Piz Buin-8) or PABA ester and benzophenone (Super Shade 15 or Total Eclipse or PreSun creamy).

There are two common and troublesome problems attending topical psoralen photochemotherapy. Casual application of the psoralen-containing solution will lead to an area of hyperpigmentation surrounding the treated vitiligo macule; this may even resemble a melanin "paint run" if application has been particularly sloppy. This psoralen-induced hyperpigmentation of normal skin is particularly slow to revert to normal skin color and is always unsightly. Second, after therapy, inadequate washing and casual sun exposure, even through window glass, may precipitate a potentially severe phototoxic eruption which may lead to blistering and even Koebnerization. The margin of safety between therapeutic dose (MMD) and the severe phototoxic dose (MPD) is narrow. Patients must clearly understand that an additional 1 or 2 min of sun exposure can result in a severe, painful, phototoxic reaction. It is this difficulty alone that restricts topical psoralen usage to those highly motivated compliant patients with one, occasionally more, very small vitiliginous macules.

Summary of PUVA Photochemotherapy of Vitiligo.

1. To achieve repigmentation, vitiligo patients need long-term therapy with oral psoralens (8-MOP or TMP) and well-controlled sunlight or artificial UVA exposures. Such patients must be regularly monitored for PUVA response.

2. Effective results may occur with either 8-MOP or TMP. Because oral TMP is much less phototoxic than 8-MOP, TMP is the preferred drug for treatment with sunlight as the source of UVA, especially for patients with Skin Types III or IV. Since many patients who treat indoors over the winter prefer the convenience of outdoor treatments over the summer and since we prefer not to switch back and forth between psoralens, we start all new patients on 0.6 mg/kg TMP and increase to 0.9 mg/kg if there is no evidence of response after 25 treatments. Serum TMP levels (when available) or the determination of a MPD should also be carried out at that time. If there is no response after an additional 15 to 25 treatments, the patient should be switched to 0.3 mg/kg 8-MOP and a MPD done to ensure absorption of drug. If sunlight is used as a UVA source, the exposures should be precise and measured. Another 25 treatments are given and thereafter, if little response, the dosage is increased to 0.6 mg/kg 8-MOP. Should this fail also after 20 to 25 treatments, combination of 0.3 mg/kg 8-MOP + 0.6 mg/kg TMP may yet be successful (after a MPD and serum levels of 8-MOP and TMP). Failure of response after 25 treatments marks patient unresponsiveness, and therapy should be abandoned. Responsiveness must be defined as development of many perifollicular macules of repigmentation. The patient who develops such macules generally is a responder; subsequent failure to continue to respond should prompt performance of a MPD and serum psoralen determinations. A patient who is undergoing reversal despite good serum levels may be Koebnerizing; therapy should be interrupted for 2 to 4 weeks and carefully resumed at a sub-MPD UV exposure dosage.

3. The patient should be informed that areas that respond poorly include the lips (mucosa), the distal dorsal hands, tips of fingers, areas of bony prominences (feet, ankles, toes, fingers, etc.), palms, soles, nipples, and gums. In the interest of minimizing the actinic changes, these areas should be shielded with broad-spectrum sunscreens during the exposure schedules.

4. The frequency of treatments should be at least twice a week, ideally on every third day. No more than three exposures a week are recommended, with at least 1 day between each treatment (alternate-day therapy).

5. If treatments are discontinued (e.g., in winter time), reversal of the induced repigmentation usually occurs *unless the macule has repigmented fully.* Therefore, no patient should begin therapy without consideration of winter maintenance treatments. A patient who repigments partially in the summer and reverses fully over the winter should not be treated unless year-round therapy is possible. Past experience reveals that totally repigmented macules may be stable for 12 to 14 years or more without any evidence of loss of color [61]. Some patients, while showing repigmentation of vitiligo macules, may also continue to develop new vitiligo lesions in the course of their treatment. This is not necessarily a harbinger of poor response or failure but should alert one to problems with light exposure or dosage schedule.

6. Patients with segmental vitiligo exhibiting one or more macules in a dermatomal or quasidermatomal distribution tend to show varying response, some macules repigmenting slowly and with difficulty. Vitiligo patients with only acrofacial distribution and lip involvement [distal extremities showing amelanotic areas at the tips of the fingers and toes and mucosal membranes (lips)] tend to show poor repigmentation response.

7. Children under age 12 are generally not treated until they are able to withstand the stress of alternate-day therapy either in the sun or in a high-intensity UVA irradiation system. Children over 12 may be treated with oral 8-MOP or TMP and proper precautionary measures, including the shielding of eyes with UVA-opaque sunglasses.

8. Treatment with oral psoralens and UVA or sunlight should be accompanied by proper shielding of eyes for 24 hr after drug ingestion if out of doors or near a bright window indoors.

9. Topical treatment with 8-MOP may prove to be effective if the treatment is carried out carefully and in cooperative and intelligent patients. Vitiligo macules, when they are small in size (2 to 5 cm in diameter or less), could be treated with topical psoralens (8-MOP, 0.1%), approximately 5 μg/cm^2, especially in children under 12 years of age who appear to respond to topical therapy quite satisfactorily. Topical therapy should be given twice or thrice a week, usually on alternate days with great caution.

Mechanism of Psoralen-induced Repigmentation.
The mechanism by which oral administration of

psoralens and subsequent exposure to UVA causes repigmentation in vitiligo skin remains mostly unknown and speculative. Certain well-documented events in pigment cell biology of normal skin may help in understanding the mode of hyperpigmentation stimulated by PUVA. It appears that the increased melanin pigmentation in normal skin is related to the photoconjugation of psoralen with pyrimidine bases in DNA to form both the monofunctional photoadducts (single-strand adducts of psoralen to pyrimidine bases) and interstrand cross-links (bifunctional adducts) between psoralen and pyrimidine bases of both strands of the DNA [62]. These events reflect damage to cellular DNA and initially retard the cell division in the preexisting functional melanocytes in the normal skin and pigmented hair bulbs and appear to prolong the availability of cell surface MSH receptor in the G_2 phase of the cell cycle [63]. This allows the MSH to activate the melanin-forming enzyme activity. Tyrosinase activity thus increases in the functional melanocytes. The inhibitory effect of sulfhydryl (SH) groups (glutathione and cystine) on tyrosinase activity is also decreased due to the oxidation of SH groups. This also may contribute to the activation of tyrosinase activity. Within 48 to 72 hr, the melanocytes appear to undergo repair of their damaged DNA by excision of the pyrimidine-psoralen adducts. Melanocytic, DNA replication and cell replication by mitosis follow. The resulting mitoses in preexisting melanocytes cause generation of new functional melanocytes with enhanced tyrosinase activity. Increased cell population and enhanced tyrosinase activity resulting from increased protein synthesis in the proliferating melanocytes leads to the increased formation of melanosomes. Thus, psoralen plus UVA irradiation influences the normal pigmentation (constitutive color) of the skin in one or more of the following ways: (1) By inducing an increase in the number of functional melanocytes as a result of a direct mitotic replication of melanocytes and also possibly the activation of the dormant or resting melanocytes existing prior to irradiation in the epidermis or skin appendages. (2) By promoting hypertrophy of melanocytes and the increased arborization of the dendrites of melanocytes. (3) By augmenting the development and the melanization of melanosomes within the hypertrophic melanocytes; this is manifested by an increase in the number of melanosomes, increased synthesis of melanosomal proteins, and the melanin-forming enzyme tyrosinase. The number of fully melanized stage IV melanosomes is increased both in the melanocytes and in the associated pool of kerati-

nocytes. Even the number of early and intermediate stages of melanosomes (premelanosomes and partially melanized stage II and III melanosomes) is increased. (4) By stimulation of tyrosinase activity, due principally to the synthesis of new tyrosinase in proliferating melanocytes and the activation of the enzyme by the availability of α-MSH receptors. (5) By enhanced migration of the activated melanocytes from skin appendages (e.g., sweat ducts and hair follicles). This is particularly evident as perifollicular repigmenting macules in patients with vitiligo undergoing repigmentation [64–66].

Depigmentation

One of the therapeutic options for patients with extensive vitiligo involves depigmentation of the remaining normally melanized skin (Fig. 10). Application of Benoquin (20% monobenzylether of hydroquinone, or MBEHQ) can result in complete depigmentation of normally melanized skin. Awareness of the effects of MBEHQ date from the observations of Schwartz et al. [67] on tannery workers who developed depigmentation—mimicking vitiligo—under gauntlet-type rubber gloves. Depigmentation remote from sites of direct exposure was initially attributed to accidental and casual MBEHQ exposure of all involved cutaneous areas. Awareness of the potential of this compound as a lightening agent led to its use for many macular hypermelanoses and inclusion in many Japanese cosmetics. Subsequently, more cases of remote depigmentation attributed to MBEHQ were reported [68,69]. It was believed that MBEHQ was responsible for antigen formation against melanin or another melanocyte faction. The inescapable conclusion is that neither the degree nor the location of MBEHQ-induced depigmentation can be predictably controlled. Furthermore, the depigmentation appears to be irreversible. Therefore, the indication for MBEHQ usage is very specific: The *only* indication for the use of Benoquin is the patient with generalized vitiligo who wants to be depigmented totally—to have what resembles vitiligo universalis.

Our criteria for patient selection for the use of Benoquin are generally the following:

1. Patient age 40 or over
2. Patient with over 40 percent vitiligo
3. Patient who has had an adequate trial of PUVA and failed or patient unwilling to commit himself or herself to 100 to 300 PUVA treatments

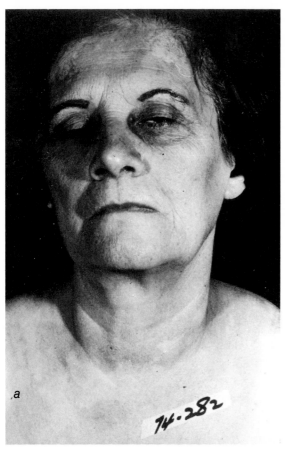 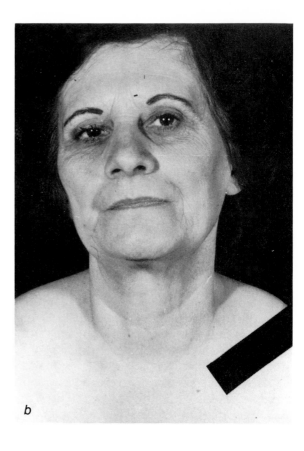

Fig. 10. Monobenzylether of hydroquinone (Benoquin) therapy to induce depigmentation of remaining pigmented skin in older patient with extensive vitiligo. (*a*) Vitiligo before MBEHQ therapy. (*b*) After 12 months the normal skin had been totally depigmented. Hair color is rarely affected.

4. Patient, for whatever reason, whose overwhelming motivation is to have a uniform color
5. Nonlactating-nonpregnant female patient
6. Patient should not be black, Asiatic, Indian, or Oriental (unless he or she understands the social implications of the color change)

Because MBEHQ-induced depigmentation is irreversible, patients must be willing to abandon forever their normal constitutive and facultative skin color; we have on occasion made exceptions to the criteria 1, 2, 3, and 6, but only after serious and protracted discussion with the patient involved. We devote particular attention to the problems potentially experienced by brown and deeply pigmented individuals; significant real or perceived cultural displacement may attend depigmentation for such people. These patients should be counseled carefully and with great sensitivity from the outset.

At least in part because of careful patient selection, those patients who have successfully used MBEHQ are the most satisfied of all patients treated for vitiligo [69]. In our recent experience (personal observations), among 25 individuals who attempted Benoquin depigmentation, two developed contact dermatitis, in both cases only on normally melanized skin, and were unable to continue therapy. A third individual developed a similar eruption which disappeared once a more dilute MBEHQ preparation was used (this being unsuccessful even at 1% concentrations in the former two patients). Patients are advised to apply Benoquin twice a day to all areas they wish to depigment but must recognize the possibility that remote areas could also be affected. Appearance of clinical change usually first becomes apparent after about 3 to 4 months of use as (1) diffuse lightening of normally melanized skin, (2) diffuse lightening and perifollicular sparing, and/or (3) development of complete hypomelanotic macules, particularly confetti macules. Complete depigmentation requires 9 to 12 months of continuous therapy. All but one individual who treated regularly for a year depigmented successfully. The one failure did not lighten appreciably despite tid usage.

All others were, however, very pleased with their results.

Problems with application are common. Over half complained of moderate to severe dryness, pruritus, and/or erythema. The problem was most marked on the face and neck; often patients had to use a reduced-strength formulation (1:1 Benoquin, Eucerin) to make usage tolerable. Except in those cases noted, the discontinuation of therapy was not required.

All who treated to completion were very pleased with their results, which are permanent. Periodic local recurrences of repigmentation in the form of brown macules should be expected in some, especially following sunlight exposure. We have seen four patients develop perifollicular macules of repigmentation (and there may be others in patients lost to follow-up) after prolonged sun exposure. However, reinstitution of Benoquin application led to loss of pigment within 2 to 3 months. After achieving desired depigmentation, patients should be advised to use sunscreens (SPF 15) daily. Several patients have been given oral β-carotene (Solatene, Hoffmann-LaRoche) (60 to 120 mg/day) to produce mild carotoderma, which occurs within 6 to 9 weeks after beginning the treatment. Some patients prefer the hue of carotoderma to the hue of amelanotic skin. The carotoderma is maintained with low doses (as little as 60 mg/day) of oral β-carotene.

The mechanism of the MBEHQ-induced depigmentation involves gradual and selective destruction of pigment-producing cells by the cytotoxic effect of MBEHQ. This occurs by one or more of the following mechanisms: (1) By generation of disruptive reactive semiquinone-like free radicals that damage cell membrane. Agents such as MBEHQ can generate diffusible OH· free radicals that can initiate lipid peroxidation of the lipoprotein membranes in melanocytes and thus destroy the functional activity of melanocytes. The cytotoxic products presumably arise from tyrosinase-mediated oxidation of MBEHQ. (2) By inhibiting melanogenesis in the follicular and nonfollicular melanocytes: MBEHQ affects the formation, melanization, and degradation of melanosomes, as well as the destruction of membranous organelles. Direct inhibition of tyrosinase activity by MBEHQ is unlikely as part of the pathogenic mechanism in vivo. (3) It is conceivable that MBEHQ conjugates with melanoprotein and this adduct becomes an antigenic substance which stimulates the formation of autoantibodies against melanin-producing melanocytes, thus causing the gradual cytotoxicity of melanocytes. This hypothesis appears most likely.

References

1. Allison JR, Curtis AC: Vitiligo and pernicious anemia. *Arch Dermatol* **72**:407–408, 1955
2. Fitzpatrick TB, Mihm MC Jr: Abnormalities in the melanin pigmentary system, in *Dermatology in General Medicine.* Edited by TB Fitzpatrick et al. McGraw-Hill, New York, 1971, pp 1591–1637
3. Nordlund JJ et al: Pigmentary changes in the eyes of patients with vitiligo (abstr). *J Invest Dermatol* **68**:241, 1977
4. Wood LC et al: High frequency of subclinical thyroid disease in older patients with vitiligo. *Proceedings of the VIIth International Thyroid Conference, Sydney, Australia, February 1980.* Australian Academy of Science, Canberra City, Australia, 1980
5. Lerner AB: Vitiligo. *J Invest Dermatol* **32**:285–310, 1959
6. Cunliffe W et al: Vitiligo, thyroid disease and autoimmunity. *Br J Dermatol* **80**:138–139, 1968
7. Perrot H et al: Vitiligo, thyreopathies et autoimmunisation. *Lyon Med* **230**:325–331, 1973
8. Lerner AB: On the etiology of vitiligo and gray hair. *Am J Med* **51**:141–147, 1971
9. Frenk E: Experimentelle Depigmentierung der Meerschweinchenhaut durch selektiv toxische Virkung von Hydrochinon-Monäthyläther auf die Melanocyten. *Arch Klin Exp Dermatol* **235**:16–24, 1969
10. Riley PA: The mechanism of hydroxyanisole depigmentation. *J Pathol* **101**:163–169, 1970
11. Jimbow K et al: Ultrastructural investigation of autophagocytosis of melanosomes and programmed death of melanocytes in White Leghorn feathers: a study of morphogenic events leading to hypomelanosis. *Dev Biol* **36**:8–25, 1974
12. Goldman PJ, Theiss AM: Berufsbedingle Vitiligo durch paratertiares Butylphenol. Eine Trios von Vitiligo, Hepatose und Struma. *Hautarzt* **27**:155–159, 1976
13. Rodermund OE, Wieland H: Vitiligo, Hepatosplenopathie und Struma nach Arbeit mit paratertiäsem Butylphenol. *Dtsch Med Wochenschr* **43**:1–3, 1975
14. Morohashi M et al: Ultrastructural studies of vitiligo, Vogt–Koyanagi syndrome, and incontinentia pigmenti achromians. *Arch Dermatol* **113**:755–766, 1977
15. Lerner AB: Neural control of pigment cells, in *The Biology of Normal and Abnormal Melanocytes.* Edited by T Kawamura et al. University Park Press, Tokyo, 1971, pp 3–16
16. Fabian G: The spread of black pigment of the denervated skin of guinea pig. *Acta Biol Acad Sci Hung* **4**:471–479, 1951
17. Voulot C: Mechanisme de controle de l'extension pigmentaire liee aux autogreffes de la peau. *Ann Dermatol Syphiligr (Paris)* **97**:549–555, 1970
18. Jachlin HN: Depigmentation of the eyelids in eserine allergy. *Am J Ophthalmol* **59**:899–902, 1965
19. Gauthier Y et al: Belan de l'activite cholinesterasique dans le vitiligo: son interet physiopathologique. Presented at the 15ᵉᵐᵉ Congrès de l'Association des Dermatologistes et Syphiligraphes de Langue Francaise, Ajaccio, May 1976
20. Chanco-Turner ML, Lerner AB: Physiologic changes in vitiligo. *Arch Dermatol* **91**:390–396, 1965
21. Koga M: Vitiligo: a new classification and therapy. *Br J Dermatol* **97**:255–261, 1977
22. Zebacha T et al: Etiopathogenesis of vitiligo. *Przegl Dermatol* **59**:507–511, 1972
23. Maiti A et al: Tactile gnosis and cold numbness in vitiligo. *Bull Univ Calif Med* **2**:32–40, 1965

24. Langhof VH et al: Melaninantiköperbildung bei Vitiligo. *Hautarzt* **16**:209–212, 1965

25. Hertz KC et al: Autoimmune vitiligo: detection of antibodies to melanin producing cells. *N Engl J Med* **297**:634–637, 1977

26. Betterle C et al: Vitiligo and autoimmune polyendocrine deficiencies with autoantibodies to melanin producing cells. *Arch Dermatol* **115**:364, 1979

27. Wasserman HP, Van der Waalt JJ: Antibodies against melanin: the significance of negative results. *S Afr Med J* **47**:7–9, 1973

28. Zelickson AS, Mottaz JH: The effect of sunlight on human epidermis. A quantitative electron microscopic study of dendritic cells. *Arch Dermatol* **101**:312–315, 1970

29. Jacobs JB et al: Halo nevus: a fine structural study of a host rejection phenomenon (abstr). *Fed Proc* **32**:870, 1973

30. Nairn RC et al: Antitumour immunoreactivity in patients with malignant melanoma. *Med J Aust* **1**:397–403, 1972

31. Lewis MG et al: Tumour-specific antibodies in human malignant melanoma and their relationship to the extent of the disease. *Br Med J* **3**:547–552, 1969

32. Bleehen SS: Quoted in Copeman PWM et al: Biology and immunology of vitiligo and cutaneous malignant melanoma, in *Recent Advances in Dermatology*, No. 3. Edited by AJ Rook. Churchill–Livingstone, London, 1973, pp 245–284

33. Ortonne J-P, Alario A: T + B lymphocytes in vitiligo. *Arch Dermatol Res* **261**:147–151, 1978

34. Brown AC et al: Alopecia areata and vitiligo associated with Down's syndrome. *Arch Dermatol* **113**:1296, 1977

35. Mishima Y: Congenital and non-congenital depigmentation, in *Modern Problems in Paediatrics,* vol 20, *Pediatric Dermatology*. Edited by R Ruiz-Maldonado. S Karger, Basel, 1976, pp 18–37

36. Copeman PWM et al: Immunologic associations of halo nevus with cutaneous malignant melanoma. *Br J Dermatol* **88**:127–137, 1973

37. Lerner AB, Cage GW: Melanomas in horses. *Yale J Biol Med* **46**:646–649, 1973

38. Millikan LE et al: Gross and ultrastructural studies in a new melanoma model: the Sinclair swine. *Yale J Biol Med* **46**:631–645, 1973

39. Boissy RE et al: The DAM chicken. A new animal model for vitiligo, in *Proceedings of the 10th International Pigment Cell Conference, Cambridge, Massachusetts, October 8–12, 1977,* vol 4, *Pigment Cell.* S Karger, Basel, 1979

40. Nordlund JJ et al: The prevalence of vitiligo and poliosis in patients with uveitis. *J Am Acad Dermatol* **4**:528–536, 1981

41. Jimbow K et al: Congenital circumscribed hypomelanosis: a characterization based on electron microscopic study of tuberous sclerosis, nevus depigmentosus, and piebaldism. *J Invest Dermatol* **64**:50–62, 1975

42. Froggart P: An outline, with bibliography, of human piebaldism and white forelock. *Irish J Med Sci* **398**:81–94, 1959

43. Woolf CM et al: Congenital deafness associated with piebaldism. *Arch Otolaryngol* **82**:244–250, 1965

44. Waardenburg PJ: A new syndrome combining developmental anomalies of the eyelids, eyebrows, and nose root with pigmentary defects of the iris and head hair and with congenital deafness. *Am J Hum Genet* **3**:195–253, 1951

45. Ziprkowski L et al: Partial albinism and deaf-mutism due to a recessive sex-linked gene. *Arch Dermatol* **86**:530–539, 1962

46. Nordlund JJ et al: Halo nevi and the Vogt–Koyanagi–Harada syndrome. *Arch Dermatol* **116**:690–692, 1980

47. Butterworth T, Strean LP: Vitiligo, in *Clinical Genodermatology*. Williams & Wilkins, Baltimore, 1962, pp 4–6

48. Gokhale BB, Gokhale TB: Corticotropin and vitiligo (preliminary observation). *Br J Dermatol* **95**:329, 1976

49. El Mofty AM: *Vitiligo and Psoralens*. Pergamon, Oxford, 1968

50. Kuske H: Experimentelle untersuchungen zur Photosensibilisierung der Haut durch pflanzliche wirkstoffe; Lichtsensibilisierung durch Furocumarine als Ursache verschied phytogener Dermatosen. *Arch Dermatol (Berlin)* **178**:112–123, 1938

51. Montgomery DW: Vitiligo treated with Finsen light. *J Cutan Dis Incl Syph NY* **2**:17–19, 1904

52. Buschke A: Notiz zur Behandlung des Vitiligo mit Licht. *Med Klin (Berlin)* **3**:983, 1907

53. Uhlmann E: Pigmentbildung bei Vitiligo. *Med Klin (Berlin)* **23**:279, 1927

54. Uhlmann E: Die Behandlung der Vitiligo und die Voraussetzungen fuer die Kunstliche Pigmentierung der Haut. *Med Welt* **8**:226–228, 1934

55. El Mofty AM: A preliminary clinical report on the treatment of leukoderma with *Ammi majus* Linn. *J R Egypt Med Assoc* **31**:651–655, 1948

56. Lerner AB et al: Clinical and experimental studies with 8-methoxypsoralen in vitiligo. *J Invest Dermatol* **20**:299–314, 1953

57. Parrish JA et al: Photochemotherapy of psoriasis with oral methoxsalen and longwave ultraviolet light. *N Engl J Med* **291**:1207–1222, 1974

58. Parrish JA et al: Photochemotherapy of vitiligo with oral psoralens and artificially produced UVA. *Arch Dermatol* **112**:1531–1534, 1976

59. Pathak MA et al: Relative effectiveness of three psoralens and sunlight in repigmentation of 365 vitiligo patients (abstr). *J Invest Dermatol* **74**:252, 1980

60. Mosher DB et al: Development of cutaneous lesions in vitiligo during long-term PUVA therapy (abstr). *J Invest Dermatol* **74**:259, 1980

61. Kenney JA Jr: Vitiligo treated by psoralens: a long-term study of the permanency of repigmentation. *Arch Dermatol* **103**:475–480, 1971

62. Pathak MA: Phytophotodermatitis, in *Sunlight and Man: Normal and Abnormal Photobiologic Responses*. Edited by MA Pathak et al; TB Fitzpatrick, consulting editor. Univ of Tokyo Press, Tokyo, 1974, pp 495–513

63. Carter DM et al: Pigment response of melanoma cell to psoralens and light, in *Proceedings of the 10th International Pigment Cell Conference, Cambridge, Massachusetts, October 8–12, 1977,* vol 4, *Pigment Cell.* S Karger, Basel, 1979

64. Pegum JS: Dissociated depigmentation in vitiligo: significance and therapeutic implications. *Br J Dermatol* **67**:348–350, 1955

65. Africk J, Fulton J: Treatment of vitiligo with topical trimethylpsoralen and sunlight. *Br J Dermatol* **84**:151–156, 1971

66. Fitzpatrick TB, Pathak MA: Historical aspects of methoxsalen and other furocoumarins. *J Invest Dermatol* **32**:229–231, 1959

67. Schwartz L et al: Occupational leukoderma. *Arch Dermatol Syphilol* **42**:993–1014, 1940

68. Klander JV, Kimmick JM: Occupational leukoderma with report of cases. *Ind Med Surg* **22**:106–110, 1953

69. Mosher DB et al: Monobenzylether of hydroquinone: a retrospective study of 18 vitiligo patients and a review of the literature. *Br J Dermatol* **97**:669–679, 1977

THE RETINOIDS

Dorothy B. Windhorst

Gary L. Peck

The retinoids, as defined by Sporn et al. [1], include retinol and its derivatives as well as a new class of synthetic compounds developed since 1968. The development of chemical analogues of retinoic acid that began in the late 1960s has ushered in a new era in the therapy for skin diseases such as cystic acne, psoriasis, and disorders of keratinization notably resistant to other remedies. Of interest is the fact that the development efforts arose primarily from observations on the ability of retinoids to affect malignant and premalignant tissues both in vivo and in vitro [2].

The increasing clinical and scientific interest in vitamin A and its analogues is well illustrated by the six international symposia from 1975 to 1981 which were limited to [3–7] or emphasized [8] these substances.

Vitamin A, Tretinoin, and Isotretinoin

Vitamin A, retinol, was known in terms of nutritional requirements to prevent night blindness by ancient Egyptians; however, it was defined in the early part of this century by Sir F. Gowland Hopkins in England and Elmer McCollum in the United States as a lipid-soluble nutritional factor essential for growth. Its first clinical application in modern medicine was in the treatment of xerophthalmia and the prevention of night blindness during World War I. As a nutrient, vitamin A has multiple functions: promoting growth; maintaining normal vision and reproduction; and maintaining the integrity and differentiation of epithelial tissue in the trachea, lungs, salivary glands, urinary bladder, ureter, and gastrointestinal tract, as well as in the skin and its appendages.

In the mammalian organism this multiplicity of biologic activities is carried out by three major compounds: retinol, retinal, and retinoic acid. Retinol (vitamin A alcohol) along with its precursor, β-carotene, is the main dietary source, as well as the transport and storage form [9]. Retinal (vitamin A aldehyde) contributes to the formation of rhodopsin, and its physiologic role is central to the visual cycle. Retinoic acid, once regarded as a mere degradation product of retinol, has been shown to be capable of replacing retinol in some, but not all, biologic functions, being ineffective in the visual cycle and in reproduction. It is not converted to retinol, it is not stored in the liver, and it is thought therefore to be less toxic than retinol. Figure 1 is a diagrammatic representation of the biologic roles and interactions of these three retinoids.

Oral vitamin A has been used in the treatment of dermatologic diseases since it was first defined chemically in the early 1930s [11]. Conditions exciting the most interest were psoriasis, the various disorders of keratinization, and acne. Initial efforts were oriented toward the possibility that disease states reflected a deficiency of intake or proper utilization of the vitamin [12]. However, higher doses rapidly became popular, reflecting the relatively low toxicity of this substance [13]. Millions of international units (IU) per day were reported in the treatment of psoriasis and mycosis fungoides by Schimpf and Jansen [14]. More recently, clinical improvement in acne vulgaris was described at 300,000 or more IU/day [15]. Except for this report and for recurring evidence of a limited efficacy in Darier's disease and pityriasis rubra pilaris (PRP), vitamin A has been disappoint-

ing as therapy in most dermatologic conditions [16].

Retinoic acid (all-*trans*-retinoic acid, tretinoin) has been found useful orally and topically as first reported by Stuttgen [17] for PRP and various ichthyoses, and by Beer [18] for psoriasis and acne. The evaluation of the efficacy of this substance topically for ichthyoses, psoriasis [19], acne [20], and actinic keratoses [21] ultimately led to its acceptance as standard therapy for acne vulgaris [22,23]. In contrast, only limited experience has been obtained with the systemic use of tretinoin and this has been obtained in Europe. The status of retinoic acid as of 1975 is well covered in the Flims symposium [4].

Isotretinoin, or 13-*cis*-retinoic acid, is thought to be a metabolite of vitamin A [24]; however, its usefulness in dermatology evolved independently of and prior to clarification of this point. Bollag published evidence of its possible usefulness in acne vulgaris [25], and the early clinical results with psoriasis and leukoplakia reported by Runne et al. [26] and by Koch and Schettler [27] were a direct consequence of the program for evaluation of synthetic retinoids developed by Bollag and Matter [2].

Synthetic Retinoids

The principal focus of the effort to synthesize new analogues of vitamin A was a search for substances that could show a better therapeutic index than retinol or retinoic acid in prophylaxis and treatment of cancer, as pioneered by Bollag [28].

Many chemical variations of the retinoic acid molecule are possible, as noted by Pawson [10]. Figure 2 illustrates the chemical structure of β-carotene, retinol, retinal, tretinoin, isotretinoin, and two synthetic retinoids that have been used

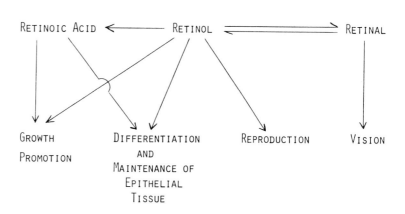

Fig. 1.   Retinoic acid, retinol, and retinal— biologic roles and interactions. *(From Pawson [10], with permission.)*

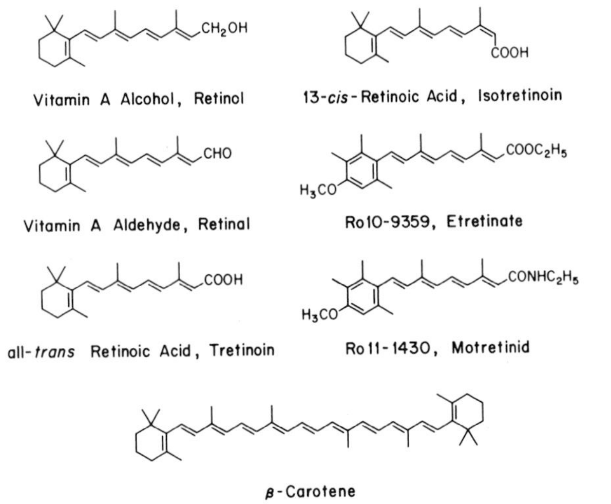

Fig. 2. β-Carotene, retinol, retinal, tretinoin, isotretinoin, Ro 10-9359, and Ro 11-1430—chemical structures.

in the clinic, Ro 10-9359 (etretinate) and Ro 11-1430 (motretinid).

For screening purposes, Bollag and Matter [2] tested the ability of various retinoids to cause regression of experimentally induced skin lesions in animal models. Sporn et al. [29] screened retinoids for their ability to inhibit keratinization in vitamin A deficiency-induced squamous metaplasia of tracheal epithelium in organ cultures. These efforts have resulted in the synthesis of many new molecules in this group.

Clinical Applications of Newer Retinoids

After the initial reports comparing isotretinoin with synthetic analogues of retinoic acid, work in Europe focused on etretinate for psoriasis and various congenital ichthyoses. In the United States, Peck and Yoder introduced studies with isotretinoin in various disorders of keratinization [30], and later, with dramatic results, in severe cystic acne.

Cystic Acne

In the study by Peck et al. [31], 13 of 14 patients receiving isotretinoin showed complete clearing of cystic acne with an average maximum dosage of 2.0 mg/kg per day. These patients did not relapse to any significant degree when treatment was stopped after 4 months of treatment. In fact, most patients whose acne had not completely involuted at the end of the treatment period continued to heal after the treatment stopped. Prolonged improvement without further therapy was observed in all 14 patients on follow-up. Figure 6 (see color

plate) shows one patient before and after isotretinoin therapy.

In a second trial by Peck et al. [32], isotretinoin was tested versus placebo in a parallel, randomized, double-blind protocol. Doses as low as 0.5 mg/kg per day were effective. Four of 33 patients developed mild relapses and required additional therapy. In a third study (unpublished) doses of 1.0 to 2.0 mg/kg per day given for only 2 weeks followed by maintenance doses of 0.25 to 0.5 mg/kg per day produced comparable therapeutic results.

The efficacy of isotretinoin in cystic acne was confirmed and extended by Plewig et al. [33], among others, who also explored possible anti-inflammatory effects of the drug. Using the potassium iodide patch test, it was found that the intensity of erythema was reduced, along with the number of pustules, within 4 weeks of beginning treatment. In addition, sebocytes were noted to retain nuclei longer than controls, suggesting that isotretinoin alters sebaceous gland differentiation.

Of interest is the demonstration by several centers that etretinate is less effective than isotretinoin in both therapeutic effects on cystic acne and in ability to decrease sebum production, illustrating the differential specificity of the two retinoids. Similarly, Gomez [34] found etretinate to be ineffective in reducing the size of sebaceous glands in adult male Syrian hamsters, up to a dose as high as 20 mg/kg per day, while isotretinoin was quite effective in this system. The other androgen-sensitive sites of the hamster flank organ, the pigment cells, were not inhibited, indicating that isotretinoin does not act as an anti-androgen.

Since retinoid therapy reduces the size and activity of sebaceous glands with a corresponding reduction in sebum production, one effect of isotretinoin in acne may be mediated by an inhibition of sebaceous differentiation. However, sebum production returns toward pretreatment values after discontinuation of therapy while the cystic acne continues in remission or even improves [32], and the possibility that the major or only action of the retinoid is mediated through inhibition of sebaceous gland function has been questioned by Plewig et al. [33].

Psoriasis

The use of large oral doses of vitamin A for psoriasis was never promising and was, in addition, always compromised by toxicity questions. Oral tretinoin appeared unpromising for related reasons, as did the studies comparing isotretinoin with an early synthetic retinoid [26].

The effectiveness of etretinate (ethyl ester of trimethylmethoxyphenyl retinoic acid) given orally in psoriasis was first described by Ott and Bollag [35] in 1975. Numerous other studies have confirmed these results, particularly the large multicenter European trial reported by Orfanos and Goerz [36]. Dosage schedules have been defined and circumstances under which other therapy may complement the retinoid therapy have been reported [6].

The multicenter study in Europe [36] described 291 patients administered an initial etretinate dose of 70 to 100 mg/day, which was reduced to 50 mg/day when significant improvement occurred, usually by 3 weeks. Thereafter, approximately 60 percent of the patients maintained good or excellent responses on a dose of 25 to 50 mg/day. Scaling, infiltration, and erythema disappeared in that order (see Fig. 7, color plate). Relapse of the psoriasis occurred in approximately 75 percent of patients within 6 months, despite maintenance therapy with etretinate with or without topical anthralin. Psoriatic arthropathy failed to respond.

Several studies have shown that the use of adjunctive therapy enhances the response of plaque psoriasis [36,37], and Fritsch and coworkers [38] observed that etretinate decreased the total amount of ultraviolet (UV) radiation needed by psoriatic patients receiving photochemotherapy (methoxsalen and long-wave UV radiation, or PUVA). The combination of retinoid with photochemotherapy has been termed *Re-PUVA*. The patients of Fritsch et al. received etretinate alone for 7 to 10 days followed by the addition of PUVA. Complete clearing was seen after an average of six PUVA treatments over 11 days. It also appeared to be effective in patients who had been PUVA failures previously, including those with palmoplantar psoriasis. Side effects to etretinate were fewer and less severe than those observed in earlier studies because of the lower doses used and the shorter duration of the therapy. One postulated mechanism was that the desquamative effect of etretinate on the psoriatic plaque facilitated the transmission of UVA radiation to the skin. Etretinate was found not to enhance photosensitivity when tested on skin not involved with psoriasis.

The results of 6 years of continuous long-term therapy of psoriasis with etretinate (10 to 50 mg/day) were reported to show that, in addition to maintaining good therapeutic responses, long-term therapy did not appear to produce chronic toxicity [39]. An initial dose of 25 to 35 mg/day was recommended in most cases of plaque psoriasis. In patients with severe disease or pustular psoriasis, higher initial doses, up to 75 mg/day, were used. In women, doses above 50 mg/day were not recommended in order to minimize the temporary thinning of hair.

Etretinate has also been said to be helpful for patients with psoriatic arthritis [40], in contrast to the report from the German multicenter study referred to previously [36]. Since a well-controlled trial has not yet been reported, the value of etretinate for psoriatic arthritis remains unclear.

Disorders of Keratinization

As reviewed by Leitner and Moore [41], keratosis follicularis, lamellar ichthyosis, and PRP were initially treated with oral vitamin A on the premise that disturbances in vitamin A metabolism might have produced the cutaneous changes. In spite of high doses, ranging from 100,000 to 1,000,000 IU/day, vitamin A was of only moderate benefit in a few patients with severe disease, showing the most promise in Darier's disease. The hypervitaminosis A syndrome frequently developed, and those patients who did respond usually relapsed upon withdrawal of vitamin A.

Both oral and topical formulations of retinoic acid have been used for disorders of keratinization. Topical all-*trans*-retinoic acid (tretinoin, 0.1% cream) has been reported to be effective for the short-term treatment of lamellar ichthyosis and ichthyosis vulgaris [42], but for palmar and plantar keratoderma a concentration of 0.3% has been recommended [43]. As noted above, European studies have reported that oral retinoic acid (tretinoin) in dosages of 5 to 200 mg/day was effective in keratosis follicularis, bullous congenital ichthyosiform erythroderma, lichen planus, PRP, and basal cell epithelioma [44]. This therapy never gained widespread acceptance, however, and its use declined as isotretinoin and etretinate became available for clinical study.

Numerous recent reports have indicated that Darier's disease, PRP, lamellar ichthyosis, and other rare ichthyoses respond to isotretinoin and etretinate. In contrast to its relative lack of effect on cystic acne, Peck et al. [45] reported etretinate to produce comparable, and possibly superior, responses to those of isotretinoin in some of these diseases. This was based on two sequential open trials in which the same 26 patients were evaluated, first with isotretinoin and then with etretinate. In diseases that respond to more than one retinoid, the choice will ultimately depend on the toxicities of each drug and on the individual patient's response. This is particularly true for patients who have rare congenital conditions that cannot be studied in well-designed clinical trials. Figures 8 through 13 (see color plates) illustrate the responses of some of these conditions to systemic retinoids. Table 1 lists the various names and indications for the two most widely studied oral synthetic retinoids.

Other Disorders

Other dermatologic disorders that have been reported to respond to oral retinoids include rosacea, gram-negative folliculitis, verrucous epidermal nevus, subcorneal pustular dermatosis, plantar warts, hereditary palmoplantar keratoderma, superficial actinic-type porokeratosis, multiple keratoacanthomas, and disseminated porokeratosis of Mibelli [12,46]. In addition, lichen planus, particularly the mucosal erosive type, has been reported to respond well to oral treatment with retinoids given for 2 or 3 months at relatively low doses. In most conditions, the disease process seems to relapse after reduction of the dose or discontinuation of therapy. Cystic acne and, in some cases, PRP are the only conditions reported to achieve long remissions.

Toxicity of Oral Retinoids

Studies of toxicity of vitamin A in animals vary regarding species, dose, and duration of drug administration. Furthermore, the human reports are anecdotal and reflect variability in thoroughness of evaluation. The International Vitamin A Consultative Group (IVAG) reviewed this matter in depth in their report *The Safe Use of Vitamin A* [13].

Two basic features affect vitamin A pharmacokinetics (and hence toxicity): It is stored in the liver and it is transported by a specific binding protein which is released from the liver partially in response to vitamin A ingestion. The former prevents individuals who have sporadic intake of vitamin A from becoming deficient, since several months may be required to exhibit symptoms. As a corollary, some data suggest that significant toxicity does not occur until the liver storage and retinol binding capacities are saturated. An apparent exception to this is the acute (within 12 to 24 hr) syndrome of somnolence, stomach pain, nausea, headache, diarrhea, vertigo, and peeling of skin associated with eating a meal of polar bear or seal liver (which is said to contain 3 to 13 million IU of vitamin A in 250 to 500 g); or with ingestion of an overdose of very high potency therapeutic preparations.

Between 1850 and 1979, 579 cases now recognized as probably hypervitaminosis A appeared in 195 reports in the world literature. About 20 of these were regarded as severe, none was associated with death, and all resolved quickly once the vitamin ingestion was stopped. For contrast, hypovitaminosis A is reported to be associated with an estimated 100,000 individuals permanently blinded and thousands dead each year [13].

Clinical Toxicity of Newer Retinoids

The clinical toxic effects reported from the systemic use of tretinoin, isotretinoin, and etretinate are similar to those of vitamin A, but are well tolerated, dose-dependent in incidence and severity, and are reversible on discontinuation of treatment. However, there is evidence that the spectrum of effects varies among the compounds, just as

Table 1 Oral synthetic retinoids

Generic name	Chemical name	Trade name	Principal indications	Other indications
Isotretinoin	13-*cis*-Retinoic acid	Accutane (USA) Roaccutane (Europe)	Cystic acne	Darier's disease Pityriasis rubra pilaris
Etretinate	Trimethylmethoxyphenyl analogue of retinoic acid ethyl ester	Tegison (USA) Tigason (other than USA)	Psoriasis	Lamellar ichthyosis, etc.

Table 2   Comparison of four oral retinoids: Frequency of adverse reactions

	Retinol, %	Tretinoin, %*	Isotretinoin, %†	Etretinate, %†
Integument and mucous membranes				
Cheilitis	37	80	100	100
Inflammation/xerosis	46	50	58	46
Pruritus	34	23	12	12
Thinning of hair	37	1	16	39
Facial dermatitis	—	—	62	42
Palmoplantar desquamation	—	—	0	47
Paronychia	—	—	0	11
Dryness of mucous membranes	—	30	50	69
Epistaxis, petechiae	—	17	35	46
Central nervous system				
Headache	40	80	6	Rare
Ataxia	12	—	—	—
Lethargy, fatigue	49	43	0	4
Psychologic changes	27	10	(1)	—
Coma	—	6	—	—
Eye				
Visual disturbances	37	30	—	—
Bulb pressure increased	—	11	—	—
Conjunctivitis	—	—	77(2)	77(2)
Musculoskeletal				
Bone/joint/muscle complaints	56	—	12	20
Gastrointestinal				
Anorexia	—	30	—	—
Nausea, vomiting	—	30	—	—
Weight loss	—	—	—	—

* Stuttgen [44].
† Peck et al [45].
Notes: (1) Meyskesn [48] observed psychologic changes in patients receiving very high doses (>3.0 mg/day) of isotretinoin for metastatic cancer. (2) Nearly all patients in this study had congenital ichthyosis and received high doses. Lower doses used for cystic acne show an incidence of one in two for conjunctivitis.

the efficacy profile varies across diseases. In the case of toxicity, different skin sites are more or less affected by different retinoids [47].

The most common clinical signs reported for the four major retinoids are compared in Table 2. Variations in terminology and in details of reporting do not permit firm conclusions to be drawn from these data, which are taken from four reports having the largest numbers of reasonably well observed patients. However, the percentages are consistent with the rest of the general literature (retinol and tretinoin) and with one well-designed double-blind study in which isotretinoin and etretinate were directly compared [49].

The most interesting feature of Table 2 is the relative prominence of central nervous system symptoms compared to effects on epithelia with retinol and tretinoin and the inverse of this distribution with isotretinoin and etretinate. The latter two substances are also different from each other in areas that are reflected in their efficacy spectrum: more facial dermatitis for isotretinoin, and more palmoplantar desquamation for etretinate. The latter also has greater effects on hair, presum-

ably a correlation with its antiproliferative action. In the majority of cases the hair loss reported with retinoids is a telogen effluvium; however, dystrophic anagen roots are occasionally found.

In patients with arthralgias, no roentgenographic evidence of arthritis was found in those reported to date, and the arthralgias are reported to disappear (as are all other clinical effects) after discontinuation of therapy. However, it should be noted that the effects of vitamin A on cartilage and bone in growing animals are complex, and must be considered, particularly if a retinoid is being given to a child. Etretinate has been reported to accelerate epiphyseal ossification in rats but not in dogs [50]. Such findings require further analysis since rat epiphyseal physiology differs from that of other animal species.

Laboratory Abnormalities

Laboratory abnormalities with the retinoids appear to be limited to infrequent elevations of liver function tests that usually return to pretreatment levels even if therapy is continued and to variable changes in blood lipids, especially hypertriglyceridemia.

The most commonly elevated liver function tests are the transaminases, but, occasionally, alkaline phosphatase and bilirubin are abnormal. Elevations of transaminases occurred in approximately 15 percent of one group of 101 patients receiving etretinate observed for 1 to 6 years. The values returned to normal within 2 to 4 weeks, remaining normal even with continued therapy. Furthermore, continuous therapy with etretinate for up to 6 years did not lead to chronic liver toxicity, as measured by liver function tests, even in patients with preexisting liver disease [39]. This is notable in view of the recognition of a prolonged elimination time for etretinate in patients who had received the drug on a chronic basis [50]. Isolated reports suggest some patients may show idiosyncratic liver reactions to etretinate [49].

Elevations of plasma triglyceride levels have occurred, which are dose-dependent and reversible on discontinuation of therapy. In rats, tretinoin produced an eightfold greater increase in plasma triglyceride levels than did isotretinoin at equal doses, and in humans, doses of isotretinoin below 1 mg/kg per day are only rarely associated with hypertriglyceridemia.

It is possible that the triglyceride reaction occurs in predisposed individuals as suggested by Katz et al. [51] in a report of 10 patients treated with isotretinoin, five of whom showed triglyceride values above 300 mg/dL on the drug. One 53-year-old male known to have type IV hypertriglyceridemia prior to therapy developed a triglyceride level greater than 1000 mg/dL on 3.0 mg/kg per day, and a 13-year-old boy whose father had died at age 34 of coronary disease went from a normal baseline to more than 400 mg/dL on the drug. Figure 3 summarizes the data on these 10 patients.

Dicken and Connolly [52] reported a patient who developed triglycerides of 4786 mg/dL and eruptive xanthomas while being treated with isotretinoin at a dose of 2.5 mg/kg per day. The serum cholesterol was elevated above normal, and the high-density lipoproteins (HDL) were below normal. These values returned toward normal after discontinuation of therapy but remained in the abnormal range 11 weeks afterwards, suggesting the presence of a preexisting hyperlipidemia. This 28-year-old male also had two sisters who developed hypertriglyceridemia while on isotretinoin. All three siblings were receiving isotretinoin for Darier's disease, all were obese, and no baseline values prior to drug therapy were available.

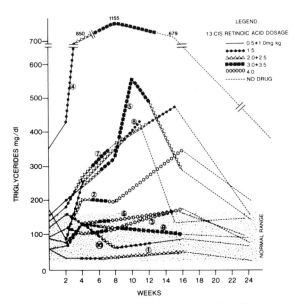

Fig. 3. Graph of triglycerides levels in 10 patients receiving isotretinoin. (From Katz [51], with permission.)

Hypertriglyceridemia has also been observed with etretinate. Five of 25 patients were reported to have had elevations into the pathologic range, and all five had at least one predisposing factor, such as obesity, high alcohol intake, diabetes, or pretreatment hypertriglyceridemia [53]. Some abnormalities in cholesterol and HDL values have been noted on occasion, but these are not as frequent, or as severe as the hypertriglyceridemias.

Reproduction

Retinoids at high doses may inhibit spermatogenesis in animals, but semen analyses from patients receiving oral retinoids have not revealed any abnormalities [54]. In fact, an increased ejaculate volume in males receiving etretinate has been noted, and cystic acne patients treated with isotretinoin have been reported to develop more normal sperm counts after showing abnormally low pretreatment values. Cytogenetic studies of lymphocytes of patients under treatment with oral etretinate have revealed no increased incidence of chromosomal aberrations.

The requirement for retinol in normal reproductive function of females is well known, as is the teratogenicity of hypervitaminosis A in experimental animals. In addition, there have been isolated reports of abnormalities in human infants born to women who had taken 25,000 or more IU/day of vitamin A during the first trimester of pregnancy. Newer retinoids vary in teratogenic potential as measured in laboratory animals [55].

Subcutaneous tretinoin is teratogenic in rats at 10 mg/kg per day; orally given isotretinoin is teratogenic at 150 but not at 50 mg/kg per day; and oral etretinate is teratogenic in rats at 8 and in rabbits at 2 mg/kg per day. Bone malformations have been observed in some, but not all, fetuses of women who had received etretinate during the first trimester, suggesting etretinate may also be teratogenic in humans.

Etretinate is excreted much more slowly than isotretinoin, substantial blood levels having been observed in psoriatic patients up to 140 days after treatment was stopped. Therefore, while the true potential for etretinate to induce teratogenic effects in humans is unknown, its long retention in the blood appears to restrict its usefulness in females of childbearing potential until more information is available.

Mechanisms of Action

Considering the apparent relative specificity of disease responses to given retinoids (cystic acne to isotretinoin, psoriasis to etretinate), no single theory of mechanism of action can explain all clinical observations. Similarly, no unifying hypothesis has been proposed to explain the diversity of effects of retinoids observed in the research laboratory. In epithelial tissues, the retinoids promote differentiation in the direction of mucous secretion while inhibiting keratinization and proliferation. Cultured cells treated with retinoids show profound changes in morphology, growth, biosynthetic activity, and membrane microviscosity [56].

Effects on Cellular Differentiation, Proliferation, and Cell Products

Lotan and Lotan reported that retinoic acid inhibited the rate of cell proliferation of murine S91 and human Hs939 melanoma cell lines while simultaneously increasing tyrosinase activity and the melanin content per cell [57]. In stem cell lines derived from teratocarcinomas, the cells differentiate upon exposure to retinoic acid [58].

Retinoic acid, topically applied, led to accelerated regression of carcinogen-induced keratoacanthomas in the rabbit ear [59]. This effect was accompanied by mucin production and changes that might be associated with regression. The amorphous, intercellular material found in the epidermis of patients with psoriasis and other diseases treated with etretinate may be analagous to the mucin induced by retinoids in experimental

systems [60]. Potassium ferrocyanide staining in psoratic plaques was more intense after etretinate therapy, suggesting increased production of this ''retinoid-stimulated material,'' or RSM [61].

Retinoids affect glycosaminoglycan (GAG) synthesis in ways that may vary with the tissue under investigation. Since these substances are central to cellular recognition and adhesion, the effects of retinoids may be closely related to the modification of differentiation [62].

Specific Binding Proteins

Vitamin A is transported in the serum by binding proteins, and the effects of retinoids on epithelial cells may be mediated by specific cytoplasmic binding proteins. In vitamin A deficiency, serum retinol-binding protein (RBP) secretion by the liver does not occur, leading to low serum levels and high liver levels of RBP. With retinol treatment there is a rapid secretion of RBP into the serum from the liver.

Cellular retinol-binding proteins (CRBP) and cellular retinoic acid–binding proteins (CRABP) are distinct proteins and show different tissue distributions (Table 3). Thus, CRABP but not CRBP are present in normal human skin fibroblasts. It may be that such receptors are critical to the biologic expression of retinoid activity [63].

Labilization of Membranes

Some of the effects of the retinoids may be attributable to their action on the lipid bilayers of cell

Table 3 Distribution of cytosol retinoid-binding proteins in normal rat tissues*

	CRBP	CRABP
Brain	+ (A,F)	+ (A,F)
Eye	+ (A,F)	+ (A,F)
Skin	+ (A,F)	+ (A,F)
Intestinal mucosa	+ (A,F)	+ (F only)
Ovary	+ (A,F)	+ (A)†
Uterus	+ (A,F)	+ (A)†
Kidney	+ (A,F)	—
Liver	+ (A,F)	—
Lung	+ (A,F)	—
Spleen	+ (A,F)	—
Skeletal muscle	—	—
Heart	—	—
Serum	—	—

* Abstracted from Chytil F, Ong DE: Cellular retinol and retinoic acid binding proteins in vitamin A action. *Fed Proc* **38**:2510–2514, 1979, by Elias and Williams [46].
† It is not known whether CRABP was present in these tissues in utero.
Notes: Abbreviations: CRBP = cytosol retinol-binding protein; CRABP = cytosol retinoic acid-binding protein; A = adult type; F = fetal type.

membranes. The viscosity of the cell membrane is dramatically decreased, and destabilization of lysosomes leads to the liberation of lysosomal enzymes. Binding vitamin A to its specific binding protein in the blood minimizes this surface-active effect on the membranes. However, the membrane destabilization seems to be dose-dependent and occurs primarily at high doses. Strikingly, at lower doses retinoids may actually stabilize biologic membranes. In a study of Darier's disease treated with isotretinoin there was no evidence of enzyme release from epidermis [64].

Effects on the Immune System

While oral retinoids act primarily on epithelial tissues, they also have effects on monocytes and lymphocytes. For example, Rhodes and Oliver reported that retinoic acid and retinol in nontoxic concentrations modulated the expression of Fc receptors and the production of arginase in macrophages [65]. The possibility that effects on the immune system may be related to the effects of retinoids in cancer has been evaluated by Medawar and Hunt [66].

Effects on Collagenase and on Prostaglandins

Retinoic acid markedly inhibited collagenase production and partially blocked prostaglandin (PGE$_2$) synthesis in monolayer cultures of rheumatoid synovial cells [67]. Another retinoid, N-(4-hydroxyphenyl)-retinamide, has been reported to be a potent inhibitor of prostaglandin biosynthesis and is also capable of inhibiting carcinogenesis of the mammary gland [68].

Retinoids in Cancer

Interest in the antineoplastic effects of vitamin A and retinoic acid has been the major motivating force in the development of synthetic retinoids [2]. The characteristic squamous metaplasia of vitamin A deficiency is rapidly reversed by active retinoids as are changes induced by carcinogens. Vitamin A deficiency in the rat enhances the susceptibility of the respiratory tract, bladder, and colon to experimental carcinogenesis, and epidemiologic studies have associated the incidence of cancer in humans with decreased serum retinol, raising the question of whether increasing retinoid intake via β-carotene or β-carotene itself could reduce cancer rates [69]. More direct evidence indicating that retinoids act to prevent some forms of cancer comes from laboratory studies. In vitro, retinoids suppress malignant transformation whether caused by chemical carcinogens, ionizing radiation, or transforming peptides from virally transformed cells. They inhibit tumor-promoting effects of phorbol esters, and have been shown to be effective in the prevention of carcinogenesis in experimental models for cancer of the urinary bladder, breast, and skin, to name only a few of the many tumors and systems that have been studied.

Tretinoin (retinoic acid) applied topically has been reported to enhance photocarcinogenesis in hairless albino mice. Some initial data seemed contradictory, and a workshop held on this topic concluded that additional data were necessary to define the effects of retinoids in photocarcinogenesis [70]. The finding was later confirmed in a second laboratory [71]. Of interest is the finding by the latter authors that topical motretinid (Ro 11-1430, the ethylamid of the trimethylmethoxyphenyl derivative of retinoic acid) and oral etretinate failed to enhance photocarcinogenesis in the same model system. Using hairless pigmented mice, Kligman and Kligman found that retinoic acid failed to enhance tumor formation measured by latent period, tumor yield, or tumor progression [72].

The retinoids have been used in the treatment of basal cell carcinomas in humans by Peck and coworkers [73], who gave isotretinoin to patients who had multiple basal cell carcinomas in the basal cell nevus syndrome or secondary to a history of excessive sunlight exposure, arsenic intake, or x-ray irradiation treatment for acne. In these 11 patients, 39 of 248 tumors (16 percent) underwent complete clinical regression. Twenty-one of 35 of these tumors examined histologically were also considered cured by this criterion. Three patients treated almost continuously for 2 to 4 years had no new tumors, while others who discontinued therapy with isotretinoin, but who continued under observation, developed new tumors 8 to 18 months after stopping therapy. The average maximum dosage in this study was 4.7 mg/kg per day and maintenance doses averaged 1.5 mg/kg per day.

A number of reports have appeared on the possible usefulness of retinoids in conditions with an increased risk of developing skin cancer: Schnitzler and Verret [74] reported variable results with etretinate given to patients with basal cell nevus syndrome, xeroderma pigmentosum, multiple keratoacanthomas of the Ferguson-Smith type, porokeratosis of Mibelli with malignant degeneration, and actinic keratosis; Haydey et al. [75]

reported that new lesions did not occur in a patient with multiple keratoacanthomas if isotretinoin was given continuously after surgical excision; Lutzner et al. [76] and Jablonska et al. [77] each reported that etretinate was effective in the treatment of the lesions of epidermodysplasia verruciformis induced by the human papilloma virus types 3 and 5. Leukoplakia of the oral cavity was reported to respond to etretinate [78].

Thus, there appears to be a significant potential for the use of synthetic retinoids in cancer prevention and therapy in addition to the profoundly important benefits they have already been shown to have for a variety of dermatologic conditions. Furthermore, the wide diversity of retinoid effects on cell systems suggests that other diseases, including nondermatologic conditions, may be found to respond to this new class of therapeutic agents. This is particularly to be expected if newer retinoids show new tissue specificities. As was true for the corticosteroids in 1950, the potential for retinoids in 1981 is only partly visible, but very exciting.

References

1. Sporn MB et al: Prevention of chemical carcinogenesis by vitamin A and its synthetic analogs (retinoids). *Fed Proc* **35**:1332–1338, 1976
2. Bollag W, Matter A: From vitamin A to retinoids in experimental and clinical oncology: achievements, failures, and outlook, in *Modulation of Cellular Interaction by Vitamin A and Derivatives (Retinoids)*. Edited by LM DeLuca, SS Shapiro. The New York Academy of Sciences, New York, 1981, pp. 9–23
3. DeLuca LM, Shapiro SS (eds): *Modulation of Cellular Interaction by Vitamin A and Derivatives (Retinoids)*. The New York Academy of Sciences, New York, 1981
4. Stuttgen G (Chairman): The Therapeutic Use of Vitamin A Acid. An International Symposium, Flims, Switzerland, January 27–29, 1975. *Acta Derm Venereol (Stockh)* **55 (suppl 74)**:7–179, 1975
5. Orfanos C, Schuppli R (Chairmen): Oral Retinoids in Dermatology, A Workshop at the XVth International Congress of Dermatology, Mexico City, October 19, 1977. *Dermatologica* **157(Suppl 1)**:1–64, 1978
6. Orfanos CE et al (eds): *Retinoids—Advances in Basic Research and Therapy*. Springer-Verlag, Berlin, 1981
7. Strauss J et al (eds): Oral Retinoids, A Workshop. *J Am Acad Dermatol* **6**:573–832, 1982
8. Farber E et al (eds): *Third International Symposium on Psoriasis, Stanford, California, July 13–17, 1981*. Grune & Stratton, New York, 1982
9. DeLuca LM et al: The metabolism of retinoic acid to 5,6-epoxyretinoic acid, retinoyl-*b*-glucuronide, and other polar metabolites, in *Modulation of Cellular Interaction by Vitamin A and Derivatives (Retinoids)*. Edited by LM DeLuca, SS Shapiro. The New York Academy of Sciences, New York, 1981, pp 25–37
10. Pawson BA: A historical introduction to the chemistry of vitamin A and its analogs (retinoids), in *Modulation of Cellular Interaction by Vitamin A and Derivatives (Retinoids)*. Edited by LM DeLuca, SS Shapiro. The New York Academy of Sciences, New York, 1981, pp 1–8
11. Windhorst DB: Evolution of retinoids as therapy in dermatology, in *Third International Symposium on Psoriasis, Stanford, California, July 13–17, 1981*, Grune & Stratton, New York, 1982
12. Peck GL: Retinoids in clinical dermatology, in *Progress in Disease of the Skin*. Edited by R Fleischmajer. Grune & Stratton, New York, 1981, pp 227–269
13. *The Safe Use of Vitamin A: A Report on the International Vitamin A Consultative Group (IVAG)*. The Nutrition Foundation, Washington, DC, 1980
14. Schimpf A, Jansen KH: Hochdosierte Vitamin A-Therapie bei Psoriasis und Mycosis fungoides. *Fortschr Ther* **90**:635–639, 1972
15. Kligman AM et al: Oral vitamin A (retinol) in acne vulgaris, in *Retinoids—Advances in Basic Research and Therapy*. Edited by CE Orfanos et al. Springer-Verlag, Berlin, 1981, pp 245–253
16. Burgoon CF et al: Effect of vitamin A on epithelial cells of skin. *Arch Dermatol* **87**:63–80, 1963
17. Stuttgen G: Zur Lokalbehandlung von Keratosen mit Vitamin-A-Saure. *Dermatologica* **124**:65–80, 1962
18. Beer P: Studies of the effects of vitamin A acid. *Dermatologica* **124**:192–195, 1962
19. Frost P, Weinstein GD: Topical administration of vitamin A acid for ichthyosiform dermatoses and psoriasis. *JAMA* **207**:1863–1868, 1969
20. Kligman AM et al: Topical vitamin A acid in acne vulgaris. *Arch Dermatol* **99**:469–476, 1969
21. Bollag W, Ott F: Therapy of actinic keratoses and basal cell carcinomas with local application of vitamin A acid (NSC-122758). *Cancer Chemother Rep* **55**:59–60, 1971
22. Baden HP: Ichthyosiform dermatoses, in *Dermatology in General Medicine*, 2d ed. Edited by TB Fitzpatrick et al. McGraw-Hill, New York, 1979, p 262
23. McLaren DS: Cutaneous changes in nutritional deficiencies, in *Dermatology in General Medicine*, 2d ed. Edited by TB Fitzpatrick et al. McGraw-Hill, New York, 1979, pp 1019–1031
24. Frolik CA: In vitro and in vivo metabolism of all-*trans*- and 13-*cis*-retinoic acid in the hamster, in *Modulation of Cellular Interaction by Vitamin A and Derivatives (Retinoids)*. Edited by LM DeLuca, SS Shapiro. The New York Academy of Sciences, New York, 1981, pp 37–44
25. Bollag W: Belgian patent 762,344, August 2, 1971
26. Runne U et al: Perorale Applikation zweier Derivate der Vitamin-A-Saure zur internen Psoriasis-Therapie: 13-*cis*-beta-Vitamin A-Saure und Vitamin A-Saure-aethylamid. *Arch Dermatol Forsch* **247**:171–180, 1973
27. Koch H, Schettler D: Klinische Erfahrunger mit Vitamin-A-Saure Derivaten bei Behandlung von Leukoplakien der Mundschleimhaut. *Dtsch Zahnaerztl Z* **28**:623–627, 1973
28. Bollag W: Belgian patent 752,924, July 3, 1970
29. Sporn MB et al: Relationship between structure and activity of retinoids. *Nature* **263**:110–113, 1976
30. Peck GL, Yoder FW: Treatment of lamellar ichthyosis and other keratinising dermatoses with an oral synthetic retinoid. *Lancet* **2**:1172–1174, 1976
31. Peck GL et al: Prolonged remissions of cystic and conglobate acne with 13-*cis*-retinoic acid. *N Engl J Med* **300**:329–333, 1979
32. Peck GL et al: Isotretinoin versus placebo in the treatment of cystic acne—a randomized double-blind study, in Oral

Retinoids, a Workshop. Edited by J Strauss et al. *J Am Acad Dermatol* **6**:735–745, 1982

33. Plewig G et al: Effects of two retinoids in animal experiments and after clinical application in acne patients: 13-*cis*-retinoic acid Ro 4-3780 and aromatic retinoid Ro 10-9359, in *Retinoids—Advances in Basic Research and Therapy.* Edited by CE Orfanos et al. Springer-Verlag, Berlin, 1981, pp 219–235

34. Gomez EC: Effects of retinoids on the sebaceous glands of the hamster flank organ, in *Retinoids—Advances in Basic Research and Therapy.* Edited by CE Orfanos et al. Springer-Verlag, Berlin, 1981, pp. 213–217

35. Ott F, Bollag W: Therapie der Psoriasis mit einem oral wirksamen neuen Vitamin-A-Saure-Derivat. *Schweiz Med Wochenschr* **105**:439–441, 1975

36. Orfanos CE, Goerz G: Orale Psoriasis-Therapie mit einem neuen aromatischen Retinoid (Ro 10-9359). *Dtsch Med Wochenschr* **103**:195–199, 1978

37. Fredriksson T: The posology of retinoids: how much, how often, how long?, in *Retinoids—Advances in Basic Research and Therapy.* Edited by CE Orfanos et al. Springer-Verlag, Berlin, 1981, pp 349–353

38. Fritsch PO et al: Augmentation of oral methoxsalen—photochemotherapy with an oral retinoic acid derivative. *J Invest Dermatol* **70**:178–182, 1978

39. Ott F: Long-term biological tolerance of Ro 10-9359, in *Retinoids—Advances in Basic Research and Therapy.* Edited by CE Orfanos et al. Springer-Verlag, Berlin, 1981, pp 355–357

40. Stollenwerk R et al: Clinical observations on oral retinoid therapy of psoriatic arthropathy (Ro 10-9359), in *Retinoids—Advances in Basic Research and Therapy.* Edited by CE Orfanos et al. Springer-Verlag, Berlin, 1981, pp 205–209

41. Leitner ZA, Moore T: Vitamin A and skin disease. *Lancet* **2**:262–265, 1946

42. Muller SA et al: Keratinizing dermatoses: combined data from four centers on short-term topical treatment with tretinoin. *Arch Dermatol* **113**:1052–1054, 1977

43. Heiss HB, Gross PR: Keratosis palmaris et plantaris—treatment with topically applied vitamin A acid. *Arch Dermatol* **101**:100–103, 1970

44. Stuttgen G: Oral vitamin A acid therapy. *Acta Derm Venereol (Stockh)* **55 (suppl 74)**:174–179, 1975

45. Peck GL et al: Comparative analysis of two retinoids in the treatment of disorders of keratinization, in *Retinoids—Advances in Basic Research and Therapy.* Edited by CE Orfanos et al. Springer-Verlag, Berlin, 1981, pp 279–286

46. Elias PM, Williams ML: Retinoids, cancer, and the skin. *Arch Dermatol* **117**:160–180, 1981

47. Windhorst DB, Nigra T: General clinical toxicology of oral retinoids, in Oral Retinoids, A Workshop. Edited by J Strauss et al. *J Am Acad Dermatol* **6**:675–682, 1982

48. Meyskens FL: Studies of retinoids in the prevention and treatment of cancer, in Oral Retinoids, A Workshop. Edited by J Strauss et al. *J Am Acad Dermatol* **6**:824–827, 1982

49. Goldstein JA et al: Comparative effect of isotretinoin and etretinate on acne and sebaceous gland secretion, in Oral Retinoids, A Workshop. Edited by J Strauss et al. *J Am Acad Dermatol* **6**:760–765, 1982

50. Paravicini U: Pharmacokinetics and metabolism of oral aromatic retinoids, in *Retinoids—Advances in Basic Research and Therapy.* Edited by CE Orfanos et al. Springer-Verlag, Berlin, 1981, pp 13–20

51. Katz RA et al: Elevation of serum triglyceride levels from oral isotretinoin in disorders of keratinization. *Arch Dermatol* **116**:1369–1372, 1980

52. Dicken CH, Connolly SM: Eruptive xanthomas associated with isotretinoin (13-*cis*-retinoic acid). *Arch Dermatol* **116**:951–952, 1980

53. Gollnick H: Elevated levels of triglycerides in patients with skin disease treated with oral aromatic retinoid. The significance of risk factors, in *Retinoids—Advances in Basic Research and Therapy.* Edited by CE Orfanos et al. Springer-Verlag, Berlin, 1981, pp 503–505

54. Schill WB et al: Aromatic retinoid and 13-*cis*-retinoic acid: spermatological investigations, in *Retinoids—Advances in Basic Research and Therapy.* Edited by CE Orfanos. Springer-Verlag, Berlin, 1981, pp 389–395

55. Kamm JJ: Toxicology, carcinogenicity and teratogenicity of some orally administered retinoids, in Oral Retinoids, A Workshop. Edited by J Strauss et al. *J Am Acad Dermatol* **6**:652–659, 1982

56. Fritsch P: Oral retinoids in dermatology. *Int J Dermatol* **20**:314–329, 1981

57. Lotan R, Lotan D: Stimulation of melanogenesis in a human melanoma cell line by retinoids. *Cancer Res* **40**:3345–3350, 1980

58. Sherman MI et al: Studies on the mechanism of induction of embryonal carcinoma cell differentiation by retinoic acid, in *Modulation of Cellular Interaction by Vitamin A and Derivatives (Retinoids).* Edited by LM DeLuca, SS Shapiro. The New York Academy of Sciences, New York, 1981, pp 192–199

59. Prutkin L: The effect of vitamin A acid on hyperkeratinization and keratoacanthomas. *J Invest Dermatol* **49**:165–172, 1967

60. Orfanos CE, Runne U: Tissue changes in psoriatic plaques after oral administration of retinoids. *Dermatologica* **157(Suppl 1)**:19–25, 1978

61. Ellis CN et al: Retinoid-stimulated material in psoriatic epidermis during Ro 10-9359 therapy, in *Retinoids—Advances in Basic Research and Therapy.* Edited by CE Orfanos et al. Springer-Verlag, Berlin, 1981, pp 93–98

62. Shapiro SS, Mott DJ: Modulation of glycosaminoglycan biosynthesis by retinoids, in *Modulation of Cellular Interaction by Vitamin A and Derivatives (Retinoids).* Edited by LM DeLuca, SS Shapiro. The New York Academy of Sciences, New York, 1981, pp 306–321

63. Goodman D: Retinoid-binding proteins in plasma and in cells, in *Modulation of Cellular Interaction by Vitamin A and Derivatives (Retinoids).* Edited by LM DeLuca, SS Shapiro. The New York Academy of Sciences, New York, 1981, pp 69–78

64. Farb RM et al. The effect of 13-*cis*-retinoic acid on epidermal lysosomal hydroxlase activity in Darier's disease and pityriasis rubra pilaris. *J Invest Dermatol* **75**:133–135, 1980

65. Rhodes J, Oliver S: Retinoids as regulators of macrophage function. *Immunology* **40**:467–472, 1980

66. Medawar PB, Hunt R: Anti-cancer action of retinoids. *Immunology* **42**:349–353, 1981

67. Brinckerhoff CE et al: Inhibition by retinoic acid of collagenase production in rheumatoid synovial cells. *N Engl J Med* **303**:432–436, 1980

68. Levine L: N-(4-hydroxyphenyl)-retinamide: a synthetic analog of vitamin A that is a potent inhibitor of prostaglandin synthesis. *Prostaglandins Med* **4**:285–296, 1980

69. Peto R et al: Can dietary beta-carotene materially reduce human cancer rates? *Nature* **290**:201–208, 1981

70. Kripke ML, Glassman HN: Retinoic acid photocarcinogenesis workshop. *J Am Acad Dermatol* **2**:439–442, 1980

71. Hartmann HR, Teelmann K: The influence of topical and oral retinoid treatment on photocarcinogenicity in hairless albino mice, in *Retinoids—Advances in Basic Research and Therapy*. Edited by CE Orfanos et al. Springer-Verlag, Berlin, 1981, pp 447–451

72. Kligman LH, Kligman AM: Lack of enhancement of experimental photocarcinogenesis by retinoic acid, in *Retinoids—Advance in Basic Research and Therapy*. Edited by CE Orfanos et al. Springer-Verlag, Berlin, 1981, pp 441–451

73. Peck GL et al: Chemoprevention of basal cell carcinoma and isotretinoin, in Oral Retinoids, A Workshop. Edited by J Strauss et al. *J Am Acad Dermatol* **6**:815–823, 1982

74. Schnitzler L, Verret JL: Retinoid and skin cancer prevention, in *Retinoids—Advances in Basic Research and Therapy*. Edited by CE Orfanos et al. Springer-Verlag, Berlin, 1981, pp 385–388

75. Haydey RP et al: Treatment of keratoacanthomas with oral 13-*cis*-retinoic acid. *N Engl J Med* **303**:560–562, 1980

76. Lutzner MA et al: Oral aromatic retinoid (Ro 10-9359) treatment of two patients suffering with the severe form of epidermodysplasia verruciformis, in *Retinoids—Advances in Basic Research and Therapy*. Edited by CE Orfanos et al. Springer-Verlag, Berlin, 1981, pp 407–410

77. Jablonska S et al: Ro 10-9359 in epidermodysplasia verruciformis, a preliminary report, in *Retinoids—Advances in Basic Research and Therapy*. Edited by CE Orfanos et al. Springer-Verlag, Berlin, 1981, pp 401–405

78. Koch HF: Effect of retinoids on precancerous lesions of oral mucosa, in *Retinoids—Advances in Basic Research and Therapy*. Edited by CE Orfanos et al. Springer-Verlag, Berlin, 1981, pp 307–312